ADVENTURE PSYCHOLOGY

In recent years a new set of psychological principles has emerged from research investigating adventure and adventurous activities. Adventure involves a special type of physical activity in natural contexts where participants voluntarily participate in experiences where the environment and activity are challenging, perhaps dangerous and potentially life threatening. To go on an adventure is to participate in an enduring event requiring sustainable effort, where effective performance is measured not only by success but also by survival. This book brings together the emerging literature in 'Adventure Psychology' that supports enduring performance and wellbeing.

The first section examines sustaining performance and wellbeing. The second section studies the transformative aspect of adventure. Adventure Psychology is of use in everyday life and the techniques and understandings can help people and business prepare for the future. This book will help us all thrive despite adversity, volatility and uncertainty.

Written for trainers, educators, researchers and students of sports, performance and organisational psychology as well as adventurers and endurance athletes, *Adventure Psychology* is designed to meet the needs of specialists across a variety of fields but importantly also to be accessible and applicable for those wanting to live life fully – to realise our full potential.

Paula Reid has a Batchelor of Education (Hons) degree and graduated with a Distinction MSc in Applied Positive Psychology and Coaching Psychology from the University of East London. Her organisation, 'Adventure Psychology', delivers the performance psychology of how to survive, cope and thrive during challenging times. She is based in the UK and is a Fellow of the Royal Geographical Society.

Eric Brymer is a behavioural scientist who specialises in researching the psychology of adventure experiences, performance in extreme environments and the reciprocal nature of health and wellbeing from nature-based experiences. He holds a PhD in Adventure Psychology, a Master's degree in Applied Sport and Exercise Psychology and postgraduate degrees in Education and Business. Eric works with and advises governments and institutional departments. He also holds research positions in health, exercise and outdoor studies in Europe, UK and Australia.

Routledge Research in Health, Nature and the Environment

The *Routledge Research in Health and Nature* series offers a multi-disciplinary forum for cutting-edge research in the broad area of nature, wellbeing and health. Showcasing the work of emerging and established scholars working in areas ranging from chronic disease, psychology and mental health to physical activity and health promotion and socio-economic and cultural aspects of interacting and engaging with nature, the series is an important channel for groundbreaking research investigating Nature and health that is fast becoming vital for the health and wellbeing of people and the planet.

Available in this series:

Nature and Heath
Physical Activity in Nature
Edited by Eric Brymer, Mike Rogerson and Jo Barton

Embodied Nature and Health
How to Attune to the Open-source Intelligence
Marcin Fabjański

Adventure Psychology
Going Knowingly into the Unknown
Edited by Paula Reid and Eric Brymer

For more information about this series, please visit: https://www.routledge.com/sport/series/RRHNE

ADVENTURE PSYCHOLOGY

Going Knowingly into the Unknown

*Edited by
Paula Reid and Eric Brymer*

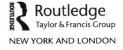
NEW YORK AND LONDON

Designed cover image: agsandrew/Getty Images

First published 2023
by Routledge
605 Third Avenue, New York, NY 10158

and by Routledge
4 Park Square, Milton Park, Abingdon, Oxon, OX14 4RN

Routledge is an imprint of the Taylor & Francis Group, an informa business

© 2023 selection and editorial matter, Paula Reid and Eric Brymer; individual chapters, the contributors

The right of Paula Reid and Eric Brymer to be identified as the authors of the editorial material, and of the authors for their individual chapters, has been asserted in accordance with sections 77 and 78 of the Copyright, Designs and Patents Act 1988.

All rights reserved. No part of this book may be reprinted or reproduced or utilised in any form or by any electronic, mechanical, or other means, now known or hereafter invented, including photocopying and recording, or in any information storage or retrieval system, without permission in writing from the publishers.

Trademark notice: Product or corporate names may be trademarks or registered trademarks, and are used only for identification and explanation without intent to infringe.

ISBN: 978-1-032-00303-0 (hbk)
ISBN: 978-1-032-00304-7 (pbk)
ISBN: 978-1-003-17360-1 (ebk)

DOI: 10.4324/9781003173601

Typeset in Bembo
by codeMantra

CONTENTS

Preface	*xi*
Acknowledgements	*xiii*
List of Contributors	*xv*

Adventure Psychology: Framing the Discipline   1
Eric Brymer and Paula Reid

Adventure Psychology: A Long Past, but a Short History   9
Peter Suedfeld

SECTION I
Sustaining Performance (While Maintaining Wellbeing)   25

1 **The Adventurer's Mind: Exploring Mindset, Mindfulness, and Wisdom**   27
Mohsen Fatemi and Paula Reid

2 **Adventures in Extreme Environments**   42
Peter Suedfeld

3 **Enduring Performance**   60
Ronald Duren Jr.

4 Dealing with the Unknown 76
Jennifer Pickett and Paula Reid

5 Adventure, Positive Psychology, and Narrative: The Wellbeing Impacts of Answering the Call to Adventure 88
Kitrina Douglas, David Carless, Paula Reid and Ruth Hughes

6 The Human–Environment Dynamic: An Ecological Dynamics Approach to Understanding Human–Environment Interactions in the Context of Adventure Psychology 104
Tuomas Immonen, Eric Brymer, Timo Jaakkola and Keith Davids

7 Fear in Extended Adventures: The Case of Expedition Mountaineering 120
Katrina Kessler and Eric Brymer

8 Success and Failure in Adventure 131
Erik Monasterio

9 Sisu: Answering the Call of Adventure with Strength and Grace 142
Emilia Elisabet Lahti

SECTION II
Transformational Impact of Adventure 157

10 How Can Adventure Change Our Consciousness? An Exploration of Flow, Mindfulness, and Adventure 159
Susan Houge Mackenzie

11 Adventure, Posttraumatic Growth, and Wisdom 172
Hanna Kampman and Petra Walker

12 Adventure and the Sublime: A Quest for Transformation or Transcendence? 187
Chris Loynes and Amy Smallwood

13 **Giving Back: An Autoethnographic Analysis of Adventure Experience as Transformational** 203
Vinathe Sharma-Brymer

Adventure Psychology: Learnings and Implications 219
Eric Brymer and Paula Reid

Index *223*

PREFACE

It was early in the pandemic, in February 2020, when we hatched our mission to write this book.

It's been a very challenging couple of years living with Covid-19, while coping with other global, local and personal adversities, uncertainties and disruption.

Our physical and mental health have been tested, perhaps found wanting, perhaps strengthened.

Adventure Psychology: Going Knowingly into the Unknown feels more relevant than ever. Not only in support of adventurers' performance and wellbeing, but for all of us as we navigate life's journey and learn how to survive, cope and thrive in challenging times.

ACKNOWLEDGEMENTS

We give our heartful gratitude to all our contributing authors. Not just for the commitment of time and workload they have given to these pages, but for their ideas and thoughtfulness, reflections and inspiration, wisdom and insights. It has been a pressurised and out of kilter couple of years for all of us as we write this after more than two years of pandemic disruption. The academic world has been hit hard, and the authors have each experienced their own adversities and personal and professional challenges. Many may have relied upon coping strategies shared in this book; many may have been ever more thoughtful about what they are writing and perhaps written from a deeper, more personally informed place. We respect and are grateful for your gift of contribution.

This reminds me of a quote ascribed to Carl Jung:

> Know all the theories, master all the techniques, but as you touch a human soul be just another human soul.

The authors in this book know their theories and have shared them with you as human souls. We hope in reading this, you are touched as a human soul, but also now know the theories.

We would also like to acknowledge the exquisite global network holding this book in its 'world wide web'. This book has motivated collaboration across the world with contributions from Alaska, Finland, America, New Zealand, England, Australia, Bali, Lapland, Cyprus, Malta and Iran. *Adventure Psychology* has epitomised a truly global, cooperative, prosocial adventure as we have co-created across the globe, across geographies, experiences, cultures and time zones.

THANK YOU.

We would like to thank our Peer Reviewers for making the content more robust, clear and strong. These include:

Amy Smallwood, Chris Loynes, Elsa Valdivielso-Martínez, Juliet L. Menager, Kate Brassington, Louise Wheeler, Maya Gudka, Petra Ann Walker, Rebecca Williams, Ruth Hughes and Sarita Robinson

Thanks also to Belinda Kirk author of *Adventure Revolution: The Life-Changing Power of Choosing Challenge* (2021). It was at Belinda's first 'Adventure Mind' conference at YHA London Lee Valley (which promotes adventure for wellbeing) in February 2020 where we hatched this book.

CONTRIBUTORS

Eric Brymer, Southern Cross University, Australia

David Carless, University of the West of Scotland, UK

Keith Davids, Sheffield Hallam University, UK

Kitrina Douglas, University of West London & Leeds Beckett University, UK

Ronald Duren Jr, Independent – Forging Mettle Podcast and Academy

Mohsen Fatemi, York University

Emilia Elisabet Lahti, Aalto University, School of Science & Technology, Espoo, Finland

Ruth Hughes, University of Cambridge, UK

Tuomas Immomen, University of Jyväskylä, Finland

Timo Jaakkola, University of Jyväskylä, Finland

Hanna Kampman, University of East London, UK

Katrina V. Kessler, Independent Researcher

Chris Loynes, University of Cumbria, UK

Susan Houge Mackenzie, University of Otago, New Zealand

Erik Monasterio, University of Otago, Christchurch School of Medicine, New Zealand

Jennifer Pickett, Independent

Paula Reid, Independent – Adventure Psychology

Vinathe Sharma-Brymer, University of the Sunshine Coast, Australia

Amy Smallwood, University of Cumbria, UK

Peter Suedfeld, University of British Columbia, Canada

Petra Walker, Independent – Petra Walker Coaching, UK

ADVENTURE PSYCHOLOGY

Framing the Discipline

Eric Brymer and Paula Reid

Adventure has emerged as an important societal and cross-disciplinary phenomenon. Examples of adventure in practice include adventure tourism, adventure travel, adventure education, adventure therapy, recreational therapy, therapeutic adventure, adventure sports, and adventure recreation. Over the years, there have been many attempts to conceptualise and define adventure either driven by the need to constrain adventure in relation to a particular field of study or in response to the developing knowledge base across the different fields of adventure. Broadly, research has posited four main frames for understanding adventure: (1) adventure as a type of activity, (2) adventure as framed through the environment, (3) adventure as within the person, and (4) adventure as a dynamic relationship. While each of the chapters in this book adhere to one or more of these frames, here we provide a structure for the reader and show how each frame has bearing on the concept of Adventure Psychology.

1) Adventure as a Type of Activity

The most common frame assumes that adventure is synonymous with a type of activity undertaken in educational, therapeutic, recreational, tourism, or sporting contexts. Adventure recreation, for instance, has been defined as, "self-initiated, nature-based physical activities that generate heightened bodily sensations and require skill development to manage unique perceived and objective risks" (Houge Mackenzie & Hodge, 2020, p. 2). Adventure therapy has been described as the deliberate engagement with adventurous physical activity for therapeutic intent. In a similar manner, adventure education has often been described as the use of outdoor and adventurous activities for educational purposes. Adventure has also been associated with activities that have uncertain outcomes, danger, and risk (Brown & Beames, 2017). In essence, the use of adventure in these contexts refers to a specific type of activity underscored by risk, physical activity, and unusual experiences. In some fields, adventure activities have been further differentiated on a continuum between soft (camping, fishing, snorkelling) and extreme (proximity flying, big wave surfing, extreme skiing). From a psychology perspective, research and practice has focused on exploring how best to design learning for technical skills, how to design activities so that the chances of mishap are minimised, and what psychological skills assist a successful adventure participant. Adventure Psychology from this perspective suggests an alignment with applied psychologies, such as sport and exercise psychology, that have been specifically created to understand and support learning, wellbeing, and the development of skills for effective performance of physical activity.

However, adventuring has a broader experiential scope than just being practiced or applied, and beyond being defined by physical activity. Adventure is not constrained by external rules, regulations, competition, time, and tightly manicured environments. It is an exploratory, dynamic activity within a certain context. Breivik (2010) for instance hints at an understanding of adventure that encompasses activity, experience, and environment:

> The term 'adventure' denotes that the activity takes place in a setting that is demanding, challenging, dangerous or exotic. An adventure is something special and valuable that sticks out from ordinary life. It is used about sports or physical activities but also about travels, in body and mind.
>
> *(p. 263)*

However, even with this more expanded appreciation of adventure incorporating "travels in body and mind", it is hard to determine what is meant by exotic, dangerous, special, and challenging settings.

2) Adventure Framed through the Environment

A different perspective on the idea of adventure hinted at by the quote above focuses more on the environment (Giddy & Webb, 2018). Proponents of this perspective point out that at a fundamental level being outdoors in nature is foundational to the notion of adventure. Nature is not pre-constructed or intentionally designed and thus presents a variable, evolving, and often hazardous newness to the adventurer. Thus, adventure is only adventure because of the interaction with the outdoor environment. Nature is key to enticing participants, as much as it is essential to the lived experience. This notion of adventure might conjure up a variety of ideas about the role of the environment as a worthy opponent in a hand-to-hand battle, or more reciprocally, a partner in a sublime dance. The characteristics of the adventure environment are described as unique. Research from this perspective examines the impact of the adventure environment on affective responses, nature connection, and pro-environmental behaviour as well as the impact of the adventure environment on immediate and long-term health and wellbeing (Hanna et al., 2019; Palmberg & Kuru, 2000). Psychologically this perspective aligns best with environmental psychology, although there is arguably crossover with health psychology as well.

3) Person-Centred Notion of Adventure

A third perspective on adventure focuses on the participant experience or characteristics. In part, this approach dates back to the early days of adventure scholarship and frameworks such as the adventure experience paradigm which focused on individual perceptions of risk and competence (Priest, 1992). In later years, the adventure participant experience has been associated with more mainstream psychological constructs such as Peak Experience and Flow and the promotion of psychological growth or "post-adventure growth", resilience, wisdom, and mastery (Reid & Kampman, 2020).

Those interested in situating adventure as person-centric often relied on deficit models of adventure and the assumption that the desire for adventure was driven by relatively consistent or innate personality characteristics such as the sensation-seeking personality trait (Gomà i Freixanet et al., 2012). Proponents of the personal characteristics' perspective have most often examined the role of personality traits in motivation for adventure, effectiveness, leadership, and teamwork during an adventure, the impact of personal characteristics on the experience of adventure, and the potential for adventure to contain harmful addictive properties (Buckley, 2015). Adventure has been categorised as both stemming from characteristics that reflect modern society and those that trigger rebellion from the constraints of modern society.

Critics of this perspective have pointed out limitations with the traditional adventure personality for its association with male, white, privilege (Warren et al., 2019), and that the variation across personality traits in adventurers is too expansive to argue a determined link (Kerr & Houge Mackenzie, 2012). Furthermore, even the more positive lived experience perspective is potentially limited as, for example, Flow and Peak experiences are found in non-adventure experiences (Houge Mackenzie & Brymer, 2018; Monasterio & Brymer, 2021; Monasterio & Brymer, 2015). For some, the "in the person" explanations might be more about how people behave during an adventure and potentially aligned with mishaps and related outcomes (Monasterio & Brymer, 2021). The psychology frames most aligned with this idea of adventure are positive psychology, humanistic psychology, transpersonal psychology, and to an extent, clinical, cognitive, and personality psychology.

4) Adventure as a Relationship

A fourth perspective on adventure recognises that adventure is bigger than each of the ideas above and in fact may be more about a dynamic relationship between all or some of the above notions. In this fourth movement, adventure is not so much an individual, environment, or activity concept but about a relationship between some or all of the individual notions within a dynamic system (Immonen et al., in press; Immonen et al., 2017; Peacock et al., 2017). Adventure could be about the person–task relationship which suggests that adventure is not a one-size-fits all notion but dependent on both task and individual characteristics. Kayaking the local Grade 2 river could be an adventure for one person but mundane for the next. Equally, setting up a new business or trying on a new leadership style could be categorised as adventures. If adventure is situated in the person–environment relationship, then the definition of adventure depends on the characteristic of the individual and environment. The relational model is dynamic, where even a mundane or ordinary experience can quickly turn into an adventure. Emerging scholarship in this area argues that adventure is an important universal phenomenon open to all and research is currently interested in the impact of the relationship on wellbeing of people and planet and new ways of understanding learning design. Adventure as a relationship fits more closely with ecopsychology and ecological psychology.

5) A Fifth Perspective

Our proposal for a fifth point of view, focusing purely on Adventure Psychology, is an encompassing description of adventure as an experiential state, drawing together the frames aforementioned. Specifically, adventure as an activity, event, or experience that plays out within an outdoors environment where nature is agentic and intrinsic to the human experience, involving a dynamic interplay between activity–person–environment that creates a unique experiential state. It is a distinctively lived experience; dynamic, variable, and evolutionary. We will revisit this fifth notion in our concluding chapter: Adventure Psychology: Learnings and Implications.

★ ★ ★ ★

While definitions may not be as precise as some would like, there is clear evidence that adventure has profound benefits for both people and planet. The idea of adventure and research into adventure is maturing. Research suggests that adventure tourism markets are growing, outcomes from adventure education and adventure therapy are profound, and adventure sports and adventure recreation participation rates seem to be outgrowing traditional recreation and sporting activities. Adventure is very accessible globally and potentially non-elitist – there are no barriers to entry that cannot be creatively resolved. Adventure Psychology is also pushing new boundaries and emerging as a new way of understanding what it means to be human. Perhaps similar to the way sport and exercise psychology emerged from the constraints of clinical and educational psychology as a distinct discipline with its own theoretical frames and applications, Adventure Psychology is coming into its own (Arijs et al., 2017).

The Content

In this book, we focus on research and scholarship that helps describe nature-based Adventure Psychology, though the ideas and descriptions are relevant for all adventures. For ease of communication, we have sliced Adventure Psychology into sections and chapters which could give the impression that the concepts described in each chapter are somehow distinct and separate. However, we see Adventure Psychology as an integrated notion and indeed the slicing could have been very different. We invite the reader to consider Adventure Psychology as a psychology that brings together environment, activity, and person factors in a unique manner and the chapters in this book reflect this.

There are two sections to this book: "Sustaining Performance (while maintaining wellbeing)", followed by "Transformational Impact of Adventure". The first focuses on teasing out Adventure Psychology in terms of the relationship between performance and wellbeing. The aim of this section is to explore Adventure Psychology as it is lived and how it relates to performance and wellbeing. Peter Suedfeld precedes this section with an enjoyable journey and historical examination of the relationship between adventure and psychology touching on the myths, folktales, and accomplishments that characterise adventure over the years. Peter traces adventure to the early human experience and links this smoothly to the stories of many more well-known adventurers. Following this, Sayyed Mohsen Fatemi and Paula Reid set out on their own adventure into the mind and mindset of the adventurer. We find that characteristics such as curiosity and exploration guide a physical and mental journey that reaches inward as much as it does outward. Peter Suedfeld takes up the mantle again this time to examine Adventure Psychology through the lens of participation in extreme environments. This chapter examines adventure in the highest, hottest, coldest, loneliest environments and provides insights into motivation, performance requirements, and emotional toll that are so tightly coupled with adventure in the extremes.

Ronald Duren follows with a considered examination of how the adventurer sustains effort enduringly despite the often intense impact of harsh environmental conditions such as severe weather. Rather than a focus on peak experience and competition, Duren crafts an argument showing that adventure is not about competition or conquering physical features such as reaching the top of Everest, instead Adventure Psychology is more about sustainability, collaboration, and getting back safely and well. Duren concludes this is best described as optimal performance rather than peak performance. Jennifer Pickett and Paula Reid go into the unknown with the psychology of navigating the unpredictability that characterises so many adventure experiences. They examine the role of personality and coping and point the adventurous reader to the crucial function of mindfulness and adaptability. Kitrina Douglas, David Carless, Paula Reid, and Ruth Hughes focus on positive psychology and narrative theory as useful frames to understand and explore Adventure Psychology. Specifically, they show how these frames help understand motivators and rewarding outcomes. However, far from the old ideas of risk and sensation-seeking, they argue for a more profound understanding that not only impacts on flourishing for the adventurer but also for those listening to and following the adventurer's journey. Tuomas Immomen, Eric Brymer, Timo Jaakkola, and Keith Davids also take a theoretical perspective to framing Adventure Psychology, stemming from ecological psychology. Using a relational scaffold, they show how adventure is a fundamental element of being human and Adventure Psychology ideally positioned to examine the human condition. Kessler and Brymer explore a much-misunderstood aspect of Adventure Psychology, the role of fear. Traditional notions of fearlessness and connotations of participants having "no fear" are rightly critiqued through the voices of mountain adventure participants. Instead, we find that fear is a benevolent guide and focusing force vital to the experience and the implications of this realisation are profound. Monasterio follows with an examination of the psychology of success and failure in adventure. Instead of traditional notions, we find that success and failure in adventure is framed by more transformative notions such as growth, self-transcendence, and pro-environmental behaviour. Emilia Elisabet Lahti's chapter wraps up this first section with a description of the links between the Finnish concept of Sisu and adventure. Sisu describes how we can go beyond our perceived limits with innate gentle power and Lahti explores how best to harness the power for good.

While on occasion, some of the chapters in the first section hint at the transformative properties of adventure, section "Transformational Impact of Adventure" sets out to explicitly examine psychological notions linked to post-adventure transformations. There are four chapters in this section each outlining important psychological outcomes from adventure. Susan Houge Mackenzie sets the scene with a description about how the natural environment inherent in adventure plays a unique role in facilitating optimal human experiences and provides an interesting insight into human potential. Similarly, Hanna Kampman and Petra Walker point to a link between adventure and optimum human experience and how adventure can facilitate growth even after considerable trauma. Taking a slightly different track, Amy Smallwood and Chris Loynes examine the role of adventure in the development of transformational and transcendent experiences. They point out the impact on society and how a transcendental notion of nature might facilitate a stronger person–nature relationship. Vinathe Sharma-Brymer takes the human–nature experience one step further and reflects on the importance of adventure for women in traditional patriarchal societies.

Finally, Eric Brymer and Paula Reid draw the chapters together to refine Adventure Psychology and propose important learnings and future development. They posit that it is time for Adventure Psychology to be recognised as an independent field of psychology.

★ ★ ★ ★

Application beyond Academia

Further, the material covered in these chapters holds strategies and tools for everyday life. Whichever 'hat' you wear while reading – as a researcher, student, in business, or in life – parallels can be drawn, and the psychological constructs held within this book can be applied.

The metaphor is that we are all on an 'adventure' – an enduring journey of challenge and uncertainty. On our journeys, we must negotiate obstacles and events and navigate environments and circumstances, with successes and trials, achievements and challenges, along the way. Adventuring requires extensive psychological adaptability due to the variability and volatility of the conditions and complexity of the interdependencies. This includes the ability to respond to change, to learn from experience, and then apply that learning to aid future performance. It requires extensive psychological agility: balance and control to deal with uncertainty and ambiguity. It demands enduring and sustainable performance via tolerance, self-regulation, and mental toughness. It challenges us, ignites our courage, and facilitates our humility. It often involves decision-making in high-pressure contexts. It demands awareness, responsibility, and autonomy. It can have transformational impact.

It is also a holistic and immersive experience, relating with the environment and the need to be perpetually attuned and sympathetically cooperative, and often also requiring us to relate with others, including our global and multifarious diversities. Adventure encourages evolution and progress, in contrast to languishing or remaining in stasis. It requires our "pre-adventure" preparedness, planning, and foresight and our "post-adventure" reflections, applications, and hindsights. Adventure can help us transform or transcend.

This book may help us all flourish and get psychologically stronger despite adversity, volatility, and uncertainty. Adventure Psychology is designed to meet the needs of specialists across a variety of fields but importantly also to be accessible and applicable for those wanting to survive, cope, and ultimately thrive in this changing, challenging, uncertain world. To Go Knowingly into the Unknown.

References

Arijs, C., Chroni, S., Brymer, E., & Carless, D. (2017). "Leave your ego at the door": A narrative investigation into effective wingsuit flying. *Frontiers in Psychology: Performance Science*, 8, 1985. https://doi.org/10.3389/fpsyg.2017.01985

Brown, M., & Beames, S. (2017) Adventure education: Redux. *Journal of Adventure Education and Outdoor Learning*, 17(4), 294–306, https://doi.org/10.1080/14729679.2016.1246257

Buckley, R. C. (2015). Adventure thrills are addictive. *Frontiers in Psychology*, 6, 1915. https://doi.org/10.3389/fpsyg.2015.01915

Giddy, J. K., & Webb, N. L. (2018). The influence of the environment on adventure tourism: From motivations to experiences. *Current Issues in Tourism*, 21(18), 2124–2138. https://doi.org/10.1080/13683500.2016.1245715

Gomà i Freixanet, M., Martha, C., & Muro, A. (2012). Does the sensation seeking trait differ among participants engaged in sports with different levels of physical risk? *Anales de psicología, 28*(1), 2012.

Gunnar, B. (2010). Trends in adventure sports in a post-modern society. *Sport in Society, 13*(2), 260–273. https://doi.org/10.1080/17430430903522970

Hanna, P., Wijesinghe, S., Paliatsos, I., Walker, C., Adams, M., & Kimbu, A. (2019). Active engagement with nature: outdoor adventure tourism, sustainability and well-being. *Journal of Sustainable Tourism*. https://doi.org/10.1080/09669582.2019.1621883

Houge Mackenzie, S., & Brymer, E. (2018). Conceptualising adventurous nature sport: A positive psychology perspective. Annals of Leisure Research. ISSN 1174-5398. https://doi.org/10.1080/11745398.2018.1483733

Houge Mackenzie, S., & Hodge, K. (2020). Adventure recreation and subjective well-being: A conceptual framework. *Leisure Studies, 39*(1), 26–40. https://doi.org/10.1080/02614367.2019.1577478

Immonen, T., Brymer, E., Davids, K., & Jaakkola, T. (in press). An ecological dynamics approach to understanding human-environment interactions in the adventure sport context – Implications for research and practice. *International Journal of Environmental Research and Public Health*. https://doi.org/10.3390/ijerph19063691

Immonen, T., Brymer, E., Orth, D., Davids, K., Feletti, F., Liukkonen, J., & Jaakkola, T. (2017). Understanding action and adventure sports participation – An ecological dynamics perspective. *Sports Medicine, 3*, 18. https://doi.org/10.1186/s40798-017-0084-1

Kerr, J. H. & Houge Mackenzie, S. (2012). Multiple motives for participating in adventure sports. *Psychology of Sport and Exercise, 13*, 649–657.

Monasterio, E., & Brymer, E. (2021). Feeding time at the zoo: Psychological aspects of a serious rock climbing accident. *Journal of Adventure Education & Outdoor Learning, 21*(4), 323–335. https://doi.org/10.1080/14729679.2020.1829494

Monasterio, E., & Brymer, E. (2015). Mountaineering Personality and Risk. In G. Musa, J. Higham, A. Thompson Carr (Eds.), *Mountaineering tourism*. Routledge.

Palmberg, I. E., & Kuru, J. (2000). Outdoor activities as a basis for environmental responsibility. *The Journal of Environmental Education, 31*(4), 32–36. https://doi.org/10.1080/00958960009598649

Peacock, S., Brymer, E., Davids, K., & Dillon, M. (2017). An ecological dynamics perspective on adventure tourism. *Tourism Review International, 21*(3), 307–316.

Priest, S. (1992). Factor exploration and confirmation for the dimensions of an adventure experience. *Journal of Leisure Research, 24*(2), 127–139. https://doi.org/10.1080/00222216.1992.11969881

Reid, P., & Kampman, H. (2020). Exploring the psychology of extended-period expeditionary adventurers: Going knowingly into the unknown. *Psychology of Sport and Exercise, 46*, 101608. https://doi.org/10.1016/j.psychsport.2019.101608

Warren, K., Mitten, D., D'Amore, C., & Lotz, E. (2019). The gendered hidden curriculum of adventure education. *Journal of Experiential Education, 42*(2), 140–154. https://doi.org/10.1177/1053825918813398

ADVENTURE PSYCHOLOGY

A Long Past, but a Short History

Peter Suedfeld

An Adventurer's Point of View: North Pole, 1909.

There is an irresistible fascination about the regions of the northernmost Grant Land that is impossible for me to describe. Having no poetry in my soul, and being somewhat hardened by years of experience in that inhospitable country, words proper to give you an idea of its unique beauty do not come to mind. Imagine gorgeous bleakness, beautiful blankness. It never seems, broad, bright day, even in the middle of June, and the sky has the different effects of the varying hours of morning and evening twilight from the first to the last peep of day. Early in February, at noon, a thin band of light appears far to the southward, heralding the approach of the sun, and daily the twilight lengthens, until early in March, the sun, a flaming disk of fiery crimson, shows his distorted image above the horizon. This distorted shape is due to the mirage caused by the cold, just as heat-waves above the rails on a railroad-track distort the shape of objects beyond.

The south sides of the lofty peaks have for days reflected the glory of the coming sun, and it does not require an artist to enjoy the unexampled splendor of the view. The snows covering the peaks show all of colors, variations, and tones of the artist's palette, and more. Artists have gone with us into the Arctic and I have heard them rave over the wonderful beauties of the scene, and I have seen them at work trying to reproduce some of it, with good results but with nothing like the effect of the original. As Mr. Stokes said, 'It is color run riot'. (pp. 66–67)

We turned in for a rest and sleep, but soon turned out again in pandemonium incomprehensible; the ice moving in all directions, our igloos wrecked, and every instant our very lives in danger. With eyes dazed by sleep, we tried to guide the terror-stricken dogs and push the sledges to safety, but rapidly we saw the party being separated and the black water begin to appear amid the roar of the breaking ice floes.

To the westward of our igloo stood the Captain's igloo, on an island of ice, which revolved, while swiftly drifting to the eastward. On one occasion the floe happened to strike the main floe. The Captain, intently watching his opportunity, quickly crossed with his Esquimos. He had scarcely set foot on the opposite floe when the floe on which he had been previously isolated, swung off, and rapidly disappeared. (p. 121)

It was during the march of the 3^d of April that I endured an instant of hideous horror. We were crossing a lane of moving ice. Commander Peary was in the lead setting the pace, and a half hour later the four boys and myself followed in single file. They had all gone before, and I was standing and pushing at the upstanders of my sledge, when the block of ice I was using as a support slipped from underneath my feet, and before I knew it the sledge was out of my grasp, and I was floundering in the water of the lead. I did the best I could. I tore my hood from off my head and struggled frantically. My hands were gloved and I could not take hold of the ice, but before I could give the "Grand Hailing Sign of Distress," faithful old Ootah had grabbed me by the nape of the neck, the same as he would have grabbed a dog, and with one hand he pulled me out of the water, and with the other hurried the team across. (pp. 130–131)

> Matthew A. Henson. Originally from: *A Negro Explorer at the North (1912), excerpts here taken from: A Black Explorer at the North Pole (1969)*

Adventure Psychology: A Long Past, but a Short History

What Do We Mean by "Adventure"?

This chapter addresses the features that are involved in adventures, considers the characteristics of adventurers, and summarises psychological theories that are relevant to the adventurous personality. It does not examine the large-scale "adventures" that groups undertake out of necessity or compulsion: the mass migrations that formed the demography of Europe, nomads and pioneers searching for new lands, refugees seeking a safe haven, or armies deployed in unfamiliar areas. The focus is on individuals or small teams facing and coping with environments that to them are novel, strange, and challenging.

"Adventure" has had many definitions. Most refer to experiences that are unusual, exciting, hazardous, exploratory (especially "unknown territory"), risky, daring, and the like. Although several expand the meanings quite broadly, including speculative financial dealings or tasting an unfamiliar cuisine, most focus on physical exploration of territory that is unfamiliar to the adventurer, and in many cases, unknown to the world at large. "To adventure" refers to the act of seeking such experiences, and "adventurers" are people who seek them. Not all definitions are positive: "Adventure is just bad planning." Thus, adventure is merely a lack of foresight. This definition is attributed to Roald Amundsen, Norwegian leader of the first expedition to reach the South Pole, famous for his meticulous, detailed, logistical, and geographical preparations (Amundsen, undated). Amundsen might have been amused by psychology's current scepticism about the possibility of accurately forecasting future needs and events (Tetlock, 2006). "When you're safe at home you wish you were having an adventure; when you're having an adventure you wish you were safe at home." – Thornton Wilder, American author who adventured in China and Italy and perhaps experienced danger and discomfort not to his liking (T. Wilder, undated).

If unfamiliarity and danger are critical criteria, the decision whether a particular act, deed, or experience is adventurous must take into account the individual characteristics of both the adventurer and the situation. Sherpas visiting a metropolis for the first time would almost definitely find crossing a major traffic thoroughfare an adventure both dangerous and strange; for lifelong Mumbaikars or New Yorkers, it would be very familiar and sometimes risky, but hardly an adventure. The reverse would be true of a climb in the Himalayas.

As in many cases, finding a suitable definition is more difficult than identifying outstanding prototypes and exemplars of the category (respectively, a mental picture of the imagined "typical member" of that category and a remembered or imagined specific example; Storms et al., 2000). We may agree on which people seek or experience adventures, while others don't (or even avoid them). Some may seek exciting, risky, unfamiliar experiences often, some only once, and others in-between, more or less frequently, or never. The category "adventurer" may be restricted to those relatively few people who seek them out again and again.

The histories and stories of such adventurers have intrigued, fascinated, and inspired generations around the world. Who, then, are these rare people, how do they differ from the rest, and what moves them to do it? Before considering scientific data, let's look at some old tales, myths, legends, fiction, and facts.

Classical Tales of Adventure

I'll begin with an early humanoid whose exact position in our evolution is unknown. I admire this person as the daring adventurer *par excellence,* facing both novelty and the likelihood of peril. No one knows when or where this person lived, but he or she was the first human being to confront, kill, and even eat a daunting, newly met animal covered in hard, segmented armor and owning large claws that it was "brandishing...like weapons" (Wallace, 2004). Imagine the courage of that very first human to deal so decisively with the bizarre, scary-looking, dangerous species we now refer to as the lobster. Was the motive merely hunger, or did curiosity play a part?

More seriously, the first explorers coming out of their African homeland were true discoverers, treading where no human or humanoid had gone before. Today, the oceans and outer space provide the last opportunities for that kind of discovery. More recent explorers usually "discovered" places hitherto unknown to their compatriots but in fact inhabited and thoroughly investigated by other human beings for centuries or millennia. Today's adventurers may innovate new routes, replicate earlier histories, or use unfamiliar environments to explore their own thoughts, emotions, competence, courage, and resilience (Davis, 2021).

The myths, folktales, and fiction of various cultures repeat themes of adventure, implying some universal substrate of content that may point to the crucial components of the concept. Many of the same features appear in the biographies of the explorers of more recent times (see, *inter alia*, Chapter 2). My choice of pronouns reflects the fact that almost all of the earlier stories are told from a male point of view, although women have been recognised as adventurers both deservedly famous (Jeanne Baret, first woman to circumnavigate the world – disguised as a male sailor; Ridley, 2010) and undeservedly obscure (Gudrun, an apocryphal Viking woman traveller in North America; Durn, 2021). There has been increasing recognition of history's female adventurers – although the definition may need to be expanded in some cases, such as Anne Bonny and Mary Read, close friends, and notorious pirates of the early 1700s (Durn, 2022).

Reluctant Adventurers

In the Greek *Odyssey*, as in the Indian *Ramayana*, the hero is forced to leave his home and wander from place to place, facing many obstacles and enemies (human, monstrous, and divine). Both heroes are in danger of losing their beloved wife, eventually to find her faithful and safe. Both use a supernatural bow to prove their identity and regain their rightful, royal place.

The parallels between the two, from opposite sides of the Earth, are striking. Neither wants to go a-venturing, but is forced to do so for a long period. Both are high-born; each has some human and supernatural supporters and enemies; each overcomes the opposing forces through bravery, fighting ability, and cleverness. Attacks on the virtue of the hero's wife, her unshakeable fidelity, and the role of a unique bow to prove his identity are other similarities.

There are many such fictional and actual biographies. A need for change, excitement, novelty, or adventure figures in some; others depict victims of accident, poverty, malevolence, or superior force. According to one observer, adventure stories became popular as they "communicated the values of bourgeois society in the 19th century: energy, tenacity, faith, and, most importantly, work and knowledge. In such tales, shipwrecked heroes rebuilt with these sole virtues the entire civilization they had lost....In the old tradition of Odysseus and Robinson Crusoe, the heroes of this literature dreamed above all else of getting back home" (Arnould, 2015).

If the decision to seek the experience or the goal is an indispensable part of being an adventurer, none of the "Reluctant" category people qualifies, regardless of what adventures they may have had.

Quests, Material, and Spiritual

Another major theme in mythical and historical adventure is that of the quest. Three components are crucial: the central character, the goal of the quest, and the adventure itself, with obstacles and perils to overcome. This omits an interesting psychological question: what motivates the adventurer? Frequently, it is an extrinsic reward: the promise of a cave full of gold, half the kingdom, the beautiful princess for a bride, the life or freedom of a beloved relative (frequent in stories of woman searchers). The hero sets out willingly, often eagerly, travels to strange places, and faces various dangers in order to win the reward.

Sometimes, the hero is motivated for an intrinsic, spiritual goal. The Knights of the Round Table are inspired by King Arthur to defend the helpless and bring order, peace, and justice to the realm; the search for the Holy Grail is an explicitly religious quest. Don Quixote de la Mancha, although deluded about reality, fights for honor and justice: attacking prison officials in a mistaken mission "to free the slaves," tilting at windmills he believes are evil giants, exalting the owner of a cheap inn as the lord of a castle. In his world, most people are either virtuous – to be respected and protected – or evil, to be thwarted. The Knights of the Jedi Order risk their lives to protect the defenseless for the sake of justice. A plethora of adventurous quest books, plays, and films are vivid in our collective memory. A quick look at any compendium of public entertainment shows similar riches from a wide variety of cultures around the world.

Spiritual quests establish a conceptual and methodological link to religion. Many indigenous cultures around the world include a "spirit quest" or "vision quest," typically a rite of passage for adolescents. Individuals isolate themselves, often abstaining from food and drink, in a challenging part of the group's territory, such as a mountain, desert, or forest. This sojourn is both a test of survival skills and immersion in the spiritual world, during which the quester may encounter ancestors, supernatural guides and advisers, totemic animals, prophetic dreams, and gods or God.

Western counterparts include religious pilgrimages and retreats. The life stories of founders and leaders of the world's major religions exemplify how solitude and natural settings serve to facilitate enlightenment, insight, and contact with supernatural beings (Storr, 1988). Contemporary commercial "vision quests" are also available (though criticised as cultural misappropriation).

Periods of contact with nature are sought by many urbanites, and research has shown their positive effects (e.g., Bratman et al., 2015). Scouting and some educational programs emphasise spiritual contact with nature and testing oneself in outdoor activities in order to supplement or counteract the sedentary artificiality of modern school curricula – e.g., Outward Bound (Hahn, 1957) and Students on Ice (Green, 2006). Up to a week in a dark, silent cabin (Darkness Therapy; Malůš et al., 2016) is used by clients as a chance to meditate, fantasise, de-stress, and – a recently fashionable formulation, not found in classical adventure tales – "find oneself."

The Adventurous *Zeitgeist*

Seekers of adventure tend to come from societies that have moved beyond subsistence efforts, from the strata in those societies that had sufficient means and leisure time to indulge in expensive, time-consuming travel and to need special opportunities to test themselves in dangerous situations. The porters and foremast sailors who support their efforts are mostly there to make a living, perhaps with some desire for novel experiences.

The 15th- to the 21st-century CE saw an outburst of exploration from European and europogenic (i.e., those derived primarily from European) nations. This resulted in the discovery of parts of the world and their populations, both hitherto unknown and mysterious to Europeans, although obviously long familiar to the folk who had wandered in and settled there millennia earlier. One important exception was the discovery and exploration of Antarctica, the only continent without any history of human population. Is (or was) there something special about European culture that imbued this fever of adventuring and the curiosity of both the travellers and their stay-at-home audiences (including governments, which very often financed the trip)? No other explorers ranged so widely to all areas of the globe.

In the language of modern psychology, some of these quests were motivated by approach motives: a search for material benefits such as land and sovereignty, precious minerals or plants, rare animals; some had significant non-material aspects, such as religious conversion, national pride, the ego of rulers, freedom, personal status and fame, or the satisfaction of curiosity. Others were avoidance quests to escape poverty, hunger, oppression, or persecution. Some were motivated by a desire for adventure for its own sake. Tourists then as now wanted to see the world, to experience excitement and suspense (and sometimes, danger). The Grand Tour of affluent British youths a few centuries ago combined some such opportunities along with exposure to unfamiliar histories and folkways, just as many young people now take a "gap year" of travel and adventure before facing extended adolescence in further schooling.

The wide variety of individuals who engaged in the early years of this Golden Age of Exploration, and their range of motives, are striking and make generalisations very difficult if not impossible. Here are capsule accounts of the accomplishments of three notable adventurers in the past few centuries. All of them spent many years in adventurous travel and the collection of naturalistic and scientific data, much of which is still of use today.

Captain James Cook started life as the son of an itinerant farmhand. At first sailing in merchant ships, he eventually joined the Royal Navy as a common seaman and rose to become a post captain (the highest rank below admiral) and a Fellow of the Royal Society. He was well known for his insistence on sanitation, ventilation, and the inclusion of antiscorbutics in his men's diet, which kept his crews unusually healthy. His expeditions explored the Pacific Ocean and its rim, from the Arctic Circle and Canada through Hawaii (where he was later killed), Tahiti, Australia, to New Zealand and the Antarctic Circle. His published journals provided the first information Europeans had about many of the peoples and areas in that vast range, contributions not only to geography, oceanography, astronomy, navigation, and cartography, but also to anthropology (e.g., Price, 1971). According to the *Encyclopedia Britannica*, "he had ... changed the map of the world more than any other single man in history" (Villiers, 2021).

In the mid-1800s, *Sir Richard Francis Burton* spent his youth in Europe, with the result that as he wrote, he ended up feeling at home everywhere except in his native England. He subsequently joined the Army and served in various regions of South Asia, undertaking missions disguised as a native merchant. Later, disguised as an Afghan, he travelled to the forbidden "holy city" of Mecca. He was wounded by a spear during an expedition to another forbidden city in East Africa. After recovering and participating in the Crimean War, he again took up exploring: first, a return to Africa and then to Utah. Next, he explored West Africa while serving as British consul in that area. His consular duties then took him to Brazil, Damascus, and Trieste, where he eventually died.

Burton was fluent in 25 languages (40 counting various dialects). He wrote 40 books in his life, covering his travels and the geography, religions, customs, myths, and histories of the cultures he encountered, as well as many translations. His magisterial 16-volume translation of the *Thousand and One Nights* (Burton, 1885) has been widely reprinted, although often condemned and bowdlerised because of its then-shocking frankness about the sexual content of the original tales.

Dr. Fridtjof Nansen was a Norwegian, university-trained zoologist who made his first Arctic sea voyage at the age of 21 and became fascinated by the Far North. His later explorations by land and sea took him across the Arctic, setting several "firsts"; but his most important achievements were technical and scientific. His contributions included *Fram*, a unique ship that could rise to the top of an ice floe rather than being crushed by it, as so many vessels had been in polar seas; the Nansen sled and the Nansen stove, improved equipment still used in polar expeditions; and many volumes of scientific material including Nansen's theory of ocean flow, later proven correct.

When Norway became an independent nation, Nansen combined science with a diplomatic career. After many high-level posts, in 1920, the League of

Nations appointed him to administer the repatriation of prisoners of war, then the food distribution in the famine-stricken USSR, and finally the rescue and resettlement of refugees from various wars, revolutions, and persecutions. The League's "Nansen passports" enabled multitudes of refugees to travel across borders and find safe countries. These accomplishments led to his being awarded the Nobel Prize for Peace in 1922, and to the League setting up a permanent office for refugee protection and naming it after Nansen.

Safetyist Adventures, Hyper-Dangerous Adventures

In recent decades, the details of adventuring have changed drastically. There is a firmer line between recreational or avocational adventurers and professional explorers, scientists, and sojourners. Their activities have been altered by sophisticated technology in transportation, communications, medicine, life-support apparatus, etc. These innovations make it possible for human beings to live and thrive in environments that were previously impossible to access safely (or at all), including of course space and the ocean depths but also high mountains, deserts, polar regions, jungles, and in fact, all parts of our globe.

These developments have led to some laughable, and some deplorable, changes in the structure of adventure tourism. "Safetyism," the worldview that safety is the supreme sacred value in all activities and circumstances (Lukianoff & Haidt, 2018), has led to so-called adventures comprised of having the "adventurer" maximally protected from all discomfort, deprivation, or danger (including unpleasant emotions). Although total safety cannot be assured in any endeavour anywhere, the goal is to keep the individual reassuringly guarded.

Professional supporters such as guides and porters traditionally did maintenance and manual chores, stood by to help in an emergency, and taught their clients how to use equipment, recognise danger, and stay as safe as possible. Present-day adventures go much further. They include safaris where the client never sets foot outside a vehicle, sky-diving and hang-gliding with the client strapped to the harness of a professional who performs all necessary tasks, underwater diving in a mini-submarine, and so on. I happened to be at the start of a trek from Resolute Bay, Nunavut (then NWT), to the North Pole, which consisted of the client sitting or lying in a comfortable sled while being towed by a local Inuk riding a snowmobile, supplies being towed by another "guide." The trip was monitored by radio from start to finish, with rescue or resupply rapidly available if needed. The result was a possibly exciting, surely interesting experience, to be recalled with pleasure and talked about with friends, but its definition as an adventure is certainly diluted.

The ultimate safetyist adventure is in sight: virtual reality (VR) will enable anyone to travel anywhere without leaving home. It's *Star Trek*'s holodeck without the USS *Enterprise*; in fact, without any enterprise at all. One visionary astrosociologist has suggested that someday, real explorers in deep space may enjoy sharing terrestrial VR adventures with their family and friends on Earth (P.J. Johnson, personal communication, June 2021).

Perhaps as a reaction to safetyism, a few adventurers take pride in arranging their exploits to be hyper-dangerous, as *un*safe as possible, some even to the point of foolhardiness. Some have climbed the highest mountains without oxygen, skied solo and unsupported across the polar icecap, sailed single-handed around the world, or spent summers living among wild predators. There are adventures that seem as though they had been designed specifically to enter the *Guinness World Records* – and, in fact, the urge to be the first to do something may play an important motivational part (Snyder & Fromkin, 1977). The same expedition outfitter who arranged the towed sled trip to the North Pole also outfitted two men who planned to ride to the Pole on motorcycles equipped with spiked tires. In a radio interview, he off-handedly quipped that people kept coming up with bizarre ideas; he would not have been surprised if someone had suggested traveling to the Pole on elephant-back. A few days later, he received a phone call from a rich person who offered to finance such an exploit, but so far as I know, it hasn't happened yet. It may come to reality when biologists use DNA retrieved from a woolly mammoth to recreate that species: the perfect ride and companion on a cold-weather trek.

What Do We Mean by "A Long Past, But a Short History"?

The title of this chapter is a paraphrase of a comment about psychology more generally (Ebbinghaus, 1908). Psychologists study and attempt to understand the mind and behaviour of both human beings and animals of other species. As such, psychological matters have been a major topic of curiosity for most people, probably since the first *homo erectus* wondered how someone else in the group would react to some gesture or communication or how a prey animal could be enticed into a trap.

Scientific psychology, however, is relatively new. In its concern with basic mental processes and the remediation of widespread mental disorders, its subject matter is among the most complex of scientific topics. In its busy concern with everyday issues, psychology has tended to downplay the unusual and esoteric. The psychology of adventure, and of adventurers, which has fascinated people for thousands of years, has barely begun to engage the organised attention of psychologists. The Adventure Psychology Network may be a door to the future, https://www.facebook.com/groups/1291472931244640/permalink/1476653389393259/, an outlet for "psychologists in related disciplines very interested in adventure and adventurers very interested in psychology."

Leading academic psychologists of the early 20th century were determined to establish the field as one of the "hard" sciences. They argued that what cannot be observed cannot be measured, and what cannot be measured has no place in science. Thus, scientific psychology was to be concerned only with observable stimuli (e.g., food deprivation) and the observable responses that follow them (e.g., eating). Although psychologists (like everyone else) wanted, feared, knew, imagined, loved, etc., these constructs were not considered to be susceptible to scientific inquiry.

This school of thought eventually hit the iceberg of what is now called "lived experience" (is there some other kind?). Clearly, people do respond to internal stimuli, psychological or physiological, that cannot be observed from the outside; and also clearly, many of their reactions are equally internal.

Eventually, the paradigm shifted (Kuhn, 1970). Research-oriented psychologists began to study the living being that has a significant role in processing a stimulus, interpreting it, responding emotionally or cognitively to it, and then choosing the response, not necessarily overt, that follows. The new theorists of the mid-20th century proposed that organisms function best and are most comfortable in a zone of moderate arousal. Both insufficient *and* excessive levels of physiological and non-physiological needs are aversive and adverse. The organism is thought to be active in seeking or becoming more responsive to additional information, novelty, or stimulation (Berlyne,1960) when its arousal level is below the moderate zone, and to be active in seeking to reduce those factors when its level is too far above the zone (Helson, 1964).

This change opened the door for a variety of new approaches in all areas of the discipline, and for new sub-disciplines. Adventure Psychology is one of those. Given sufficient food, water, rest, etc., there is no obvious reason for people to explore dangerous places, engage in risky sports, or endure unnecessary hardship and discomfort. Those behaviors can be explained by the desire for the optimal level of arousal, optimal being a function of personality, health, age, culture, life experience, and social group.

The adventuring personality may have changed with changes in the nature of adventure itself. Expeditions no longer rely on recruiting members through advertisements such as the famous (and apocryphal) newspaper notice attributed to Shackleton's search for Antarctic crewmates (cited in Elmore, 1944, p. 53 and frequently elsewhere):

> Men wanted for hazardous journey. Low wages, bitter cold, long hours of complete darkness. Safe return doubtful. Honour and recognition in event of success.

The advertisement supposedly attracted a long queue of volunteers. One need not be a psychologist to draw some inferences from this. It is clearly aimed at men only, no surprise in a polar expedition around the early 1900s. Moreover, it seeks men motivated to face uncertainty, extreme discomfort, and danger, in the pursuit of intangible rewards. These could be external, such as social recognition, as well as internal, the potential experience of excitement and novelty and feelings of achievement, hardiness, and courage.

Does motivation matter in defining the adventurer? The difference between adventuring for the sake of intangible versus material rewards is one of the major (although fuzzy) dividing lines between two large categories of participants. We can compare, as somewhat random examples, Marco Polo and Lady Hester Stanhope.

Marco Polo was a 13th-century Venetian merchant who followed his family tradition by searching strange lands and peoples to find new commercial opportunities. Accompanied by relatives, he travelled through what are now Israel, Turkey, Iran, Afghanistan, Pakistan. In China, he became an administrator for the Mongol Emperor Kublai Khan. Amassing riches, after a quarter century, he eventually reached home, suffering robbery, war, and imprisonment before settling down to a quiet old age.

Lady Hester Stanhope was a socialite and one of the most famous travellers of the early 19th century. She travelled, often in male disguise, through the Near and Middle East in a seemingly insatiable search for new experiences. She made important archaeological discoveries in what is now Israel. To assure the Ottoman government of her selfless dedication to pure discovery, she destroyed a large statue, the first relic of Greek and Roman antiquity ever found in the area. She experienced fame, celebrity, and influence, shipwreck, factional strife, and both the admiration and the suspicion of powerful people. Finally, she died alone and poor, far from home.

Most psychologists accept the influential view – in my opinion, an axiom — that behaviour is generally a function of the interaction between person and environment [$B = f(P \times E)$] (Lewin, 1946). The life circumstances of the early Renaissance Venetian merchant and the Georgian-era British noblewoman were widely different, as were their motives and personalities. How, then, did both end up among the most famous adventurers of their time and place?

Anecdotes Aren't Data; Descriptions Aren't Theories

Basic values and motives are important aspects of personality. We can consider them from two points of view. One is that human beings in general have an innate need or combination of needs that leads them to engage in the behaviours that are involved in adventuring. Studying this motivation is difficult because adventuring takes such varied forms, attracts so many widely different personalities, and offers so many kinds of possible rewards, that drawing widely applicable conclusions seems an impossible task.

Psychologists to a great extent have not faced this task. Studies of the personality and motivational characteristics of adventurers are overwhelmingly idiographic and inductive. We test or interview one or a few aspiring or actual (or retired) adventurers, or content analyse their logs and diaries. Then, we analyse the results and draw inferences about the personality, motives, values, etc. of those particular people. We seldom create testable generalisations.

To progress, adventure psychology needs theory-based, hypothesis-testing research. It should begin with formulating a theory of factors that are likely to characterise adventurers and differentiate them from non-adventurers, create one or more measures of those factors, and administer the measures to representative samples of both groups. The results should enable us to identify the degree to which the measures actually do differentiate. Next, refine the measures by analysing the power of each component to discriminate.

The process can be repeated until the measures yield clear results. The measures can then be administered to current and past adventurers, prospective adventurers, and people with no interest in adventure. Eventually, the researchers would recruit large groups of people in situations where going on an adventure is optional, and using the now well-tested and refined measures, predict which of them will volunteer, go, and succeed.

At this point, no such research has even been started. Still, social and personality psychologists have studied some seemingly relevant traits and motives, which might be a place to begin. The list below is very selective and limited; I picked a few concepts that seem to be appropriate to the task. I only briefly mention each theory and leave details and further reading to those whose interest is aroused. I omit formulations based on depth psychology, which are often creative, interesting, and persuasive, but also often untestable.

Psychology's Relevant Concepts: A Selective Sampling

1. *Maslow's hierarchy of needs* (1962, first version 1943) is a theoretically hierarchical sequence (a controversial idea, not fully supported by data) of important needs. Beginning with the basic things needed for *physiological survival*, such as food, to *safety*, it moves to the future assurance of those things; then, *belonging* and acceptance in a social group; next, the *esteem* and respect of other members of the group; and when all of those are satisfied, the need for *self-actualisation*, becoming all one can be. Later, Maslow added *transcendence*, the need to become one with something greater than oneself: humanity as a whole, our planet, history, the spiritual sphere. The first four needs are likely to be relevant to adventuring, as to life more widely; the drive to test oneself against challenge may be related to self-actualisation, and transcendence has been discernible in the way that explorers have written about the new emotions they have felt in space, the polar regions, and other vast natural environments.
2. *"The Big Five"* are five clusters of personality traits, the patterns of which influence one's reactions to different situations and other people. There are several versions of a psychometrically well-established test to measure them (e.g., McCrae & Costa, 2008). The trait dimensions are:

    Openness to Experience, which includes curiosity, stimulation-seeking, and enjoyment of new experiences and ideas – a good description of adventurousness;

Conscientiousness, meaning organisation, dependability, planning ahead, and focusing on goals, a useful set of traits for expedition organisers and leaders unless it rises to obsessive-compulsive disorder;

Extraversion, liking to be with others, enjoying conversation and cooperative activities, impulsiveness traits that are good in moderation, but can become negative in an uncomfortable and confined environment, especially if people are tired or stressed;

Agreeableness, which includes empathy, trust, and helpfulness, all generally good characteristics if not carried too far; and

Neuroticism, meaning mood swings, irritability, anxiety, and high susceptibility to stress, obviously not desirable traits in an adventurer.

Incidentally, note the acronym, OCEAN. An alternative way of arranging the letters gives us CANOE, both showing an association with the theory to exploration.

3. *Thrill-Seeking* (Farley, 2010) and *Sensation-Seeking* (Zuckerman, 2009) personalities exhibit preferences for high levels of arousal and stimulation, excitement, and risk. The scales that measure the different components can help selectors for adventure teams to rule out applicants who are high in the undesirable characteristics. The two personality types are related to each other and also show some correlation with Openness in the Big Five. They may seem to be a perfect basis for taking on adventurous activities, and to some extent, the seekers seem to live up to their billing. Type T's crave excitement; they are also self-confident, creative, optimistic, self-reliant, and courageous. Their self-confidence, if carried to an extreme, can lead them to value their own opinions above anyone else's and to take unwise risks, especially when combined with high courage and need for excitement and risk.

High Sensation seekers like excitement and adventure, as well as new experiences of other sorts, but their trait cluster also includes what Zuckerman called "disinhibition," a preference for uncontrolled emotion and wild behaviour. This can negate the positive aspects of the other components of the trait, making the individual a dangerous and unpopular group member.

Another component is "boredom susceptibility." A high score on that should indicate the undesirability of a person for adventures that involve long periods in restricted environments such as a small hut or tent, or long stretches of trekking in monotonous places such as an icefield. Antarctic jobs often attract applicants who are high on this trait and then immure them in monotonous habitats and repetitive work duties for the long winter. This strategy is self-defeating, but sometimes unavoidable because of restricted availability of some specialists.

4. *Need for Uniqueness* (Snyder & Fromkin, 1977) is not as obviously related to adventurousness, but perhaps it explains the often surprising and even appalling forms that adventuring sometimes takes. It seems intuitively obvious that people want to be recognised as individuals, not just as members of a faceless crowd, and to be valued and appreciated. Maslow's esteem need

and various theories of need for achievement agree on the importance of this motive; cultures around the world recognise and honour outstanding accomplishment, and individuals in all of those cultures strive for that outcome. This need, too, has its dark side, not only in hyper-dangerous adventuring but also in distortions where the individual expresses the need for uniqueness by committing unusual and widely publicised atrocities.

5. *Reversal Theory* (Apter, 2007) is a much wider-ranging set of concepts than the previous ones discussed, with a variety of ideas concerning human motivation, personality, and emotion. However, in the context of Adventure Psychology, its main application is in the distinction between seriousness and playfulness (telic versus paratelic orientation, respectively). The telic state is marked by seriousness and goal orientation, especially the achievement of long-term goals. The paratelic state emphasises the enjoyment of the process that might lead to such achievement, but the positive affect is experienced along the way and is thus real even if in the end the goal is not reached. Although the theory emphasises the fluidity of these two states, with motivation changing from one to the other (thus, "reversal theory"), the distinction seems to me to apply centrally to adventurers. One important question seldom asked of them, either during the event or after it ends, is: "What did you enjoy about it?" The answer to that question may point to the core of whether the person sees the adventure as something to be got through to reach some desired end or as a progression that is interesting, challenging, and appreciated from start to finish.

6. *Problem-Oriented versus Emotion-Oriented Coping* (Folkman & Lazarus, 1988). This is not really a theory, and coping behaviour may not reflect stable personality differences. But the difference is real. I have experienced and observed it through many years of research, including considerable travelling and conducting field studies. The basic distinction is between people who in an uncomfortable situation, such as an isolated, confined environment (ICE), deal with discomforts and inconveniences by trying to adjust the environment to *make* it more benign ("problem-oriented coping"), versus people who deal with it by adapting their own expectations and standards to *make it feel* more benign ("emotion-oriented coping") (Folkman & Lazarus, 1988).

The core example for me was a summer field season in the High Arctic Psychology Research Station on Ellef Ringnes Island, then part of the Canadian Northwest Territories but more recently of Nunavut. A half-dozen people, mostly psychologists or students, were conducting studies on each other and exploring the surroundings in our spare time. We lived and worked in an abandoned weather station, where only the lab/dining area was heated. We had plenty of food, but it was not very interesting; we took turns cooking, which was even less so.

One of our crew was Roberto Vallverdu, a now deceased and much mourned veteran of Argentine Antarctic expeditions. He addressed the problem of the uninspired menu by thoroughly cleaning a used fuel drum and with a few hand tools converting it into a baking oven. We then had greatly appreciated pizza, home-baked bread, and muffins. Any of us could have improvised various amenities to make our sojourn more pleasant, but we merely adjusted our emotional reactions rather than the environment. It was probably a personality and occupational difference: Roberto was a biologist with polar experience as well as technical and mechanical skills; the rest of us were a physician and a bunch of academic social scientists.

There is a plethora of other potentially relevant theories and measures; their role, if any, in the study of adventurers is waiting to be assessed. By using archival methods, changes across the centuries of exploration and adventure could be tracked as well, inviting opportunities for both "psychologists interested in adventure and adventurers interested in psychology."

Acknowledgments

I am grateful to the many adventurers, including colleagues and students, who have participated in my research on isolated, confined environments, and to the agencies, including the Social Sciences and Humanities Research Council of Canada, Environment Canada, and the Canadian Space Agency, that have provided funds and field support in kind to make it possible. My thanks also to Dr. Phyllis J. Johnson for her meticulous assistance in preparing this manuscript for publication.

References

Amundsen, R. (ascription, undated). *Roald Amundsen quotes.* BrainyQuote.com. Accessed May 10, 2021 from https://www.brainyquote.com/quotes/roald_amundsen_179783
Apter, M. J. (2007). *Reversal theory: The dynamics of motivation, emotion and personality*, 2nd ed. Oneworld.
Arnould, J. (2015, March 1). Man transcends man. In *The history and philosophy of adventure. Public Books.* Accessed March 10, 2021 from https://www.publicbooks.org/author/jacques-arnould/
Berlyne, D. E.(1960). *Conflict, arousal, and curiosity.* McGraw-Hill.
Bratman, G. N., Daily, G. C., Levy, B. J., & Gross, J. J. (2015). The benefits of nature experience: Improved affect and cognition. *Landscape and Urban Planning, 138*, 41–50.
Burton, R. F. (1885). *The book of the thousand nights and a night.* Privately printed.
Davis, W. (2021, July 12). Exploration, then and now. *Royal Canadian Geographical Society Newsletter.* Accessed July 12 2021 from newsletter@rcgs.org
Durn, S. (2021, March 3). Did a Viking woman named Grudrid really travel to North America 1000 years ago? *Smithsonian Magazine.* Accessed March 3, 2022 from https://www.smithsonianmag.com/history/did-viking-woman-named-gudrid-really-travel-north-america-1000-years-ago-180977126/
Durn, S. (2022, 10 March). 9 female adventurers who ventured into the unknown. Atlas Obscura. Accessed March 10, 2022 from https://www.atlasobscura.com/articles/women-adventurers-explorers
Ebbinghaus, H. (1908). *Psychology: An elementary textbook.* Heath.

Elmore, C. H. (1944). *Quit you like men.* Charles Scribner's Sons.
Farley, F. (2010). *Heroes and heroism.* Paper presented at the meeting of the American Psychological Association, San Diego, CA.
Folkman, S., & Lazarus, R. S. (1988). *The ways of coping questionnaire.* Consulting Psychologists Press.
Green, G. (2006). Students on ice: Learning in the greatest classrooms on Earth. In M. Lück, P. T. Maher, & E. J. Stewart (Eds.), *Cruise tourism in polar regions: Promoting environmental and social sustainability.* Routledge.
Hahn, K. (1957). *Outward Bound.* Address given to a conference at Harrogate. Outward Bound Trust.
Helson, H. (1964). *Adaptation-level theory: An experimental and systematic approach to behavior.* Harper and Row.
Kuhn, T. S. (1970). *The structure of scientific revolutions.* Chicago, IL: University of Chicago Press.
Lewin, K. (1946). Behavior as a function of total situation. In D. Cartwright (Ed.), *Field theory in social science: Selected theoretical papers* (pp. 238–304). Harper & Row.
Lukianoff, G., & Haidt, J. (2018). *The coddling of the American mind.* Penguin.
Malůš, M., Kupka, M., & Dostál, D. (2016). Existential meaning in life, mindfulness and self-esteem in the context of restricted environmental stimulation. *Psychologie a Její Kontexty, 7*(2), 59–72.
Maslow, A. H. (1962). *Toward a psychology of being.* Harper.
McCrae, R. R., & Costa, P. T. Jr. (2008). The five-factor theory of personality. In O. P. John, R. W. Robins, & L. A. Pervin (Eds.), *Handbook of personality: Theory and research* (pp. 159–181). Guilford.
Price, A. G. (1971). *The explorations of Captain James Cook in the Pacific: As told by selections of his own journals 1768-1779.* Dover Publications. ISBN 0-496-22766-9
Ridley, G. (2010). *The discovery of Jeanne Baret.* Crown. ISBN 978-0-307-46352-4.
Snyder, C. R., & Fromkin, H. L. (1977). Abnormality as a positive characteristic: The development and validation of a scale measuring need for uniqueness. *Journal of Abnormal Psychology, 86*(5), 518–527. https://doi.org/10.1037/0021-843X.86.5.518
Storms, G., De Boeck, P., & Ruts, W. (2000). Prototype and exemplar-based information in natural language categories. *Journal of Memory and Language, 42,* 51–73.
Storr, A. (1988). *Solitude: A return to the self.* Free Press. ISBN: 978-0-00-654349-7
Tetlock, P. E. (2006). *Expert Political judgment: How good is it? How can we know?* Princeton University Press.
Villiers, A. J. "James Cook." *Encyclopedia Britannica.* Accessed May 31, 2021 from https://www.britannica.com/biography/James-Cook
Wallace, D. F. (2004, August). Consider the lobster. *Gourmet: Summer Reading Issue.* Accessed May 22, 2021 from http://www.gourmet.com.s3-website-us-east-1.amazonaws.com/magazine/2000s/2004/08/consider_the_lobster.html
Wilder, T. (undated). *Thornton Wilder Quotes.* (n.d.). Accessed May 10, 2021 from BrainyQuote.com, https://www.brainyquote.com/quotes/thornton_wilder_391427
Zuckerman, M. (1979). *Sensation seeking: Beyond the optimal level of arousal.* Erlbaum. ISBN: 978-0-470-26851-3

SECTION I
Sustaining Performance (While Maintaining Wellbeing)

1
THE ADVENTURER'S MIND
Exploring Mindset, Mindfulness, and Wisdom

Mohsen Fatemi and Paula Reid

From an Adventurer's Point of View: Switching On and Switching Out

I always say, like Scuba diving saved my life, you know. I'd already saved my life before. I'd got to that point – you know what I mean. I'd turned my life around, but the physical aspect of your head going under water … everything else shuts off … a couple of the symptoms of PTSD I had were hyper-vigilance, self-worth and anxiety … and putting myself in an arguably high stress situation where you are surrounded by water and if your air runs out you die, if you get trapped you die, if you are not controlling your buoyancy, and you shoot up too fast, or you go down too far you can be in trouble very quickly. You know there's a million things that could go wrong. So, although I find it therapeutic and peaceful, you, you are putting yourself into a stressful situation where you need to be switched on.

It's almost like a firefight, you know. If you don't do what you are supposed to do then you can become injured and you could die. If you stay switched on and do as you've been taught, that's how you enjoy yourself … so you have to switch on as soon as your head goes under the water. Because you switch on, you're automatically faced with a situation that becomes all encompassing, and that then subconsciously switches out the rest of my mind so all the worries that I had, all the anxieties, everything like that, gets overtaken by the need to be in the moment with the scuba diving.

I went on a shipwreck safari and that was amazing, but it was no better than when I first went underwater, because of the adventure. You know it doesn't matter if I am diving in Wraysbury or diving in the Red Sea. As soon as my head goes into the water, and I am living that adventure it doesn't matter where I am. I could be in the pool. The fact that I am breathing underwater, that's enough for me. I remember the first time when we were in the Red Sea and we were first going into the water, and we were going to follow the guide down who was going to take us out to the reef and just being on that line, being underwater, feeling the tide, sort of pulling you back and having to haul yourself across the rope … it was like an action movie, you know and that's what I find addictive, not "Oooh, look at that fish", "Oooh look at that piece of coral". It's more for me like "Look at me I'm underwater!" That sense of adventure, mixed with that calm you get, which is very similar to the sort of calm you get before a firefight, that's enough for me.

"Ben" – ex-UK serviceman with PTSD

The Adventurer's Mind: Exploring Mindset, Mindfulness, and Wisdom

Switching On and Switching Out

Because you **switch on**, you're automatically faced with a situation that becomes all encompassing, and that then subconsciously **switches out** the rest of my mind …

Ben, the ex-serviceman with post-traumatic stress disorder (PTSD), talks about the need to "switch on" while scuba diving (and while in a fire fight). We suggest that he means being fully present or mindful, including mindful of his body and context. His situational awareness demands that he attends, otherwise there may be serious consequences, such as running out of air or diving too deep.

One may assume that switching on requires some sort of work load, or cognitive burden, and thus contra-intuitive to Ben finding therapeutic peace; however, he goes on to say that it was the switching on that allowed for the enjoyment and the "calm": "If you stay switched on and do as you've been taught, that's how you enjoy yourself." This supports the concept of "going knowingly into the unknown" (Reid & Kampman, 2020) where the "knowing" (i.e., training, knowledge, skills, past experiences) allows for the "into the unknown" exploration to be more enjoyable (and potentially less stressful). At the same moment, the "switching on" can engender mindfulness, focus, or flow, for instance, to help the adventurer cope with the discomfort of uncertainty, extreme conditions, or adversity (see for example Boudreau et al., 2020; Brymer, 2005; Reid & Kampman, 2020; Walker & Kampman, 2021).

Paradoxically, despite the PTSD symptom of hyper-vigilance, Ben chose to place himself underwater, in "an arguably high stress situation" as a recovery intervention which brought him the opportunity to "switch out the rest of [his] mind." The underwater experience meant that his otherworld concerns got "overtaken by the need to be in the moment with the Scuba diving." In this example, we observe that: Ben has a mindset that enables him to go scuba diving in the first instance despite his PTSD, that the adventurous activity engenders mindfulness, and that it allows him to switch off from his wider concerns and anxieties. Indeed, it provides calm, joy, therapy, and peace in contrast with his PTSD symptoms. As Walker and Kampman noted in their research of Post Traumatic Growth in veterans: "This combination of mindful presence and tranquility underwater appears to lead to two main experiences: relief from everyday worries, negative thoughts and anxieties; and the relief from symptoms of PTSD such as hypervigilance" (Walker & Kampman, 2021, p. 6; see also Chapter 11).

Situational demand for attention would be a common experience for adventurers as they negotiate variable, unknown, and challenging territory, whether above or below the water. The adventurer's "presence" could be lifesaving as well as therapeutic. In addition, "green" or "blue" experiences, such as forest bathing or wild swimming, often naturally elicit therapeutic mindfulness or meditative states (Methley et al., 2020). Thus, the demands of the environment and the natural out-of-doors setting can have a positive impact on the mind or state of the adventurer. Of course, the reverse may also be true. Trauma, adversity, and stressors can be experienced on adventures resulting in PTSD or other debilitating responses.

So what do we mean by "switching on" and "switching out"? Arguably switching on is about being fully present and mindful in the moment: hyper-aware of one's environment and situation, perhaps experiencing flow or an "adventurous mindset." Switching out could be described as shutting off from the rest of life's thoughts and worries, perhaps, akin to a meditative state. Either not being aware, or not permitting oneself to think about, anything outside of the present place and time.

In this chapter, we explore the mind of the adventurer, especially in relation to mindsets and mindfulness. We firstly review mindfulness, mindlessness, and presence in general and with specific regard to adventuring. We then define mindsets and look at the fixed and growth mindset model, along with neuroplasticity. We next review some mental limitations which may hinder our adventuring, before moving on to motivations and potential tendencies that may encourage us towards adventuring. Finally, we look at the concepts of curiosity and exploration, in relation to epistemology and knowledge acquisition, and in association with journeying, wayfaring, and pathways to enlightenment.

We acknowledge that there is a long path yet to be travelled with regard to the psychology of adventuring and exploration, and much that is yet to be researched or understood. Is there for instance, an adventure persona such as Campbell's "hero" (1949), Jung's "explorer" archetype (1964), or Ingold's "wayfarer" (2011) who has a certain mindset? Do adventures facilitate a mental uplift towards transcendence (see Chapter 12)? Does adventure force a mindfulness in the adventurer as they grapple with conditions that require them to be fully present? Is the mental capacity to adventure "successfully" a personality trait or acquired through experience? Further research into the psychology of adventuring – and adventure psychology – is welcomed.

Mindfulness and Mindlessness

Mindfulness is about being fully present and aware. Kabat-Zinn defined it as: "moment-to-moment, non-judgmental awareness" which through mindfulness meditation can be: "cultivated by paying attention in a specific way, that is, in the present moment, and as non-reactively, as non-judgmentally, and openheartedly as possible" (Kabat-Zinn, 2005, p. 4). The word mindfulness is used in a few different ways, including mindful meditation, a psychological process or trait, and – more relevant to adventuring – a mode or state of awareness (Germer et al., 2005). The concept akin to mindfulness – presence – is about being present, in the here and now. Eckhart Tolle, who wrote *"The Power of Now,"* described it thus: "your entire life only happens in this moment. The present moment is life itself" and that once found, "life begins to flow with joy and ease" (Tolle, 2004). Tolle also described life as a journey towards enlightenment and pertinently to the adventurous mind: "If everything was clear to you now, everything was already mapped out, there would be no evolution of yourself as a human being" (Winfrey, 2022). The path to enlightenment may well be physical as well as spiritual.

In contrast, *mindlessness* corresponds with automatic behaviour. It is a state of mind in which we act and do things without so much awareness or attention. Have you ever read a page and had no idea what it said at the end? Although you are reading, there is no awareness. We may walk to the end of a path and suddenly realise where we are; one does not walk when mindless but is instead walked. Mindlessness is also described as a state of mind where one can depend on past conclusions and specific categorisations; where one is locked within a particular way of thinking and views are more permanent. In terms of personal development, the biggest conflict is with oneself, there is an inadequate amount of awareness and mindfulness about one's own potential. Mindlessness can diminish and overshadow capabilities and agency; as a mindless individual locks into information, there is less attention to alternative modes of knowing. Anyone determined by mindless or automatic mindsets are less likely to explore the possibility of going on an adventure or have an open mind towards the adventure experience itself, including the choice of which path to take. A mindless adventurer would be less aware of themselves and their relationship with an ever-fluxing environment. Their travels may be more automatic, and the traveller less present. Alternatively, this singular-minded mode, lacking awareness or attention, may indeed be a useful mindset when adventurers are faced with periods of boredom, inactivity, or enduringly unstimulating contexts, such as skiing to the South Pole.

Harvard University psychologist Ellen Langer has suggested that the concepts of mindlessness and mindfulness are associated constructs which greatly influence our living and achievements and in turn act like mindsets (Langer, 1989).

Mindsets

Mindset has been defined as "a mental frame or lens that selectively organises and encodes information, thereby orienting you toward a unique way of understanding an experience and guiding you toward certain actions and responses" (Crum et al., 2013, p. 717). A mindset can be defined as the way we perceive the world, upheld by our beliefs, and shaping how we make sense of the world and ourselves within it. Our pragmatic view of life and performances are inspired by our mental overview and are the implications of our mindsets. These implications and practical outcomes of our thoughts lead to results, which settle our point in life. Our mindsets influence our achievements and abilities and the extent to which we believe in possibilities or a "self-theory." Mindsets drive our actions, shape our view and philosophy of life, and impact our paradigms and thoughts. Our thoughts affect our actions, and this relationship vividly depicts how what we think becomes our reality.

One of the most often cited mindset theories is Dweck's fixed and growth model which we shall explore shortly in relation to mindlessness and mindfulness. There are other mindset concepts and theories, however, which broaden the field beyond Dweck's work. Crum et al., for instance, have researched the "stress mindset" and whether stress is perceived as enhancing or debilitating (Crum et al., 2013). Similarly, the explanatory style of optimism and pessimism may be attributed to mindset. Our appraisal of whether a situation is perceived as a "challenge or threat" may stem from mindset (Turner et al., 2014). Mindsets may be collective (i.e., worldview), systemic (i.e., politics or religion), or individualistic – all of which may impact on the adventurer's phenomenological lived experience.

After years of research, Dweck proposed two types of mindsets: fixed and growth. A fixed mindset is when capabilities are deemed to be fixed, inflexible, and constant. The mind is indeed "set." A fixed mindset holds us in a more stationary position. Dweck says "In a fixed mindset, people believe their basic qualities, like their intelligence or talent, are simply fixed traits" (Dweck, 2007). A fixed mindset does not expect change; potentials are constant.

Fixed mindsets have low limits with regard to abilities – resources and possibilities are considered scarce and restricted. This is due to the mindless scope one has of one's own potential. Due to categorisation, automatic behaviour, and single perspectives, there is little space for development. If something does not work, it is categorised as a failure and other perspectives are not sought or heeded. Automatic responses to life do not allow deeply reflected decisions to improve. If failures were used for improvement, they could help with development, growth, insight, and wisdom.

In contrast, growth mindsets hold the belief that skills can be developed. Studies by Dweck and her students supported the hypothesis that mindsets affect success and performance differently. Throughout life, we grow and change physically; however, that is not always the case for our mindsets. This leads us to the concept of neuroplasticity.

Neuroplasticity

Physiologically, brains can change and have the power to transform from their initial formation at birth. The existence of mindsets and their roles in our lives can also be supported biologically. Our physiological being may change without any outer manipulations, but rather by the internal world of thinking. The brain's structure and functioning provides evidence for mindsets as our brains change throughout our lives and we gain psychological flexibility. This is due to the phenomenon known as neuroplasticity. Neuroplasticity can be defined as:

> ... the brain's ability to reorganise itself by forming new neural connections throughout life. Neuroplasticity allows the neurons (nerve cells) in the brain to compensate for injury and disease and to adjust their activities in response to new situations or to changes in their environment.
>
> *(Marks, 2021)*

A study by Pittenger and Duman (2008) suggests that stress and depression can affect the neurological pathways of the brain and in turn influence the brain's neuroplasticity. This indicates that our brain can be altered by our living. Another study by Merzenich et al. (1984) showed that when the third fingers of owl monkeys were cut off, after 62 days, cortical remapping took place and the sensory area in the brain that was for the third finger was covered by the areas of the adjacent fingers. This is an example of how the brain can physically change. Studies also show that relieving suffering and improving the quality of life, or palliative care, can impact mood and suggest that these conditions can lengthen survival, specifically tested in patients with non-small-cell lung cancer (Irwin et al., 2013). This shows how environment and mood can impact one's mindset and, consequently, our health and lifestyle.

We can change our brain by personal thinking and living. Christopher Bergland states that "through neurogenesis and neuroplasticity, it may be possible to carve out a fresh and unworn path for thoughts to travel upon" (2014). One could speculate that this process opens up the possibility to reinvent oneself and move away from the status quo or to overcome past traumatic events that evoke anxiety and stress. Hardwired fear-based memories often lead to avoidance behaviours that can hold one back from living life to the fullest, then again, fear also has the benefit of keeping one alive (see Chapter 7).

Our mindsets develop and how they develop is not always mindful. Typically, the way in which one thinks, or one's vision of life and possibilities, is impacted by society and surroundings. These can consist of family, teachers, and culture one is surrounded by, or simply how one socially interacts within a system. In addition, our engagement with life and how we encounter and re-encounter situations can shape our mindset. Mindsets that form without much reflection are "premature cognitive commitments" (Langer, 1989). The scope we have of our abilities, or our mindset, can be formed by many interactions we have within different contexts. "In 1972, Martin Seligman proposed that when an organism perceives a loss of control in a situation and faces repeated failures, that organism may abandon any future attempt to achieve related goals" (Popov et al., 2017, p. 338). This can be termed as "learned helplessness," thus fixed mindsets can cause re-failure (since challenged by McGonigal and Audio, 2022). Additionally, within a social group, people mindlessly adopt mindsets. This is a reasonable explanation for why many fail to try hard and use phrases such as "it's impossible," simply because "no one's ever done it before" (bring on the explorer, the innovator, and the "world firsts" adventurers).

Mindsets and Adventuring

Approach to Challenges

Whatever goals one has – to achieve financial success, become famous, invent something revolutionary, sail around the world, or climb a mountain, it is challenging work. Adversities may occur and hardships are likely to be perceived as obstacles. With a fixed mindset, one can tend to avoid challenges: "People with a fixed mindset avoid risks, challenges, and failures, because it threatens their sense of identity – I'm smart and I failed can become I thought I was smart, but I failed" (Cameron, 2018, p. 133). Avoiding challenges can limit improvement, resilience, and knowledge acquisition garnered through hard graft and self-development through tests and tasks. Avoiding challenges and risks may also prevent people from embarking on challenging adventures or adventurous challenges.

Single Mindedness

In an adventurous mode of mindlessness, travellers may act from a single perspective that does not allow them to see other possibilities except the ones in which they are enmeshed. The trip may become arduous both in the process and the outcome without giving rise to a sense of liveliness. Mindlessly lived journeys do not leave room for attention to variability. Helping travellers understand how perspectives can be limiting – or liberating – would allow them to see the implications of their phenomenologically lived journeys.

Then again, single mindedness can also lead to achievement. Above average achievements take an extreme, singular focus and thus a fixed mindset can be advantageous to some (even if the cost is lack of insight, harm to relationships, isolation, and so on). In addition, the assessment or opinion of one's own potential – not necessarily limited – can be overinflated. Those with narcissistic personality disorder (NPD), for instance, may be grandiose and overestimate abilities but great feats of endurance or expedition can be achieved with a singular determination.

Stereotypical Limits

It is reasonable to say that people with fixed mindsets abide by stereotypical limits. Even research can be stereotypical: Langer says "research in general tells us something about 'most' people." This suggests how we could limit ourselves based on norms. In the movie "The Shawshank Redemption," prisoners are mindlessly categorised and succumb to regular limits. However, one of the prisoners, Andy Dufresne, does the "impossible" and escapes. This is because he did not abide by stereotypical boundaries. Susceptibility to agreeing with norms and not responding to setbacks from a different perspective make us prone to failure. When something has not happened yet, it seems impossible for us. We fail to think outside the box and try something new: "… the fact that something has not yet happened doesn't mean it cannot happen; it only means that the way to make it happen is as yet unknown" (Langer, 2009, p. 24). Going on an adventure is not a stereotypical way of living life, it disrupts the norm. It requires a pioneering mindset to choose to break away from the common place and participate in something unusual, beyond typical daily life limits.

Cognition

"It is not primarily our physical selves that limit us but rather our mindset about our physical limits" (Langer, 2009, p. 11). It is not the physical outside world that limits us, but the way we think about it. In other words, our inner world may limit (or liberate) us. The outer world we live in and how much we achieve in this outer world greatly depends on our inner world. Life is surrounded by manifold variables. Mindset is not the sole determining factor. Environmental, societal, and biological components are also influential factors.

Mindsets are unique to individuals. There is nothing that can make one thrive and succeed like one's own mind can. Revisiting one's mindset may begin with the courage to take an adventure deep into the hills and valleys of one's mind.

Adventure and the Position of Not Knowing

An adventurer starts from a position of not knowing the path ahead; from where the adventurer experiences mysteries, intricacies, and complexities as they become more steeped into the process of exploration.

"In more than thirty years of research, I've discovered a very important truth about human psychology: certainty is a cruel mindset" (Langer, 2009, p. 24). Adventure incorporates embracing uncertainty and exploring possibility. The psychology of possibility is akin to having a growth mindset and allows for an open mind, or relaxation, towards not knowing.

Adventurous exploration may unfold with unique stages of awe, bewilderment, exhilaration, liveliness, and vivacity. The experience is phenomenologically aligned with emotional (and maybe physical) ups and downs; a dark path may suddenly transform from disillusionment and despair to the searing light of sunrise or hope. The adventurer may be relentless in their quest for experiencing the spirit of discovery: the endeavour to embrace the splendour of an epiphany.

The psychology of an adventure provides an inner dialectical back and forth between the realm of possibility and inventiveness, where the fixed façade of realities and actualities strain their rigour into convincing the impossibility of a movement beyond the topographical boundaries of defined postulations. Epistemic fusion may transpire as the flux of discoveries keep on presenting their novelty.

Adventures are fraught with newness, freshness, and exquisiteness. They may steer away from the perception of fixations and the illusion of stability. They presage the cynosure of novelty and reveal the nuances of rapture amid, experiencing rupture from the established mindsets. Adventures may serve as a panacea for the malaise of freezing in one's entanglement, one's mindsets, and one's problems. Rigidity may give way to liberation. Dogmatism, belongings, and attachments may be replaced by openness, simplicity, and naturalness.

Deep down in the nature of an adventure, there lies the magnificence of flexibility in seeking the novel features that may be hidden from the senses stuck in the ordinary perspective. This may allow us to understand the interconnectedness of mindfulness and adventures.

A change of perspective can create a new course of action where responsibility, responsiveness, proactivity, choice, and empowerment can give rise to a novel mode of being. This is understandable in the process of experiencing a mindful journey with an adventurous tone where the path is integrated with connectedness.

Mindfulness helps the adventurer notice perspectives that may not be available in the repertoire of the person with fixation, entanglement, and enmeshment. The adventurer is encouraged to explore possibilities of alternative modes of perspectives.

Journeys entail *a what and a how*. In discussing the "what" of journeys, travellers examine the events, their sequential order, their syntagmatic analysis, and focus on what is it that has occurred – namely, the content of their journeys. In focusing on "how" journeys unfold, travellers are encouraged to fathom the discourse of their trips. How the journeys are experienced and their modes of presentation are pronounced here.

This can be of great significance for travellers who aspire to walk along the meanders of a path and look for liminal spots and spaces (Fatemi, 2016b). Liminality unfolds itself in an adventurous mode where mindful perspicacity celebrates the exploration of novel zones of being and meaning in the process of an adventure.

This helps the observing traveller to mingle with the gift of mindfulness through each step that they take. The dyadic observation and action – namely the bilateral interaction of an observer and an actor in the process of making a journey – may bring the traveller to an in-depth examination of spaces that are unknown to the eye of the beholder even during the experiential process of launching the adventure.

A brook that ceases to flow loses its riveting exhilaration just as a bystander loses their creativity through lingering in the deterministic view of one perspective. A mindful adventurer creates the panacea of growth through proactive engagement and reflective observation. The essence of a mindful adventurer incorporates receptiveness, flexibility, care and compassion, and an expressiveness with an infinite expectation of the dawn.

Going Knowingly into the Unknown

"*Going Knowingly into the Unknown*" – the subtitle of this book, was selected mindfully. The phrase arose from the research analysis of Reid and Kampman's interpretative phenomenological study into the purpose and benefits of expeditionary adventuring (2020). Whilst one traditional assumption is that adventurers are risk-seeking or thrill-seeking, as they spontaneously leap into the unknown, the data revealed another, more considered and mindful, narrative. Experienced adventurers were risk aware, conscientious and prudent before they "leapt." They did their homework, and chose to go knowingly into the unknown:

> In a seeming contradiction, or a tension of opposing needs, adventurers go knowingly into expeditions and prepare hard to be "lazy", and then consciously choose to step off from the known into the unknown world. In defining adventure, all participants chose to define it by describing the uncertainty: "Not knowing what's round the corner" (Joanna, 14/490), "pushing boundaries" (Sean, 8/255), "unpredictability, where it's not regimented and rigid and expected" (Lara, 16/614-5), "where there are no rules, things can change" (Dora, 2/64).
>
> This theme describes the aspects of adventure that are outside of knowing. Participants described newness, variety, discovery, exploration (of self and the environment), possibilities, chaos and unpredictability. Thus, according to these participants, a core defining element of adventure is the unknown.

Thus, rather than going mindlessly into an adventure, many adventurers go mindfully; knowingly. Here, "knowingly" represents three states of mind: in the first instance mindfully choosing to go on an adventure through conscious decision making rather than luck; secondly, adventuring mindfully rather than mindlessly; and thirdly, referring to pre-acquired knowledge and wisdom to adventure knowingly, i.e., to make decisions en route informed by experience. This then extends to having more knowledge and wisdom the next time in an iterative process of self-development. Wisdom is a way of using knowledge practically as we negotiate life and in Glück and Buck's research wisdom was thought to be gained "from: 'a broad spectrum of positive and negative experiences'" (Glück & Bluck, 2011, p. 2). Adventures certainly incorporate this.

Adventurers are not typically rash or risky in their choices, in fact, we posit that they are possibly some of the most risk experienced people on the planet. Twenty-four-hours-a-day, whilst on expedition, adventurers need to be risk aware, risk analysing and risk managing, to help them be effective, avoid failure or trauma, and in extremis, stay alive.

Some adventurers perhaps transcend, to a higher awareness and "leave their ego at the door"; "knowing self, skills, environment and taming one's 'inner animal'" (Arijs et al., 2017, p. 8). This was eloquently described in a narrative study of wingsuit flying, perhaps one of the most extreme, "risky" adventurous activities one could choose to do. Participants described themselves as being fully present and mindful, hyper-aware of conditions, and directing their awareness and attention skilfully towards the factors that would enhance or endanger their flying experience:

> I'm noticing everything around me, if there's clouds, I'm noticing the trees, and if there's wind blowing, noticing if the birds are flying, where they're flying, how they're flying because that can give me a good idea if there are any thermals in the air or a decent breeze. Because all of this is going to affect me once I actually jump.
>
> *(Arijs et al., 2017, p.37)*

They then choose to fly or not, based on their rapid cognition, intuition, situational awareness, proprioception, mindfulness, or wisdom, garnered from past and present mindful experience. They may use three sources of wisdom: hindsight (from past experience), insight (from present awareness) and foresight (through future assessment). The decision is conscious, stepping off from the safety of land into the uncertainty of their future flight, knowingly.

Going Knowingly into the Unknown thus provides an interesting juxtaposition of mind states. The *knowing* provides mindfulness, wisdom garnered from experience (the more/deeper experiences we have, the more experienced we are) or even a sense of certainty, to which we are drawn (see Chapter 4). The *unknown* allows for the freedom of possibility and not being fixed or enmeshed in cognitive certainty. This is perhaps a splendid and natural symbiotic equilibrium.

This book is a form of the same narrative. *Adventure Psychology: Going Knowingly into the Unknown* is an accumulation of theories and ideas in a new collection to aid the reader's knowledge, so that they may go more knowingly into the future. The knowledge is "correct" at the point of publication but will evolve and develop over time and potentially be superseded or made redundant with new research, concepts, or data. Similarly, an adventurer can only set off with the knowledge, skills, qualities, and wisdom they have thus far acquired. By mindfully exploring the "unknown," they acquire fresh knowledge and wisdom and can go more knowingly next time. Their knowledge is volatile and realised moment by moment. This is the path towards enlightenment of the *"wayfarer"* rather than the traveller. According to the anthropologist Tim Ingold, the wayfarer forges knowledge as he or she journeys through life (whereas the traveller is more concerned with the destination rather than the journey). Knowledge is organically woven, grown and accumulated, rather than assembled: "along such paths, lives are lived, skills developed, observations made and understandings grown" (Ingold, 2011).

The Psychology of Possibility

An adventure is oftentimes a dynamically novel experience and thus the adventurer cannot help but be in their *stretch zone* (which is sometimes referred to as the growth zone), beyond their secure and familiar environment or *comfort zone*. The dynamic and demanding context requires the adventurer to be present and mindful for fear of a mismanaged move or mistake which may result in failure, injury, or death (Brymer, 2005). We suggest that because adventurers are dealing with uncertainty, in their exploration of newness – newness of external environment or internal self – they are more likely to be vulnerable, humble, or open to experience. Working on the assumption that adventures may contain peak experiences (Maslow, 1962) in a dynamic environment conducted while the adventurer is in a state of uncertainty or openness, the "porosity" of the adventurer is likely to be high – they are inclined to be "sponge-like" or penetrable by the experience and thus receptive to possibility, potential and growth. This psychology of possibility creates ontological expansion, epistemological enhancement and cognitive elevation (Fatemi, 2016a). Where "knowing" closes us down, or "fixes" our view, "possibility" may open us up or broaden our view. We may gain perspective. Further research into this receptive state while undergoing peak adventurous experiences would be welcome.

Adventurers explore *terra incognita* and are required to manage uncertainty and challenge, which would suggest a tendency towards a growth mindset, and the "Big Five" trait of *openness to experience*. What is "the right stuff" (Kjærgaard et al., 2014; Steel et al., 1997) for adventurers' mindsets? Todd Kashdan and colleagues have been working on a scale to measure curiosity and exploration (Kashdan et al., 2009). With reference and appreciation for their work, if we adopt and adapt this, then an Adventure Mindset Scale could look something like this:

Please rate the extent to which you agree or disagree with the following statements, from Strongly Disagree to Strongly Agree:

1. Experiencing adventure facilitates my learning and growth.
2. Experiencing adventure enhances my performance and productivity.
3. Experiencing adventure improves my health and vitality.

4. The positive effects of adventure should be utilised.
5. Being present and in the moment is useful to me.
6. I believe a level of discomfort can be good for me.
7. Engaging in new experiences enhances my wellbeing.
8. Seeking out new experiences creates possibilities.
9. I believe it's good to push myself out of my comfort zone
10. Being flexible improves my agility.

These are suggestions for a measurement scale based on Kashdan et al.'s more rigorous inventory (and second version) and includes some qualitative feedback from an adventurer-psychologist network (Adventure Psychology Network, 2021). Further research and evidence again is welcomed.

An Experiential State

Adventure is an experiential concept as well as an adjective (to be adventurous), verb (they adventured into the woods) and noun (her recent adventure in Java). Can adventure also be described as a state of mind? Is an adventurous mindset also an experiential state of being, such as flow? Flow is defined as being in the zone, fully immersed and engaged in the process of an activity in which one may lose oneself or sense of time (Csikszentmihalyi, 1990). Emotions or feelings may pass through – some may be co-valanced, dialectical or seemingly in-coherent (such as "survivors' guilt"), but the mindset or state endures. If the concept of flow is a state wherein there is mid-high challenge and mid-high skill, can adventure be considered to be an experiential state as well as a mindset?

Let's leave the final words to an Australian adventurer, Sarah Davis:

> I believe adventure is a state of mind as much as a physical undertaking. For me adventure is my greatest teacher. It teaches me about who I am, what I am capable of both physically and mentally as well as teaching me about the world around me. It stretches and shapes me and gives me new perspectives. It gives me a future that excites me and a now that exhilarates me. It's what lights me up! (Sarah Davis, personal communication, February 3, 2021).

References

Adventure Psychology Network. (n.d.). *Home*. Facebook. Retrieved February 22, 2021 from https://www.facebook.com/groups/1291472931244640

Arijs, C., Chroni, S., Brymer, E., & Carless, D. (2017). "Leave your ego at the door": A narrative investigation into effective wingsuit flying. *Frontiers in Psychology, 8*, 32–41.

Bergland, C. T. (2014, February 6). How do neuroplasticity and neurogenesis rewire your brain? *Psychology Today*. https://www.psychologytoday.com/gb/blog/the-athletes-way/201702/how-do-neuroplasticity-and-neurogenesis-rewire-your-brain

Boudreau, P., Houge Mackenzie, S., & Hodge, K. (2020). Flow states in adventure recreation: A systematic review and thematic synthesis. *Psychology of Sport and Exercise*, 46. 10.1016/j.psychsport.2019.101611

Brymer, G. E. (2005). Extreme dude! A phenomenological perspective on the extreme sport experience, Ph.D. thesis, Faculties of Education and Psychology, University of Wollongong. http://ro.uow.edu.au/theses/379

Cameron, L. (2018). *The mindful day*. National Geographic.

Campbell, J. (1949). *Joseph Campbell's The hero with a thousand faces*. Princeton University Press.

Crum, A. J., Salovey, P., & Achor, S. (2013). Rethinking stress: The role of mindsets in determining the stress response. *Journal of Personality and Social Psychology, 104*(4), 716–733. https://doi.org/10.1037/a0031201

Csikszentmihalyi, M. (1990). *Flow: The psychology of optimal experience*. New York: Harper and Row.

Dweck, C. S. (2007). *Mindset: The new psychology of success*. Gildan Media Corp.

Fatemi, S. M. (2016a). Psychology of possibility. [Presentation]. European Conference on Positive Psychology, Angers, France.

Fatemi, S. M. (2016b). Langerian mindfulness and liminal performing spaces. In A. L. Baltzell (Ed.), *Mindfulness and performance (Current perspectives in social and behavioral sciences)* (pp. 112–124). Cambridge University Press.

Germer, C. K., Siegel, R. D., & Fulton, P. R. (2005). *Mindfulness and psychotherapy*. Guilford Press.

Glück, J., & Bluck, S. (2011). Laypeople's conceptions of wisdom and its development: Cognitive and integrative views. *The Journals of Gerontology: Series B: Psychological Sciences and Social Sciences, 66B*(3), 321–324. https://doi.org/10.1093/geronb/gbr011

Ingold, T. (2011). *Being alive: Essays on movement, knowledge and description*. Routledge.

Irwin, K. E., Greer, J. A., Khatib, J., Temel, J. S., & Pirl, W. F. (2013). Early palliative care and metastatic non-small cell lung cancer: Potential mechanisms of prolonged survival. *Chronic Respiratory Disease, 10*(1), 35–47. https://doi.org/10.1177/1479972312471549

Jung, C. G. (1964). *Man and his symbols*. Dell Publishing Group.

Kabat-Zinn, J. (2005). *Coming to our senses: Healing ourselves and the world through mindfulness*. Hyperion.

Kashdan, T. B., Gallagher, M. W., Silvia, P. J., Winterstein, B. P., Breen, W. E., Terhar, D. and Steger, M. F. (2009). The curiosity and exploration inventory – II: Development, factor structure, and psychometrics. *Journal of Research in Personality, 43*, 987–998.

Kjærgaard, A., Leon, G. R., & Venables, N. C. (2014). The "Right stuff" for a solo sailboat circumnavigation of the Globe. *Environment and Behavior, 47*(10), 1147–1171. https://doi.org/10.1177/0013916514535086

Langer, E. J. (1989). *Mindfulness*. Addison-Wesley.

Langer, E. J. (2009). *Counterclockwise*. Ballantine Books.

Marks, J. W. (2021). MedicineNet. *Medical definition of neuroplasticity*. https://www.medicinenet.com/neuroplasticity/definition.htm

Maslow, A. H. (1962). Lessons from the peak experiences. *Journal of Humanistic Psychology, 2*(1), 9–18.

McGonigal, J., & Audio, P. (2022). *Imaginable: How to See the Future Coming and Be Ready for Anything*. Transworld Digital.

Merzenich, M. M., Nelson, R. J., Stryker, M. P., Cynader, M. S., Schoppmann, A., & Zook, J. M. (1984). Somatosensory cortical map changes following digit amputation in adult monkeys. *Journal of Comparative Neurology, 224*(4), 591–605.

Methley, A., Vseteckova, J., & Jones, K. (2020, October 12). *The benefits of outdoor green and blue spaces.* https://www.open.edu/openlearn/health-sports-psychology/mental-health/the-benefits-outdoor-green-and-blue-spaces

Pittenger, C., & Duman, R. (2008). Stress, depression, and neuroplasticity: A convergence of mechanisms. *Neuropsychopharmacology, 33*, 88–109. https://doi.org/10.1038/sj.npp.1301574

Popov, A., Parker, L., & Seath, D. (2017). *IB psychology.* 2nd ed. Oxford University Press.

Reid, P., & Kampman, H. (2020). Exploring the psychology of extended-period expeditionary adventurers: Going knowingly into the unknown. *Psychology of Sport and Exercise, 46*, 101608.

Steel, G. D., Suedfeld, P., Peri, A., & Palinkas, L. A. (2007). People in high latitudes: The "Big-Five" personality characteristics of the circumpolar sojourner. *Environment and Behaviour, 29*, 324–347.

Tolle, E. (2004). *The power of now: A guide to spiritual enlightenment.* Namaste Pub.

Turner, M. J., Jones, M. V., Sheffield, D., Barker, J. B., & Coffee, P. (2014). Manipulating cardiovascular indices of challenge and threat using resource appraisals. *International Journal of Psychophysiology: Official Journal of the International Organization of Psychophysiology, 94*(1), 9–18. https://doi.org/10.1016/j.ijpsycho.2014.07.004

Walker, P. A., & Kampman, H. (2021). "It didn't bring back the old me but helped me on the path to the new me": Exploring posttraumatic growth in British veterans with PTSD. *Disability and Rehabilitation.* https://doi.org/10.1080/09638288.2021.1995056

Winfrey, O. (2022). "Host", A New Earth: Awakening to your Life's Purpose. Audio Podcast. Super soul conversations. OWN podcasts.

2
ADVENTURES IN EXTREME ENVIRONMENTS

Peter Suedfeld

From the Point of View of an Adventurer: Lessons in Navigation

When I was 10 years old, my dad brought home a go-cart for my two brothers and me. It was a little surprising; he wasn't a go-cart kind of guy. My brothers didn't take much interest, but I loved that thing. We took the governor off and I went speeding around the neighbourhood.

It was fast. It was freedom. It was just ... fun.

That go-cart was the start of a lifetime of memorable experiences for me. World travel. A professional racing career. Skydiving. Aerobatic stunt flying competitions. Summits of Mt. Rainier and Mt. Kilimanjaro. The first white-water descent of a remote river in the Himalayas. An expedition to the bottom of the deepest ocean. Serving as the pilot on the first all-private crew to reach the International Space Station.

I've been fortunate.

People call me a thrill-seeker or an adrenaline junkie. But I disagree. Even as a kid I understood the difference between acceptable and unacceptable risk. I take risks, but not unacceptable risk. An adrenaline junkie may be out for the biggest high they can get irrespective of risk. That's a recipe for a short lifespan. I've always wanted a long life – filled with challenging and interesting experiences and relentless self-improvement. That's why I do these things. And along the way I've learned a lot.

I've learned how to learn.

I wasn't a great student growing up. A traditional classroom setting and traditional subjects never appealed to me, I guess. When I got into racing and then skydiving and then flying and all kinds of other endeavours, I created a methodology that worked for me. Whatever the activity, I'd find a knowledgeable and believable teacher or coach and take an experiential

DOI: 10.4324/9781003173601-5

approach to learning. After every session, I'd take notes. What I did well, and what I didn't do well. Then I'd review my notes before the next session. I've refined that system over the years and gotten pretty good at a number of new things – both adventurous and mundane.

I've learned how to mitigate risk and keep my cool amid chaos.

I've had three what I would consider "close calls." I almost drowned twice and there was a skydiving "incident." I was jumping with two guys I didn't know and someone else's parachute. Everything that could go wrong did. One of the guys deployed his chute right into me. I ended up tumbling and by the time I stabilised I couldn't find my rip cord. I only had one chance at it. I deployed my chute at 800 feet; it fully opened at 300 feet. Another second or two and I was done. In all those cases, I could have avoided the issues I had with better forethought and preparation. Like they say in flying, "keep your problems on the ground." Still, I stayed calm and in control; and that's what saved me.

I've learned how to navigate adversity.

In racing, wrecks are inevitable. You can't control everything that happens on the track; you can only control how you respond. So when there's a wreck, I've learned to always look for the escape route. Don't focus on the wreck. Get your eyes up and look long. The wreck won't happen with the car in front of you. It usually starts way ahead. And if you can identify it early on and find the solution, you're going to be all right. Whatever bad happens or what adversity you find yourself in, there is almost always an opportunity embedded in it. But you have to find it. That's been key for me in any endeavour – sports, adventure, business, my personal life. Whatever.

And yet, I've had plenty of wrecks in my life. It's something people ask me about quite often. They'll say, "Remember that time in that race when you got wrecked …" And to be totally honest, I never do. I guess I have a selective memory. I don't remember wrecks – actual ones on the track or metaphorical ones in life. Once the actual incident is over, it's gone.

When bad things happen, I forget them. But I always remember the good thing – and that's the lesson.

Larry Connor

Adventures in Extreme Environments

Labels and Definitions

Environmental psychologists, and others familiar with studies of people who seek out (or find themselves in) extremely challenging environments, have encountered many phrases, abbreviations, and acronyms used as labels for such situations. These include *Isolated, Confined Environments (ICE)*, and *Extreme, Unusual Environments (EUE)*; less frequently, exotic environments, dangerous environments, hostile environments, etc. None of those terms are quite appropriate.

Large expeditionary groups are not necessarily isolated or confined. The Lewis and Clark expedition (1803–06) included more than 70 men and at least one, now famous, woman: Sacagawea. The members of the group, who came into contact with an estimated 50 indigenous tribes along the way, were certainly not isolated; and their journey of about 8,000 miles, from St. Louis, Missouri, to the Pacific coast, and back, imposed no sort of confinement.

"Extreme" and "unusual" are fully defined only as compared with a baseline: the "normal" environments of the specific people involved. "Exotic" evokes beaches and palm trees, definitely not very common in this kind of situation, except for adventurers in the tropics. Not all such environments are particularly dangerous, and even those that had been so are becoming less so (polar stations, for example). "Hostile" implies malevolent enmity on the part of natural forces and phenomena that have no known mental or emotional processes.

I have participated in spreading some of those labels and abbreviations around the literature. But now, having considered and been dissatisfied with the above options, I suggest "EST" as a useful temporary label for this chapter. In English, "est" is the suffix most often added to an adjective to indicate that it is the most extreme of at least three levels of a particular quality. Thus, we refer to "the fastest runner," "the tallest building," "the sweetest dessert," and so on. The topic of this chapter is "Adventure in the Extremes": "EST" designates the most extreme of those. EST environments may, of course, also be ICE or EUE environments; but if they are, they are the ultimate exemplars of their particular type.

Extreme and EST Environments

Extreme environments pose serious threats to human life and well-being. Many possess EST features. The highest altitudes and the highest latitudes, the deepest oceans, the longest rivers, the farthest distances, the loneliest deserts, the lands with the "strangest" animals and cultures—these are the magnets that draw explorers. To reach them takes resources not every adventurous soul can command. Consequently, most exploits are quite brief, inexpensive, close to home, low-tech, and accomplished by people for whom adventuring is a recreational or spiritual sideline. Those adventures are dealt with in other parts of the book; this chapter concentrates on voyages to and in the EST.

Dangerous Adventures

That said, less extreme adventure sites are no less exciting, and mastering them no less satisfying, than their EST counterparts. Their spiritual and emotional benefits can be just as great and are accessible to people for whom the extreme environment may be unreachable. It is also true that less extreme environments do not lack challenge or danger. For example, in 2017, 162 recreational divers world-wide died in SCUBA accidents (Denoble et al., 2019). Between 2000 and 2021, there were 72 fatalities in hot-air balloon accidents around the world (Wikipedia, 2022).[1] Mountain hiking (not mountain *climbing*) has involved an average of 170 deaths annually in just the Austrian Alps, France (Gatterer et al., 2019), and American national parks (Carroll, 2021). Non-lethal injuries are probably numerous, and include almost unimaginable events such as Aron Ralston's self-amputation of his arm, using a pocket knife, to free himself from a fallen boulder (Simon & Kennedy, 2003). In considering these and similar figures, we must remember the importance of baselines: i.e., fatalities and injuries as fractions of the total number of people and events in each category of adventures, a number that is seldom known.

This Chapter

The next section of the chapter examines psychological aspects of three prototypical EST adventures that are manageable without complex, highly technical life support technology or an elaborate organisational structure. The three environments offer unpredictable excitement, harsh but beautiful panoramas, and the opportunity to overcome discomfort and danger with courage, competence, determination, and a modicum of luck. The three adventures are explorations in Antarctica, solo sailing in the great oceans, and climbing Earth's highest mountains.

Adventure Is Where You Find It: General Considerations

The Earth offers infinite places for adventure. This chapter does not deal with such questions as how to survive in dangerous circumstances, what supplies to stock, how to dress, what technical skills must be learned, and so on. That kind of information can be found in many publications (e.g., Kamler, 2004; Leach, 2011; Towell, 2020). Rather, we consider psychosocial matters that can have serious impact on expeditioners.

When discussing adventurers, one frequent question concerns why they seek out the dangers and deprivations involved. What are the psychological benefits of participating in risky adventuring? The list is similar across various EST sites, including adventures this chapter does not cover, such as deep ocean diving, spelunking (caving), wilderness and desert trekking. The rewards also come from more mundane and less esoteric activities. A risk to life and limb is not always crucial; as the skier graduates from the bunny slope to the black diamond runs, or as strolls give way to hikes, people can experience peak and flow experiences (Csikszentmihalyi, 1996), the thrill of having challenged oneself and succeeded, the feeling of competence, and the satisfaction of joining a group of similar achievers (Suedfeld, 2012).

Personality Factors

The desire for adventure can be a focused determination to immerse oneself in one particular place or activity; but it can also be more generalised and diversified. It would be interesting to measure the personality characteristics of inveterate adventurers, those whose desire for such exploits seems to be insatiable and who embark on them repeatedly. Fluctuations in their motivational profile, adaptation level, and optimal arousal level would be worth studying. There certainly are short-term changes: many adventurers returning from ICEs take a week or more to acclimatise to temporarily excessive stimulation—parties, loud music, or even driving in traffic. Whether the basic trait itself changes, perhaps with increasing experience or age, is an interesting question.

Published psychometric studies (as opposed to anecdotal narratives) of the personality of adventurers have concentrated on those employed by large organisations such as space and polar agencies (e.g., Steel et al., 1997). Those have found well-adjusted individuals, with practical approaches to solving problems, positive values (such as caring for those near the person, seeking stimulation, and autonomy), concern for group functioning, high goal-directedness, and a stoic attitude toward hardship and discomfort (Brcic, 2013). Measures of neuroticism and of conscientiousness respectively showed negative and positive relationships adjustment and social cohesion in Antarctic crews (Van Fossen et al., 2021). Sociable introverts, who enjoy the company of other people but are also quite comfortable in solitude, are best suited for most adventures. Kiko Matthews, a woman who on her first long solo row set a new trans-Atlantic record, put it well "I love socializing but I'm also OK on my own and quite like the unknown" (Chadband, 2018).

Salutogenesis and Post-Experience Growth

How do adventurers reminisce about their experiences? Reading their memoirs or listening to their interviews, audience members are usually struck by the privations, difficulties, and dangers confronted and overcome. Most participants are open about discussing their negative emotions: fear, uncertainty, homesickness, loneliness, and the psychological concomitants of physical problems such as fatigue, hunger, heat or cold, pain, and illness. It is difficult not to agree with Apsley Cherry-Garrard, whose 1922 book about exploring Antarctica with Sir Robert Scott was entitled *The Worst Journey in the World*.

Considering all of those adversities, we might expect that post-traumatic stress disorder (PTSD) would be widespread and severe. There has been no evidence pointing to such a pattern. Some temporary emotional disturbances have been found (Palinkas & Suedfeld, 2021), and there have been dramatic episodes of major behavioral problems (Spielmann, 2022); but EST environments show both negative and positive emotions and effects (Mocellin & Suedfeld, 1991; Palinkas & Suedfeld, 2021; Stuster et al., 2000; Zimmer et al., 2013).

The negative aura reflects the unequal levels of attention paid to the two kinds of emotional responses. The suggestion that a widened focus, encouraging interest in positive outcomes, might be appropriate (Suedfeld, 2001, 2005) has resulted in more consideration of salutogenic (health-enhancing; Antonovsky, 1987) impacts and positive post-adventure changes in emotions, values, self-perception, social relations, etc. (Ihle et al., 2006; Smith et al., 2016; Suedfeld, 2012). This could be termed as "Post-Adventure Growth." Adventurers in EST environments are very likely to want to go again, try to go again, and in fact, many do go again. This is true of both those who serve in formally organised groups such as ship's crews and astronauts, and individual venturers who, alone or together, design and carry out their own exploits rather than filling prescribed roles within an established social structure.

Even those who encountered severe problems and failures to reach their goal usually looked back on the experience with pride and satisfaction. Charcot (1911), for example, described in great detail the "agonizing" aspects of his 1903–05 Antarctic expedition, and his determination never to repeat the experience. Yet, a few weeks after he returned home, he started organizing another trip to the ice, and in 1908, he was embarking on it. He later engaged in Arctic exploration, and eventually died in a shipwreck off Iceland. Incidentally, as we shall see, this kind of "the pitcher returning too many times to the well" is not uncommon for adventurers in extreme environments.

Another example was Maurice Herzog, leader of the first team to reach the summit of an 8,000-m mountain (Annapurna). Herzog's fingers and toes eventually had to be amputated because of frostbite, but in his memoirs he wrote of the rapture of being on the summit, the "perfect joy," and the feeling that his team's success was an achievement for "mankind itself" (Herzog, 1953). There is a striking parallel with Neil Armstrong's "That's one small step for man; one giant leap for mankind," uttered as he first stepped onto the surface of the Moon.

The reactions are not always so ecstatic, but can nevertheless be impressively positive. One study of women who had been in the Antarctic concluded that:

> … most women felt they had benefited from going to the Antarctic, usually in terms of personal growth, self-reliance, and independence … In fact the hardest part of the experience was often settling in back home, and so some women continued to travel or applied to go back to the Antarctic.
>
> *(Rothblum et al., 1998, p. 9)*

This is probably the most common kind of evaluation by those who spend time in EST sites, regardless of gender.

Post-adventure reminiscences also document feelings of having benefitted from and experienced changes in personal values (e.g., Ihle et al., 2006; Kjærgaard et al., 2013; Suedfeld, 2018; Suedfeld et al., 2012; Suedfeld, Johnson, et al., 2018; Suedfeld, Legkaia, & Brcic, 2010). The motives that animate adventurers have had limited scientific attention; some studies have been described earlier in this volume. The roles of intrinsic drives—curiosity, thrill-seeking, uniqueness, need for novelty or stimulation—and extrinsic motivators—fame, money, honors, national glory—are difficult to untangle. In most if not all cases, motives are probably mixed in complex and changing ways.

Team Size and Composition

In many cases, the size and composition of the group are predetermined. Spacecraft and submersibles have limited capacity; polar stations need experts in a number of specific areas. In other ventures, the organiser(s) have choices. One of the most famous examples is Admiral Richard Byrd, trying to decide the size of the complement for an Antarctic winter-over in 1934. He was concerned that if two men (female crewmembers were not considered) were isolated in the small, ice-covered habitation, their personal habits and preferences could eventually lead to animosity and even violence; if the crew consisted of three people, two of them could form a partnership hostile to the third; and the shelter could not accommodate more than three. Consequently, he decided to winter over by himself. That decision almost led to his death from a combination of carbon monoxide poisoning (from his stove) followed by disorientation outside the shelter and frostbite from the exposure (Byrd, 1938).

Although there have been many successful solo adventures of all sorts – polar treks, single-handed sailing, mountaineering - some deaths might have been avoided if another person had been present to help. Personality assessments have found nothing surprising: successful protagonists tend to be well adjusted, open to new experiences, self-confident, realistic and flexible copers, and hardy enough to carry on despite injury, illness, and adversity (Kjærgaard et al., 2015; Suedfeld et al., 2017). Despite the fame and admirable qualities of the loners, many, perhaps most major discoveries of historical exploration and adventure have involved teams. Currently, adventurers who want to accomplish a "first" may need to do something alone that had previously been accomplished by groups of two or more. To be unique, to be featured in *Guinness World Records*, doing it solo may be mandatory. Those who undertake such a feat should be people who even in risky situations are comfortable in the absence of others and several extended practice or analogue experiences are advisable.

It is safer to have at least one competent and compatible companion. The selection of that companion should pay attention to competence in the required tasks, but also to resilience, cheerfulness, personal compatibility, and perhaps a construct relatively new to psychological research, *grit* (Duckworth et al., 2007). Grit is the combination of high motivation and dogged perseverance in pursuing a long-term goal. Grit may be beneficial, as for polar explorers slogging to shelter through ice storms and whiteouts, or fatal, as for Captain Scott's party returning from the South Pole and refusing to abandon the heavy loads of mineral samples exacerbating their hunger and fatigue and slowing them down until bad weather trapped them in the tent that became their tomb.

Interpersonal friction and sometimes, hostility, in groups is not unusual. Although Byrd's gloomy forecast of murder within a two-person team has not come true, a similar comment was made later by Valery Ryumin, a *Mir* cosmonaut. Several years later, a couple of *Mir* crewmates spent over 200 days of their mission almost never speaking to each other except when pretending friendship as a show for others (Mundell, 1993). I was once consulted by an adventurer whose less experienced and less competent companion so resented being instructed and guided that by the end of the venture the senior partner was afraid for his life.[2] Other reports of conflict and hostility, as well as of friendship and mutual support, between members of adventurous dyads have emerged from anecdotes of dual military patrollers in the Arctic (Kjærgaard et al., 2015) and in other highly challenging expeditions.

Larger groups offer more chances for friction, but also for timely intervention by other members and for finding potential friends. Some requirements for teammates are unchanging: occupational competence, emotional stability, and sociability without intrusiveness. Decades of research in various ICEs have generated useful selection guidelines for anyone wishing to create an effective adventure team (e.g., Palinkas & Suedfeld, 2021).

Engineering issues are not relevant to this chapter; but in designing the project, expedition planners must take into account the impact of different crew numbers on needed supplies, probabilities of injury or illness, and habitable or transportable shelter—and their psychosocial effects (see, e.g., Salotti et al., 2014).

One source of possible problems is a crew composed of two or more mutually suspicious or unfriendly subgroups, such as a military support force and scientists depending on such support (see the reference to Finn Ronne, later in this chapter). This is a special concern when the two groups disrespect each other: for example, scientists condescending to tradespeople as uneducated and less intelligent, and workers ridiculing researchers as impractical know-it-alls unfit to deal with real-life difficulties.

There have been fist-fights in polar stations (in recent decades, sometimes ameliorated, but at other times exacerbated, by the growing presence of women) and other ICEs. Romantic relationships develop, some ending with the deployment and others leading to long-term bliss or eventual disaster. In a few overpublicised cases of the latter, the media had to be reminded that bizarre behaviour by star-crossed lovers is not limited to former explorers and adventurers. There has been one event in a spaceflight simulator that was interpreted by some, including the victim, as a sexual assault; and one Antarctic scientist who was officially considered to have been guilty of sexual harassment. There is a list of conflicts and derangements in Antarctic stations (Spielmann, 2022); but in general, peccadillos have been no worse (and perhaps less frequent) than in daily life back "home."

The Sensed Presence Phenomenon

More frequently than one might expect, a phantom companion appears to the adventurer (Suedfeld & Mocellin, 1987). This has occurred during solo voyages and to small groups. Perhaps most importantly—and challenging hypotheses of mental derangement, hallucination, or mirage—the sensed presence frequently provides guidance, instruction, or physical assistance to the adventurer who has a problem. That problem may be illness, injury, fatigue, lack of food, excessive cold or heat, or being lost. The apparition may help by offering encouragement, performing needed tasks, pointing out the direction to safety, or even providing food. For example, an Antarctic trekker felt her late grandmother's presence and heard her voice encouraging her to keep going despite her fatigue (Kahn & Leon, 1994). An extensive analysis of this phenomenon, in which it is called *The Third Man Factor* (Geiger, 2009), describes many such anecdotes, including some from famous explorers such as Joshua Slocum, the first man to sail around the world single-handed, Sir Ernest Shackleton, and Charles Lindbergh, and examines theories of their origin.

Leadership

In team projects, the personality and behaviour of the leader is of major importance. Although adventure leadership is a complex role, there are some generally important attributes without which the success of the enterprise is shaky. The leader must, of course, have expertise in the basic skills involved. Depending on the specific situation, these may include map reading and orientation, fieldcraft, first aid, small-boat handling, SCUBA diving, spelunking, rock climbing, etc. In some cases, communication in a local language may be crucial, as may the ability to find water, food, and shelter and to make field repairs to equipment.

Besides that, leaders of small groups of adventurers need to be flexible, patient, and open-minded. Their team members are likely to have their own opinions about decisions, be quite sure about their own expertise, and in some cases inclined to criticism and rebelliousness. These traits may be exacerbated when the group is under stress, especially if the leader shows indecisiveness, uncertainty, or self-doubt. Ideally, the leader should master a repertoire of approaches: flexible when decisions are about matters that are not urgent or critical, respectful to expertise outside the leader's own knowledge, and decisive, definite, assertive in emergencies. The hierarchy of EST groups is flat: unlike leaders in ordinary circumstances, most expedition leaders have no special distinguishing marks, no particular privileges, little or no power to punish or reward, no buffers (aides and secretaries, private offices, etc.). They live and work among their group members and endure the same stressors plus the additional burdens of leadership and must maintain their equanimity and poise when others panic or shirk.

Good leaders must try to adapt and carry on with the mission. Grit, determination, has not been measured as a selection criterion, but it might be a good predictor for both leaders and followers. Leaders must know when *not* to be flexible, when determination provides an example for the group as a whole to proceed toward the goal without quailing.

A set of case studies (Suedfeld, 2010) showed some examples of poor leadership in polar situations: indecisive tolerance of negativism and rivalry (Henry Hudson), military stiffness and hierarchical dominance (Finn Ronne), and a combination of inadequate preparation and rigidity in planning (Robert F. Scott). These traits preceded mutiny, impaired mission performance, and lethal failure in the three expeditions, respectively; and they exemplify the difficulties of leadership under extreme conditions.

Having discussed some of the most important aspects of EST psychology in general, we now look at three of the most rigorous EST adventure sites. Much of what we know about the people who have responded to the challenge those sites pose, and some of the outcomes that may serve as lessons for the future, are considered. The focus is on Antarctica, long-distance solo sailing, and climbing the highest mountains in the world. Knowledge and implications from other ESTs are cited when relevant, but not analysed in detail.

Antarctica, the EST-est Place on Earth

After centuries of sightings, the late 19th and early 20th centuries saw an outburst of exploratory expeditions launched to Antarctica. Many of these were failures. Ships disappeared, men died by the dozens, and readers wondered at the courage and dedication of the volunteers. A plethora of memoirs and histories appeared, and continue appearing.

What was overlooked for a long time, and neglected until quite recently, were the toughness and resilience of the crews and their inventiveness in devising ways to survive and even thrive during multi-year voyages under what might seem to us intolerable conditions. Officers and crews of whaling and exploration ships, powered by sail, frozen into the ice, kept their sanity and disciplined order with lectures, games, diaries, theatrical and musical performances, and ships' newspapers (Johnson & Suedfeld, 1996).

Antarctica is special, unique, and awesome. The diaries of early explorers are replete with references to the grandeur, beauty, and enchantment of its ice-and-sea-scape (see Mocellin & Suedfeld, 1991). Early explorers described dangers and privations, but nevertheless bonded with the environment. Antarctica is the champion EST environment: the highest, coldest, driest, windiest, barest, and loneliest of the continents. It is a desert, mostly covered with ice, and its average altitude is that of high mountains, 2500 m; some visitors pass out as they exit the plane. A T-shirt reads: "Ski South Pole: 9,000 feet of base, ¼" of powder." Weather in the interior of the continent includes Earth's lowest temperatures, whiteouts, blizzards, and katabatic winds that can reach 300 km/hr.

Antarctica is the only continent that has never had any indigenous or permanent human population. None of it officially belongs to any country, and all bases are accessible to anyone.

Sojourners can be roughly divided into four categories. People in the first two can be further divided into 4,000 summer personnel and about 1,000 "winterers." Most scientists and support people rate the experience as positive and wish to return, some annually for many years.

1. Scientists working in the dozens of bases, stations, and camps, concentrated in the Antarctic Peninsula but scattered across the continent as well. Most

scientists get (or make) opportunities to visit outlying camps, interesting natural or historical sites, penguin rookeries, seal colonies, etc. They also have unique research opportunities.

2. Support personnel needed to keep those bases and scientists operational and in good order. They include flight and ships' crews, radio operators, weather technicians, search and rescue experts, medical professionals, plus all the usual trades—plumbers, electricians, vehicle operators, etc. Many first-time ("newbie") support workers hope for an adventurous year. For the most part, they are disappointed because of the limitations and demands of the work and the environment. They may find sufficient compensation in the camaraderie, the good pay that is easy to save, and the relaxed pace and fewer demands. Some also appreciate the escape from unpleasantness at home.

    If risk-taking is part of adventuring, these sojourners qualify. Accidental deaths are not rare. Most of them are due to air crashes with multiple fatalities; others are industrial accidents, ordinary or unusual such as collapsing ice, crevasses, and becoming disoriented in a whiteout. There are maritime accidents, such as a boat overturning or a vehicle crashing through thin ice over the sea; and one snorkeling scientist was killed by a leopard seal. Frostbite and hypothermia occur when working or travelling outdoors. Medical care is mostly basic, and evacuation during the depth of winter is chancy.

    Among syndromes with local names (Palinkas & Suedfeld, 2008, 2021) are "Big Eye," chronic insomnia, and "Long Eye" ("the 20-foot stare in the 10-foot room"), a temporary fugue state in which the person, with eyes open, is totally unaware of events. A polar counterpart of "space fog" or "the space stupids" is a state of reduced cognitive alertness and efficacy.

    The other two categories cover short-term visitors, for whom the list of dangers is shorter, and the list of adventures much longer.

3. Tourists in ever-increasing numbers (up to 56,000 in the year before the COVID pandemic) typically spend a week or two, mostly in the Peninsula. Some packages offer Zodiac or helicopter excursions, kayaking, glacier climbing, or hiking. Tourists experience grandeur, awe, a spiritual unity with an environment of overwhelming panoramas. The expanse of ice and sky seems to go on forever. Various species of penguins and seals can be seen, although visitors are now prohibited from approaching the native fauna too closely. This is not a problem with most species, but some small penguins seem to invite a friendly pat. Alas, it is not to be.

4. Roving "explorers" or independent researchers. As the history of exploration testifies, Antarctica is a prime site for adventurers seeking a place of hardship and challenge. One person or a small team strives to accomplish something unique or at least unusual, such as replicating a historical exploration. Such an enterprise requires considerable planning, organisation, and funding.

The Loneliest: Solo Long-Distance Sailing

Several extreme environments could lay claim to loneliness. As a general rule, solo adventurers tend to be the most self-confident and perhaps the toughest personalities, and perhaps the least risk-averse. The remoteness of help or relief makes the solo's situation considerably more perilous and daunting.

Of the many solo voyagers in deserts, mountains, icefields, and ocean depths, single-handed circumnavigators seem among the loneliest of the lonely. Sailing alone over long distances will almost definitely take sailor and boat through changeable and dangerous winds and waves, as well as extremes of temperature. Those conditions, and a plethora of possible accidents, may destroy or irretrievably damage the craft; errors in navigation may take it off course to the point of exhausting the sailor's strength or supplies. Rescue arrangements can fail. So can self-steering equipment, intended to allow periods of safe sleep, perhaps the most common need of solo sailors. Steering the boat and adjusting the sails are crucial; either falling asleep or performance decrements resulting from lack of sleep are salient perils facing maritime adventurers.

Food and, especially, potable water are difficult to replace if used up, contaminated, lost through accident, or inadequately supplied to begin with. However, it is possible to survive on sources from the ocean itself, and the well-known rapid onset of death among uninjured shipwreck survivors may be due more to psychological factors than physical privation (Bombard, 1953; Lindemann, 1998). Psychology's task in this context is not to identify a "survivor personality," but rather to understand why so many survivors (in many situations, not only after shipwreck) so quickly lose the will to live (Leach, 2011).

One of the best-known examples of single-handed sailors is Captain Joshua Slocum, the first solo circumnavigator (1895–98). He was a highly experienced sailor and ship's captain, having commanded many sail and steam vessels in different oceans and having coped with shipwrecks, mutiny, pirates, and outbreaks of cholera and smallpox. He was an excellent navigator, competent to find his way without some of the instruments that others relied on.

His book describing the circumnavigation (Slocum, 1900) was extremely popular, and he became world famous. Like many sailors, he retired to a farm as the ideal haven and lived for some time ashore with his family. But Slocum eventually got restless. He went back to sea to explore the course of the Amazon, and disappeared, joining the many casualties of repeated expeditions. Adventure psychologists may wonder about the possible roles of, for example, adrenaline addiction (Odunton & Deras, 2005), Type T personality (Farley, 2010), high and insatiable need for achievement (McClelland, 1961), and/or repetition compulsion in service of an unconscious death instinct (Freud, 1920).

The next lone sailor to reach world-wide fame was Francis Chichester, a successful businessman, cartographer, and long-distance pilot. He became interested in single-handed sailing and completed several trans-Atlantic races. At age 65, he entered an around-the-world race for solo sailors. Despite several close calls and the failure of his self-steering gear (thus depriving him of any prolonged sleep), he won the race (Chichester, 1968). When knighting him, Queen Elizabeth II used the same sword that Elizabeth I had used to knight Sir Francis Drake, England's first circumnavigator.

Like Slocum, Chichester was well suited to his adventures. An expert yachtsman and navigator, used to equipment failures and setbacks, he was strongly self-reliant in the face of setbacks. His father was sparing of praise, never satisfied with the son's achievements, and domineering about his life choices. This may have influenced Sir Francis's later preference for doing things alone, and sparked his ambition to be the first and best in his various endeavours. The elder Chichester is reminiscent of the father of the highly achievement-focused Colonel Buzz Aldrin, the second man on the Moon and later, a prolific author and public speaker (Suedfeld & Weiszbeck, 2004).

More than fifty people have tried *rowing* solo across the Atlantic, in most cases accompanied by supporters in other boats. Of those, two dozen have succeeded and six have died in the attempt. John Beeden, one of the very few who have rowed alone across both major oceans without support, argued that even those who die in the attempt show the "indomitable human spirit that will break before it bends. To test what we are made of, that is our pursuit" (Beeden, 2015). Kiko Matthews (2018), who set a speed record (49 days) for a woman rowing solo across the Atlantic, reported flights of imagination, strange questions that came to her mind, fantasies about fresh food (a common dream topic of early polar explorers), fear when conditions were unusually daunting, talking aloud, learning to go without much sleep, changes in musculature, but also the state of total psychological immersion in one's activity that psychologists refer to as *flow* (Csikszentmihalyi, 1996).

The Highest: Climbing the Giant Mountains

There are various kinds of adventures in and above the highest terrestrial altitudes, but the pursuit most generally considered as an adventure sport is rock- and mountain climbing. Many people enjoy climbing local heights, to feel the exultation of challenge and success. But the EST version of mountain climbing is to reach the summit of the highest mountains on Earth, the "eight-thousanders": peaks of at least 8,000 meters above sea level, the so-called "Death Zone." Climbing there is unique among the three EST ventures in this chapter: it is by far the shortest in duration, and it is the only one whose adventurers, with few exceptions, are dependent on groups of paid professionals (the Sherpas of Tibet and Nepal) to help them reach their goal and then return to safety.

This is truly pure adventuring: no practical benefits are obtained from getting to the summit, and the risks are extreme. As in many ESTs, the scenery is awesome; but high climbers must focus on the task, and except for their short time on the summit itself, during clear weather, don't get to enjoy the panorama.

The annals of climbing are replete with deaths and injuries everywhere in the world. Falls are perhaps the most frequent cause; but there are also avalanches, high winds, sudden changes in weather conditions, oxygen deprivation, altitude sickness (*soroche*), snow blindness and severe sunburn caused by ultraviolet radiation, frostbite, dehydration, and physical and mental exhaustion (e.g., US National Park Service, 2021). After having reached the summit, the climber faces the need to return to safety. More people have died during their descent from the summit than in climbing to reach it. Among the causes are sheer fatigue and reduced vigilance, carefulness, and motivation.

In recent years, the glory of having reached the top of Mount Everest, the highest peak on Earth, has diminished. There are more climbers (900 summiteers in 2019, 55% of them Sherpas; Arnette, 2019). Many of the "clients" are inexperienced and unfit, needing to be heavily supported by their Sherpa guides, who comprise about 1/3 of the fatalities (Preiss, 2018). Garbage litters the slopes, and long queues cause more exposure, fatigue, and impatience (Woodward, 2019). Countering these trends is "free climbing," using a minimum of equipment and having as little impact on the mountain environment as possible. Advocated by the pioneering mountaineer Hermann Buhl, this method has been a hallmark of the legendary Reinhold Messner, the holder of dozens of climbing records including being the first to make a solo ascent of Everest, the first to summit all 14 eight-thousanders—and for variety, a man who crossed over the South Pole on skis and explored the Gobi and other deserts as well. Obviously much more dangerous and demanding, the free climbing ethos could reduce both the crowds and the damage to the environment (Messner & Höfler, 2000), although it would certainly reduce the economic benefits of mountaineering for governments, suppliers, guides, and tour companies.

Conclusion

This has been an excursion into areas, psychological and conceptual as well as geographical, that are remote from the adventures that most people ever experience. The perils, difficulties, and complexities of these and other EST environments are great, and many who dared face them paid dearly. But they can be thought of as prototypes of the mixture of excitement and trepidation, the confrontation of novelty and hazard followed by learning how to cope with both and the pride and satisfaction of succeeding, that adventures in other venues and contexts also offer to varying degrees.

One other point should be considered. As time goes on and there are changes in technology and techniques, some of the EST situations have become less daunting and more safe, comfortable, and familiar. Someday, they may become psychologically less alien; skiing in Antarctica may be thought of as no more extraordinary than a cross-country skiing vacation in the nearest park (or on Mars).

When that happens, where will we go for an extreme adventure?

Acknowledgments

I am grateful to the many adventurers, including colleagues and students, who have participated in my research on isolated, confined environments, and to the agencies, including the Social Sciences and Humanities Research Council of Canada, Environment Canada, and the Canadian Space Agency, that have provided funds and field support in kind to make it possible. My thanks also to Dr. Phyllis J. Johnson for her meticulous assistance in preparing this manuscript for publication.

Notes

1 There was an ominous precedent. A French scientist, Jean-François Pilâtre de Rozier, became one of the first two aviators in human history when he and a colleague were the first persons to fly in a free balloon (Nov. 21, 1783). Ironically and tragically, on June 15, 1785 he also became the first aviator killed in an air crash (if we discount Icarus).
2 To protect the privacy of the individuals involved, and of my sources, I am not able to provide specific details.

References

Antonovsky, A. (1987). *Unraveling the mystery of health: How people manage stress and stay well*. Jossey-Bass.

Arnette, A. (2019, June 7). Everest 2019: Season summary: The year Everest broke. Accessed December 9, 2021 from https://www.alanarnette.com/blog/2019/06/07/everest-2019-season-summary-the-year-everest-broke/

Beeden, J. (2015). Website @*solopacificrow*. Quoted in M. Kullman. This man just completed world's first solo row from California to Australia. *EcoWatch Daily Newsletter*, December 28, 2015. Accessed September 12, 2021 from https://www.ecowatch.com/this-man-just-completed-worlds-first-solo-row-from-california-to-austr-1882138557.html

Bombard, A. (1953). *The voyage of the "Heretique."* Simon & Schuster.

Brcic, J. (2013). *Extreme teams: Coping and motive imagery of small, mission-oriented teams in extreme and unusual environments*. Ph.D. dissertation, University of British Columbia.

Byrd, R. (1938). *Alone in the Antarctic*. Putnam. (Many subsequent editions).

Carroll, V. (2021). What's killing America's hikers? *Sky above us*, March 11. Accessed September 18, 2021 from https://skyaboveus.com/climbing-hiking/Whats-Killing-Americas-Hikers

Chadband, I. (2018, May 22). Rogue waves, a near capsize and 49 days alone on the Atlantic, what could stop Kiko Matthews? Accessed September 25, 2021 from ESPN.com

Charcot, J. B. (1911). *The voyage of the "Why-Not?" in the Antarctic: The journal of the second French South Polar expedition, 1908–1910*. Translated by P. Walsh. Stodder & Stoughton.

Cherry-Garrard, A. (1922). *The worst journey in the world*. Doran. (Many subsequent publishers/editions).

Chichester, F. (1968). *"Gipsy Moth" circles the world*. Coward McCann.

Csikszentmihalyi, M. (1996). *Creativity: Flow and the psychology of discovery and invention.* Harper Perennial.

Denoble, P. J., Chimiak, J., Moore, A., et al. (2019). In P. J. Denoble (Ed.), *DAN Annual Diving Report 2019 Edition: A report on 2017 diving fatalities, injuries, and incidents.* Durham, NC: Divers Alert Network. Accessed September 18, 2021 from https://www.ncbi.nlm.nih.gov/books/NBK562534/

Duckworth, A. L., Peterson, C., Matthews, M. D., & Kelly, D. R. (2007). Grit: Perseverance and passion for long-term goals. *Journal of Personality and Social Psychology, 92*(6), 1187–1101.

Farley, F. (2010). *Heroes and heroism.* Paper presented at the meeting of the American Psychological Association, San Diego, CA.

Freud, S. (1920). *Beyond the pleasure principle.* Republished by Penguin, 1991.

Gatterer, H., Niedermeier, M. Pocecco, E., et al. (2019). Mortality in different mountain sports activities primarily practiced in the summer season – A narrative review. *International Journal of Environmental Research and Public Health, 16*(20). Accessed September 18, 2021 from https://www.ncbi.nlm.nih.gov/pmc/articles/PMC6843304/

Geiger, J. (2009). *The Third Man Factor.* Penguin. ISBN 10: 0143017519ISBN 13: 9780143017516

Herzog, M. (1953). *Annapurna: First conquest of an 8,000-meter peak.* Dutton.

Ihle, E. C., Ritsher, J. B., & Kanas, N. (2006). Positive psychological outcomes of spaceflight: An empirical study. *Aviation, Space, and Environmental Medicine, 77*(2), 93–101.

Johnson, P. J., & Suedfeld, P. (1996). Coping with stress through microcosms of home and family among Arctic whalers and explorers. *History of the Family, 1*(1), 41–62.

Kahn, P. M., & Leon, G. R. (1994). Group climate and individual functioning in an all-women's Antarctic expedition team. *Environment and Behavior, 26,* 669–697. Reprinted in *Journal of Human Performance in Extreme Environments* (2000), *5,* 35–43.

Kamler, K. (2004). *Surviving the extremes: A doctor's journey to the limits of human endurance.* St. Martin's Press.

Kjærgaard, A., Leon, G. R., & Fink, B. A. (2015). Personal challenges, communication processes, and team effectiveness in military special patrol teams operating in a polar environment. *Environment and Behavior, 47,* 644–666.

Kjærgaard, A., Leon, G. R., Venables, N. C., & Fink, B. A. (2013). Personality, personal values and growth in military special unit patrol teams operating in a polar environment. *Military Psychology, 25*(1), 13–22. https://doi.org/10.1037/h0094753

Leach, J. (2011). Survival psychology: The won't to live. *The Psychologist, 24*(1), 26–29.

Lindemann, H. (1998). *Alone at sea.* Pollner Verlag.

Matthews, K. (2018). *KIKO: How to break the Atlantic rowing record after brain surgery.* Polperro Heritage Press. ISBN: 0995736820

McClelland, D. C. (1961). *The Achieving Society.* Free Press.

Messner, R., & Höfler, H. (2000). *Hermann Buhl: Climbing without compromise.* Mountaineers Books.

Mocellin, J. S. P., & Suedfeld, P. (1991). Voices from the ice: Diaries of polar explorers. *Environment and Behavior, 23*(6), 704–722.

Mundell, I. (1993, April 16). Stop the rocket, I want to get off. *New Scientist Newsletters.* Accessed September 3, 2021 from https://www.newscientist.com/article/mg13818693-700/

Odunton, A., & Deras, D. (2005). *Confessions of an Adrenaline addict.* Synergy Unlimited.

Palinkas, L. A., & Suedfeld, P. (2008). Psychological effects of polar expeditions. *The Lancet, 371,* 153–163.

Palinkas, L. A., & Suedfeld, P. (2021). Psychosocial issues in isolated and confined extreme environments. *Neuroscience and Biobehavioral Reviews, 126*, 413–429.

Preiss, D. (2018, April 14). One-third of Everest deaths are Sherpa climbers. *Parallels: Many Stories, One World.* Accessed September 20, 2021 from https://www.npr.org/sections/parallels/2018/04/14/599417489/one-third-of-everest-deaths-are-sherpa-climbers

Rothblum, E. D., Weinstock, J. S., & Morris, J. (Eds.) (1998). *Women in the Antarctic.* Haworth.

Salotti, J.-M., Heidmann, R., & Suhir, E. (2014). *Crew size impact on the design, risks and cost of a human mission to Mars.* Presented at the 2014 IEEE Conference, Big Sky, MT, USA.

Simon, S., & Kennedy, J. M. (2003, May 3). Trapped hiker had one way out – with his knife. *Los Angeles Times.* Accessed September 19, 2021 from https://latimesblogs.latimes.com/thedailymirror/2010/11/aron-ralston-the-real-story.html

Slocum, J. (1900). *Sailing alone around the world.* Century.

Smith, N., Kinnafick, F., Cooley, S. J., & Sandal, G. M. (2016). Reported growth following mountaineering expeditions: The role of personality and perceived stress. *Environment and Behavior, 49*(8), 933–955.

Spielmann, P. J. (2022). *Darkest Antarctica: Greed, madness, and mayhem.* Unpublished MS in preparation.

Steel, G. D., Suedfeld, P., Peri, A., & Palinkas, L. A. (1997). People in high latitudes: The "Big Five" personality characteristics of the circumpolar sojourner. *Environment & Behavior, 29*(3), 324–347. DOI: 10.1177/001391659702900302

Stuster, J., Bachelard, C., & Suedfeld, P. (2000). The relative importance of behavioral issues during long-duration I.C.E. missions. *Aviation, Space, and Environmental Medicine, 71*(9, Sect2, Suppl), A17–A25.

Suedfeld, P. (2001). Applying positive psychology in the study of extreme environments. *Human Performance in Extreme Environments, 6*, 21–25.

Suedfeld, P. (2005). Invulnerability, coping, salutogenesis, integration: Four phases of space psychology. *Aviation, Space, and Environmental Medicine, 76*, B61–73.

Suedfeld, P. (2010). Historical space psychology: Early terrestrial explorations as Mars analogues. *Planetary and Space Science, 58*, 639–645.

Suedfeld, P. (2012). Extreme and unusual environments: Challenges and responses. In S. Clayton (Ed.), *The Oxford handbook of environmental and conservation psychology* (pp. 348–371). Oxford University Press.

Suedfeld, P. (2018). Antarctica and space as psychological analogues. *REACH: Reviews in Human Space Exploration, 9–12*, 1–4.

Suedfeld, P., Brcic, J., et al. (2012). Personal growth following long-duration spaceflight. *Acta Astronautica, 79*, 118–123.

Suedfeld, P., Johnson, P. J., Gushin, V., & Brcic, J. (2018). Motivational profiles of retired cosmonauts. *Acta Astronautica, 146*, 202–205.

Suedfeld, P., & Mocellin, J. S. P. (1987). The "sensed presence" in unusual environments. *Environment and Behavior, 19*, 33–52.

Suedfeld, P., Shiozaki, L., Archdekin, B., Sandhu, H., & Wood, M. (2017). The polar exploration diary of Mark Wood: A thematic content analysis. *The Polar Journal, 7*(1), 227–241 (also published online).

Suedfeld, P., & Weiszbeck, T. (2004). The impact of outer space on inner space. *Aviation, Space and Environmental Medicine, 75*(7), C6–C9.

Towell, C. (2020). *The Survival Handbook.* Penguin.

US National Park Service: Denali Dispatches (2021). *Troubling trends.* Accessed September 24, 2021 from https://www.nps.gov/dena/blogs/troubling-trends.htm

Van Fossen, J., Olenick, J., Ayton, J., Chang, C.-H., & Kozlowski, S. W. J. (2021). Relationships between personality and social functioning, attitudes towards the team and mission, and well-being in an ICE environment. *Acta Astronautica, 189*, 658–670. https://doi.org/10.1016/j.actaastro.2021.09.031

Wikipedia (2022, January 7). List of balloon accidents. Accessed January 23, 2022 from https://en.wikiipedia.org/wiki/Listof ballooning accidents

Woodward, A. (2019). What happens to your body in Mount Everest's "death zone," where 11 people have died in the past week. *Insider,* May 28. Accessed September 20, 2021 from https://www.businessinsider.com/mount-everest-death-zone-what-happens-to-body-2019-5

Zimmer, M., Rodrigues Cabral, J. C. C., Czarneski Borges, F., Gonçalves Côco, K., & da Rocha Hameister, B. (2013). Psychological changes arising from an Antarctic stay: Systematic overview. *Psychological Treatment and Prevention, 30*(3). Accessed September 16, 2021 from https://doi.org/10.1590/S0103-166X2013000300011

3
ENDURING PERFORMANCE

Ronald Duren Jr.

An Adventurer's Point of View – One More Step

My day had started at 4:00am in Leadville, Colorado. It was now early afternoon. I had already run 38 miles, and was less than halfway into the iconic Leadville 100-mile running race. I was sitting down for the first time all day with my support crew tending to my needs. I was doing my best to eat some food to nourish my exhausted body. As I shovelled food into my mouth, I couldn't take my eyes off the large mountain in front of me. It was Mt. Hope, my next challenge. I knew this is where the race takes on a new dimension. This is where most runners lose the fight and the will to continue moving forward.

The next 12 miles would take me over Hope pass at 12,600′ elevation to the halfway point of the abandoned mining town of Winfield. To get there requires a steep 3400′ ascent in 3.5 miles. On tired legs that had already given me 38 miles of mobility. I knew if I could survive this climb, I might be able to stay in the game. As I left the cosy atmosphere of the aid station, I felt a little sad to be leaving my friends and facing this beast of a mountain alone. I was soon aware no one was coming to my rescue. It was now up to me. I crossed several rivers. With soggy wet shoes I started my climb. The calories I had just consumed were not yet providing the caloric energy I needed. I started to acutely feel the fatigue of the previous miles as the terrain dramatically changed and my pace slowed considerably.

Up the mountain I climbed. Slow and steady at first. Soon I found myself stopping more frequently to catch my breath in the thin air as my lungs gasped for precious oxygen. My legs didn't want to continue. They now felt heavy, like lead. My body was failing, and my mind was in agreement. It pleaded with me, "let's just quit, this is dumb." As I listened to this inner dialogue, I used my trekking poles to lower myself down to one knee to rest.

I bowed my head and looked down. I focused my gaze on a 6-inch circle of earth directly in front of my face. I examined every detail of that patch of dirt and became lost in another world. It was beautiful. I felt delirious, nauseous and light-headed, which contributed to an out of body experience. At that moment, that circle of earth was all that mattered in my world. The outside world no longer existed. I heard other runners vomit from exhaustion, but I never looked up as I continued to hang my head. It was just background noise. No one was laughing anymore, as we were earlier in the race. Pain, struggle, and discomfort had taken over our minds. This was now about survival. It was a scene stolen from 'The Walking Dead.'

I wondered, "should I quit?" In my mind a battle raged. I felt like I was on the witness stand being interrogated in a courtroom by my inner critic as the prosecuting attorney. The voice was making a compelling case, pleading with me to make the pain stop. All I have to do is quit, and it will all be over. No one is forcing me to continue, I am here at my choosing. Why keep going? What do I have to prove?

I laboriously forced myself into a standing position, and took another step up the mountain.

Ronald Duren Jr.

Enduring Performance: Keep Moving Forward

Adventuring often requires enduring performance while also dynamically coping with unknown, challenging and variable conditions. This chapter examines how the adventurer sustains effort, attitude and energy to optimally perform while immersed in dangerous, extreme or rapidly changing environments. All the while responding to volatile conditions such as weather and fluctuating landscapes or seascapes.

What does it take to keep moving forward when your inner dialogue is begging you to quit? Where does the commitment come from to keep going in a voluntary endeavour? When is the desire to quit stronger than the desire to seek comfort? How does the subjective perception of effort – or perceived limits – come into play? Most adventures are voluntary activities, and quitting can be easy, but psychologically a very subjective concept. Each adventure has the possibility to have moments when progress becomes difficult, or seemingly impossible.

Quitting is often a viable option. Contrary to popular memes, winners do quit. Knowing when to quit, and when to push on, is not an easy decision for the adventurer in the thick of the experience. This judgement and decision-making process is just one of many challenges facing the endurance performer. In the context of adventure, quitting is sometimes the only option that will prevent an adventure from transitioning into a survival situation, or even death. Sound judgement can keep the adventurer alive. This is an incredibly important skill to possess, as your life and the lives of your team may depend on making the correct choice at the correct time.

There are many variables in an adventure context that are factors impacting enduring performance. Rapidly changing weather conditions, unforeseen challenges, human dynamics, broken or malfunctioning equipment all must be accounted for. An adaptive, pragmatic, flexible mindset is needed to maintain a calm demeanour and self-control as situations dynamically, and oftentimes rapidly and repeatedly change.

★ ★ ★ ★ ★

How we define endurance is important to our discussion. A review of the literature in similar fields provides a starting point. Endurance in sport often defines it as performance lasting one hour or more. In the world of *ultra-marathon running*, it is typically any activity beyond 26.2 miles (42.2 km) covered, or six hours duration (Waldvogel et al., 2019). Suffice to say, an adventure activity (expeditions, travels, experiences), can be any duration in length. There is no regulation time or scoreboard clock. Many adventures are multi-day, multi-week or even multi-month durations.

There does not seem to be consensus on how long an endurance activity is within the context of adventure. Many of the definitions for endurance mention "prolonged" periods but fail to define where the threshold lies. For the purposes of this chapter, I will describe it as at least six hours of physical activity in a 24-hour period, oftentimes occurring over multiple days.

In this chapter we will examine current research that looks at endurance performance in various contexts inside and outside the world of adventure. First, let's acknowledge that there are many components to endurance performance. Far more than we can cover in this chapter. Enduring performance is a multi-variable challenge. There exist no easy recipes or methodology to follow since each situation, each participant, is different. Physiological and psychological aspects both play a part. They are intertwined and difficult to separate.

Psychophysiology is the study of the relationship between physiological signals recorded from the body and brain to mental processes and functions. Endurance performance sits squarely in the area of psychophysiology. The scope of this chapter will limit most of the discussion to the psychological aspects of endurance. The reader may choose to explore the physiological elsewhere for a more complete picture of how to perform at optimum.

More precisely, how to perform optimally in variable, dynamic conditions. Optimal performance, as opposed to peak performance that is often coveted in organised sport. Life, and adventure, are not well-controlled, 90-minute matches with set rules and regulations. During an adventure, sometimes optimal performance is just putting one foot in front of another and continuing to move forward. Optimal performance, to be sustained, often falls far short of peak performance when burn-out can be the downfall of many elite athletes exhausted from attempting to maintain peak performance over long periods of time.

Additionally, how do we interpret endurance that is more mental or cognitive in nature? Anyone who has finished a gruelling calculus test can attest to mental endurance that is not physical, but nonetheless exhausting. Although we lean heavily on research for endurance athletes and physical nature, adventure can take on less physical aspects as well. Much of what is covered in this chapter is directly or indirectly applicable to these aspects too.

Beyond the question of duration, the Oxford dictionary defines *endurance* as "the fact or power of enduring an unpleasant or difficult process or situation without giving way" (Oxford English Dictionary, 2022). It is often described as the ability to endure hardship or adversity over a long period of time. The ability to keep going when the journey is difficult. Endurance in the context of sport is an athlete's psychophysiological resistance to fatigue.

The American Psychological Association (APA) dictionary of psychology defines "endurance activity" as, "a physical activity that depends on aerobic capacity, that is, the ability to produce energy for muscles by using oxygen for long periods of time. Sport performances that are endurance activities include marathons, runs over 10,000 m, and triathlons" (APA, 2022). Interesting that a *psychological* association uses *physical* capacity for its definition, when research – as we shall see below – suggests that aerobic capacity, energy production, muscles and oxygen are not necessarily the core enabling or limiting factors. Motivation, perception of effort, self-regulation, and other "mind over muscle" talents are also legitimate considerations.

Personally, I am sceptical of a single variable that holds the secret to endurance performance. Performance will be diminished without sufficient caloric intake for example, but may not stop the adventurer in their tracks. And although not every adventure is about survival, it walks a precarious line between life and death at times. Perhaps it would be wise to label a survival situation as *optimal* performance, rather than peak performance, which has a strong focus on athletic achievement. Nonetheless, the ability to endure and continue moving forward is rather difficult to tidily define. It is not as simple as caloric intake or metabolic rate (Donnell, 2012) or VO2 max. Beyond the physiological, into the psychological, we find that perseverance, in the context of achievement motivation, is associated with better endurance performance (Röthlin et al., 2022). This serves as a good segue into the next section of psychological skills training.

Psychological Skills Training: Managing your Headspace

In sport psychology, the concept of psychological skills training (PST) is a catch-all term for many skills that have been shown to increase performance in endurance athletes (McCormick et al., 2015). Some of these skills include: self-talk

(Blanchfield et al., 2014; Hatzigeorgiadis et al., 2011, 2018); self-efficacy (Brace et al., 2020; Desharnais et al., 1986; Howle et al., 2016; Martin & Gill, 1991); self-belief (Leach & Ansell, 2008); self-regulation (Brick et al., 2015, Molden et al., 2016); cognitive reappraisal, metacognition (Brick et al., 2015); decision-making (Collins et al., 2016, 2018; Collins & Collins, 2013; Maier & Taber, 2007; Mees et al., 2021; Pageaux, 2014); goal striving (Bueno et al., 2008; Howle et al., 2016); perceived effort (Marcora et al., 2008; Marcora & Staiano, 2010; McCormick et al., 2015; Pageaux & Lepers, 2016; van Cutsem et al., 2017); attentional focus, arousal regulation (Cooper et al., 2020); humour (Brcic et al., 2018; Rice & Liu, 2016; Sliter et al., 2014); gratitude, awe, self-compassion (Röthlin et al., 2022); acceptance and mindfulness.

For the sake of brevity, we will narrow our focus on perhaps the most salient for adventure psychology: self-talk, self-efficacy, self-regulation, self-belief, cognitive reappraisal, metacognition and humour. Many of these skills focus on increasing motivation and/or reducing perception of effort in line with the psychobiological model of endurance. You will also notice that many of them overlap.

Perceived Effort: Changing the Story

The psychobiological model of endurance proposed by Samuel Marcora is an effort-based decision-making model centred on motivational intensity theory (Marcora et al., 2008). The model looks closely at the psychological factors that influence endurance performance. Essentially the concept of "mind over muscle" (Marcora & Staiano, 2010). In this model, the decision to keep moving forward is primarily determined by two factors: *perception of effort* (how hard does it feel) and *potential motivation* (commitment to keep going) (Röthlin et al., 2022).

How we appraise our effort levels will dictate how well we perform for prolonged periods. Marcora describes the perception of effort as "the conscious sensation of how hard, heavy and strenuous a physical task is" (Marcora & Staiano, 2010). His model postulates that this is one of two limiting factors for endurance (the other being motivation to keep going).

There has been shown to be a connection between perceived effort and mental fatigue. Perhaps contrary to intuition, mental fatigue has a direct impact on physical performance (Clarkson et al., 2016; Inzlicht & Marcora, 2016; Pageaux & Lepers, 2016; Schiphof-Godart et al., 2018; van Cutsem et al., 2017). There appears to be a direct coupling; each directly influences the other.

How we assess and interpret our energy states (mental and physical) is largely dependent on cognitive appraisal. This is the narrative we tell ourselves, an interpretation of our current situation. Preferably adventurers are able to tell positive, optimistic stories, without ignoring harsh realities. If an adventurer feels (real or perceived) mental fatigue, it stands to reason that they will feel physically depleted as well. Motivation to continue will wane. This perceived exertion has been shown to be a limiting factor, and perhaps the factor most responsible for "the negative impact of mental fatigue on endurance performance" (van Cutsem et al., 2017). Indeed, mental fatigue has a multi-factorial nature, and different types of mental fatigue may produce different styles of task performance (Shigihara et al., 2013).

Evidence suggests that elevated dopamine allows athletes to continue moving forward and exert effort, reducing the effects of impaired cognitive functioning. This will positively impact the decision to not quit in the face of adversity, pain and discomfort (Roelands et al., 2008; Schiphof-Godart et al., 2018). It's clear that finding ways to increase dopamine production can be an effective strategy to reduce perceived effort and thereby increase endurance performance. For instance, mental fatigue can be minimised purely by rinsing the mouth with a carbohydrate and/or caffeine drink, even in the absence of swallowing (van Cutsem et al., 2017). Other studies show a cup of coffee or monetary rewards can also reduce mental fatigue (Barte et al., 2017; Hulleman et al., 2007; Skorski & Abbiss, 2017; van Cutsem et al., 2017). One dopamine delivery vehicle, which we will discuss later, is humour. This leads to a decrease in perception of effort.

Self-Talk: Managing Inner Dialogue

As pain and/or discomfort increase, the frequency and urgency of our inner dialogue often increases proportionally with it. How we manage this inner dialogue has direct implications on how we perform during prolonged, difficult activity. Attentional focus plays a part in this calculus. If we are experiencing internal pain or discomfort in our body, like a tender ankle or blistered foot, focusing on external stimuli has been shown to be effective in shifting our attention away from our discomfort. If you are experiencing physical pain, savouring a beautiful sunrise or experiencing awe can offset the pain. Conversely, if the weather unexpectedly turns bad (an external factor), focusing inward can ease our emotional distress. Instead of focusing our attention on the poor weather conditions, we should focus on how our body and breathing feels. Or perhaps listening to music, repeating a mantra, or counting steps. All of which can distract our mind from the negative external variable.

Attentional focus, along with self-talk can be effective to reduce perception of effort. There are three types of self-talk that can facilitate learning and enhance performance: self-regulated positive self-talk, assisted positive self-talk, and assisted negative self-talk (Hamilton et al., 2007; Hatzigeorgiadis et al., 2011, 2018). Of the three, assisted positive self-talk (positive encouragement with reinforcement) showed the biggest gains. However, all three can increase performance (Hamilton et al., 2007). Which strategy to employ will depend on each individual. The author responds best to positive self-talk, but some athletes respond favourably to negative self-talk.

Self-talk has been shown to significantly reduce rating of perceived effort (RPE) and enhance endurance performance. These findings suggest that psychobiological interventions designed to positively influence perception of effort are beneficial to endurance performance (Blanchfield et al., 2014).

Self-control/Self-regulation: Resisting Negative Thoughts

Roy Baumeister identifies four components of self-regulation: standards, monitoring, strength and motivation. Standards are needed to establish a baseline, or target, for behaviour. Oftentimes these are core values and a personal ethos defined by the adventurer in reflection. Monitoring is a necessary component of the feedback loop. Monitoring and adjusting behaviour, as needed, is required to self-regulate. Self-regulatory strength, often colloquially referred to as willpower, is vital. Behaviour change is difficult, and mental strength is required to facilitate this change. This has been shown to be an exhaustible, replenishable resource. Lastly, we have motivation. A desire and commitment to regulate ourselves is foundational. Without motivation, self-regulation would not exist (Baumeister & Vohs, 2007).

Often self-control and self-regulation are used interchangeably but have subtle differences. Dr. Stuart Shanker states, "Self-control is about inhibiting impulses; self-regulation is about identifying the causes and reducing the intensity of impulses and, when necessary, having the energy to resist" (Shanker & Barker, 2017).

For the adventurer, the ability to resist negative thoughts about discomfort and pain and a compelling urge to quit the pursuit is critical to making forward progress toward the goal. This is particularly true for activities that require prolonged physiological, as well as psychological efforts at moderate to high intensity levels. Overriding the urge to quit when things get hard can be the difference between achieving the goal, or not. This "keep moving forward, whatever it takes" mindset is largely driven by the notion of self-control or self-regulation (Taylor et al., 2020).

It is helpful to think of self-control as a muscle which can be exercised to exertion or fatigue. When self-control is fatigued, performance will decline and eventually fail. Once rested, it will be restored. Mental exhaustion is one factor that can affect self-control. Continuing the metaphor, our self-control muscle can also be strengthened with repeated use. The adventurer can train this muscle to be strong when called upon to perform in an endurance environment (Baumeister, 2016). There is ample research to suggest that self-control is an exhaustible resource. *Ego depletion*, the state following exertion of self-control, and a loss of motivation are sure to follow. This concept forms the basis for the strength model of self-control (Baumeister & Vohs, 2007). Going beyond adventure, those with good self-regulation have been shown to have more satisfying relationships, achieve more in academia and their careers, have higher subjective wellbeing and suffer fewer mental and physical health maladies (de Ridder et al., 2012).

A useful tool to strengthen our self-control and assist performance despite depletion, is forming *implementation intentions*. An implementation intention is a pre-described plan to mitigate unfavourable situations when they occur. These plans to direct our behaviour have been shown to be effective for goal pursuit when things get hard. An implementation intention will take the form of "if X, then I will do Y." For example, "If I do not reach the summit by 2:00pm, then I will terminate my ascent and descend back to the safety of camp."

Another strategy to strengthen our muscle is by incorporating helpful habits. These automatic behaviours can carry the day when willpower is low. Thus, trait self-control can produce desirable outcomes by way of habit formation. Trait self-control can be thought of as an ability to resist temptation or have good impulse control. It has also been shown to help us tolerate pain for longer periods of time (Schmeichel & Zell, 2007). These habits create a sort of autopilot when our reserves are low or depleted. When motivation deserts us, as it often will, we can fall back on habits and systems that are cognitively less demanding (Neal et al., 2013).

Somewhat surprisingly, the benefits of good self-control appear to be linear with no upper bound. There is no evidence to suggest that there is a downside to more self-control. Contrary to many things in life, with self-control, more actually appears to be better (Baumeister, 2016).

There is also evidence that a positive mood, or good attitude, continues to yield dividends. *Going knowingly into the unknown* requires a positive attitude towards future uncertainty. Positive mood has been shown to have a positive impact on self-control and, more specifically, an individual's self-control recovery. When we become depleted, having a positive attitude will help us get back on track quicker (Tice et al., 2007).

Again, there is interplay between mental fatigue and self-regulation. The perception of mental fatigue may impact agency, allocation, and/or efficacy of our resources to self-regulate and continue moving toward our goal (Clarkson et al., 2016). Many top sport psychologists have started to assess athletes' stress levels outside of sport before a competition. If an athlete has high stress levels and mental fatigue from personal relationships, it can affect their athletic performance. Before starting an adventure, it would be useful to be aware of external (to the expedition) stressors before and during the adventure. I like to use a *backpack metaphor*. What stress are you carrying in your imaginary backpack? What can you offload so you can travel light? Discarding unnecessary stress is vital to perform at your best. Having an allocated person to take care of stressors while you are in the field will help keep your mental resources strong and on point and not worried about paying the utility bill.

Humour and Laughter: Bolstering our Mood

Humour and laughter have been shown to be effective coping mechanisms in extreme environments like high altitude mountaineering, firefighting and space travel (Brcic et al., 2018; Harrison et al., 2021; Sliter et al., 2014). Humour contributes to psychological resilience (Harrison et al., 2021) and creates dopamine to counteract high stress levels by cognitively reframing stressors as less severe, thereby minimising their impact. Humour bolsters one's mood by changing the way we appraise our situation. It is thought impossible to be angry or sad when laughing. It will also lessen, or even briefly eliminate sensations of pain. Even chronic pain sufferers have been shown to forget about their pain while laughing.

All these benefits can happen even though the external, objective situation itself has not changed. Countless survival stories portray survivors who have used humour to maintain their mental faculties when facing massive levels of uncertainty, suffering, pain and a constant fear of death. Ancient Spartan soldiers knew the power of humour and were known to use it expeditiously. They were famous for their *laconic humour* to lighten the mood as they were marching into battle. This distinctive tactic is described as speaking in a blunt and succinct manner with a dry, witty sense of humour. It gets its name from a region in Greece called Laconia, which included the city of Sparta.

> The Humour Coping Scale (HCS) was devised to assess five categories of humour: Affiliative (designed to enhance interpersonal cohesiveness and liking), Enhancing (expression of a humorous outlook on life), Aggressive (tendency to express critical or sarcastic humor that may have negative impact on others), Self-defeating (excessive use of self-disparaging humor), and Problem-oriented (humor used to cope with specific stressful events).
> *(Brcic et al., 2018)*

Each category can be effective in the right context. Perhaps the greatest adventure for humankind is space travel. Astronauts often use positive humour to make light of stressful situations, build team camaraderie and increase motivation (Brcic et al., 2018). Adventure racers also routinely used humour to appraise their situation as a challenge (rather than a threat) (Harrison et al., 2021). When things suck, sometimes all you can do is laugh. It may not fix the situation, but it will make us feel better. Indeed, in the adventure world, "type two fun" is described as not fun at the time, but enjoyed after the event.

Mental Toughness: Forging Mettle

One of the most important aspects of endurance performance is steeling the mind for the adversity that is sure to visit during adventures. There are many descriptors, with some commonality, of this steely resolve: mettle, fortitude, perseverance, hardiness, grit, resilience, sisu (see Chapter 9), mental toughness and others. We will focus our attention on mental toughness and psychological resilience.

Mental toughness began as a construct in the world of sport but has begun to gain a foothold in many areas of life including business and academia. It has many definitions that are similar, and again, no consensus. Some are sport specific, but most are more inclusive of all areas of life.

"Mental toughness is a collection of values, attitudes, behaviours and emotions that enable you to persevere and overcome any obstacle, adversity, or pressure experienced, but also to maintain concentration and motivation when things are going well to consistently achieve your goals" (Gucciardi, 2017). Someone with a high level of mental toughness has "a high sense of self-belief and an unshakeable faith that they control their own destiny, these individuals can remain relatively unaffected by competition or adversity" (Clough et al., 2002).

I once interviewed a U.S. special forces soldier who shared the mindset of their teams. They possessed an "irrational" belief they could win in any situation. This is a trait mentally tough individuals often share. They have a strong self-belief they can be successful that may appear irrational to outside observers. This strength of self-belief can be incredibly powerful to get the job done and return safely. However, too much mental toughness, and self-belief, can be detrimental. Knowing when to be humble, and keep your ego in check, is also important for good, sound decision-making. There has to be a counterbalance. Countless souls have lost their lives because they pressed on, driven by incredibly high levels of mental toughness and self-belief that was perhaps irrational, delusional or even, narcissistic. Cultivating self-awareness, a strong sense of situational awareness and emotional intelligence can help adventurers understand when it's not their day, and retiring is the best option.

From these descriptions, one can imagine mental toughness as a capacity that would benefit many areas of our lives beyond adventure. Our business, personal lives, academia, and athletic endeavours could be enhanced. Each day, we may encounter challenges and adversity that require mental toughness to navigate successfully.

Although some believe mental toughness is generally set, there is evidence that it is a plastic personality trait that can be developed, including within-person variability (Cooper et al., 2020). Mental toughness can ebb and flow and has been shown to be a dynamic variable that changes with time. Again, much like a muscle, we must exercise our mental toughness to keep it strong and capable. We can use it, or lose it.

Psychological Resilience: Positive Adaptation in the Face of Adversity

Closely related to mental toughness is psychological resilience. The traits common for resilience include a sense of control or internal locus of control, strong problem-solving skills, strong social connections, a survivor mentality, emotion regulation and self-compassion or grace.

The ability to positively adapt in the face of adversity is vital to successful adventuring. Although, like mental toughness, there is not a widely accepted definition of resilience, most definitions have a common theme of "positive adaptation in the face of adversity." One of the more widely cited definitions of psychological resilience is a "dynamic process encompassing positive adaptation within the context of significant adversity" (Luthar et al., 2000). How quickly we can bounce back or adapt when plans are disrupted can mean the difference between life and death.

If we examine the roots of the word, there is an evident theme. The word resilience originates from the Latin verb *resilire*, or "to leap back," and is defined in the Oxford Dictionary of English as being "able to withstand or recover quickly from difficult conditions" (Fletcher & Sarkar, 2013). For an in-depth look at this concept, see: Bryan et al., 2019; Fletcher & Sarkar, 2013.

Competition vs. Cooperation: Working Together

In sport, there is evidence to suggest that competition can be helpful and increase performance levels. Does this hold true for adventure scenarios? Most adventures, unless part of an organised race, are not competitive in nature. In the world of ultrarunning that I frequent, outside of the elite athletes scrambling for the podium there is very little outward competition to be found. In fact, even among the top racers a sense of community support and cooperation is prevalent. Is cooperation and collaborative effort more beneficial than competition for endurance performance? Is competition the best model? This is a debate that borders on a form of blasphemy in many cultures, as competition starts to resemble a religion.

This is a complex issue that is difficult to sort from existing research. Namely, in most western democratic societies, capitalism and an element of competition are foundational to existing culture and sociological structure. We are taught to compare, rank and compete with others from an early age. Because we are indoctrinated into being competitive from our youth, it is difficult to separate nature from nurture. However, there is evidence to suggest that our biological nature, passed down from our ancestors, is actually one of cooperation rather than competition.

I would offer this as a thought experiment. If we allow our minds to go back in time to our ancestors on the plains of the Serengeti - would cooperation or competition ensure survival of the tribe? If your answer is competition, how would that scenario ultimately end? In the extreme, one person would eventually be the "victor" and likely all others would be deceased. In time, this victor would also cease to exist and propagate the species. This, by my way of thinking, is not a good system of survival! Cooperation – or prosocial collaboration - was key to our ancestors enduring survival in a hostile environment. (For more on this see: Evolutionary Psychology, Prosocial Principles and the work of Paul Atkins and his chickens - Atkins et al., 2019). The endurance of the human *race* – ultimately the longest endurance race of all – is perhaps more reliant on cooperation rather than competition.

Does competition imply someone has to "lose" or otherwise be defeated? Most modern definitions would say yes. Sport is usually a zero-sum game. Is that a problem? Alfie Kohn defined the essence of competition as "mutually exclusive goal attainment (MEGA)" adding that "one person succeeds only if another does not" (Kohn, 1992). Perhaps the word "competition" has a bad reputation?

With its roots in middle French *compéter* meaning "be in rivalry with" and the early 17th century Latin word *competere* from *com* meaning "together" and *petere* meaning "to strive for or seek," we can see origins of striving for excellence and working together. This sounds positive and healthy. Indeed, competition can be viewed through a different lens. "Competition can also be conceived primarily as the human struggle in a challenging ecological environment, which in turn serves as a major catalyst for extensive human cooperation" (Blanchard, 1995). In this view, we can start to envision a catalyst for growth and excellence that does not necessitate conquering an opponent.

Perhaps competition could more accurately be viewed as a mastery mindset. Mastery is defined as "comprehensive knowledge or skill in a subject or accomplishment" (Oxford English Dictionary, 2022). A mastery mindset refers to having a goal of mastering certain subjects, skills, or materials, and a belief that this can be done. This is an inner journey. Much like going on an adventure. "Understanding competing as pursuing an objective through trying to surpass others does not presume the importance of the end result (winning or losing) over the condition of pursuing. People can be equally competitive while their modes of competitiveness differ" (Kajanus, 2018). Perhaps then, the emphasis in adventuring is on mastery. The mastery of self rather than mastery of the other. It would be interesting to research the endurance effect of competition versus collaborative performances.

Further Research

As endurance performance in an adventure context is a new area of research, there is ample opportunity to advance our understanding of endurance performance across the board. In fact, there is very little research that focuses primarily on endurance in the adventure environment. We are left to use other contexts, like endurance sport, to apply to adventure. One area that is developing interest for example, is in gender differences in endurance performance. There has been some evidence that has indicated that women close the performance gap on men as distances and durations get longer. Where do women excel? Are they as mentally tough as men, or more so? Do they have advantages over men in long distances and durations? If so, how?

Conclusion

We have only scratched the surface of endurance. I have outlined areas that might be beneficial, but there is far more to explore in the quest for sustainable, healthy performance. Among those we have covered: perception of effort, motivation, managing self-talk, reappraising our narratives, practicing reflection and metacognition to learn and grow, using humour and laughter to ease discomfort, building mental toughness and psychological resilience, and considering different ways to look at competition vs. cooperation. Clearly psychology has a significant contribution to how we sustain optimum performance, not just VO2 max, muscles and Mars bars, and not just on adventures.

Bibliography

American Psychological Association (APA). (2022). *Dictionary of psychology.* https://dictionary.apa.org/endurance-activity

Atkins, P. W. B., Wilson, D. S., & Hayes, S. C. (2019). *Prosocial: Using evolutionary science to build productive, equitable, and collaborative groups.* Context Press/New Harbinger Publications.

Barte, J. C. M., Nieuwenhuys, A., Geurts, S. A. E., & Kompier, M. A. J. (2017). Fatigue experiences in competitive soccer: Development during matches and the impact of general performance capacity. *Fatigue: Biomedicine, Health & Behavior, 5*(4), 191–201. https://doi.org/10.1080/21641846.2017.1377811

Baumeister, R. F. (2016). Limited resources for self-regulation: A current overview of the strength model. In *Self-regulation and ego control* (pp. 1–17). Elsevier. https://doi.org/10.1016/B978-0-12-801850-7.00001-9

Baumeister, R. F., & Vohs, K. D. (2007). Self-regulation, ego depletion, and motivation. *Social and Personality Psychology Compass, 1*(1), 115–128. https://doi.org/10.1111/j.1751-9004.2007.00001.x

Blanchard, K. (1995). *The anthropology of sport: An introduction* (Rev.). Bergin & Garvey.

Blanchfield, A. W., Hardy, J., De Morree, H. M., Staiano, W., & Marcora, S. M. (2014). Talking yourself out of exhaustion. *Medicine & Science in Sports & Exercise, 46*(5), 998–1007. https://doi.org/10.1249/MSS.0000000000000184

Brace, A. W., George, K., & Lovell, G. P. (2020). Mental toughness and self-efficacy of elite ultra-marathon runners. *PLOS ONE, 15*(11), e0241284. https://doi.org/10.1371/journal.pone.0241284

Brcic, J., Suedfeld, P., Johnson, P., Huynh, T., & Gushin, V. (2018). Humor as a coping strategy in spaceflight. *Acta Astronautica, 152,* 175–178. https://doi.org/10.1016/j.actaastro.2018.07.039

Brick, N., MacIntyre, T., & Campbell, M. (2015). Metacognitive processes in the self-regulation of performance in elite endurance runners. *Psychology of Sport and Exercise, 19,* 1–9. https://doi.org/10.1016/j.psychsport.2015.02.003

Bryan, C., O'Shea, D., & MacIntyre, T. (2019). Stressing the relevance of resilience: A systematic review of resilience across the domains of sport and work. In *International review of sport and exercise psychology* (Vol. 12, Issue 1, pp. 70–111). Routledge. https://doi.org/10.1080/1750984X.2017.1381140

Bueno, J., Weinberg, R. S., Fernández-Castro, J., & Capdevila, L. (2008). Emotional and motivational mechanisms mediating the influence of goal setting on endurance athletes' performance. *Psychology of Sport and Exercise, 9*(6), 786–799. https://doi.org/10.1016/j.psychsport.2007.11.003

Clarkson, J. J., Otto, A. S., Hassey, R., & Hirt, E. R. (2016). Perceived mental fatigue and self-control. In *Self-regulation and ego control* (pp. 185–202). Elsevier. https://doi.org/10.1016/B978-0-12-801850-7.00010-X

Clough, P. J., Earle, K., & Sewell, D. (2002). Mental toughness: The concept and its measurement. *Solutions in Sport Psychology,* 7(12), 32–43.

Collins, L., Carson, H. J., Amos, P., & Collins, D. (2018). Examining the perceived value of professional judgement and decision-making in mountain leaders in the UK: A mixed-methods investigation. *Journal of Adventure Education and Outdoor Learning, 18*(2), 132–147. https://doi.org/10.1080/14729679.2017.1378584

Collins, L., Carson, H. J., & Collins, D. (2016). Metacognition and professional judgment and decision making in coaching: Importance, application and evaluation. *International Sport Coaching Journal*, *3*(3), 355–361. https://doi.org/10.1123/iscj.2016-0037

Collins, L., & Collins, D. (2013). Decision making and risk management in adventure sports coaching. *Quest*, *65*(1), 72–82. https://doi.org/10.1080/00336297.2012.727373

Cooper, K. B., Wilson, M. R., & Jones, M. I. (2020). A 3000-mile tour of mental toughness: An autoethnographic exploration of mental toughness intra-individual variability in endurance sport. *International Journal of Sport and Exercise Psychology*, *18*(5), 607–621. https://doi.org/10.1080/1612197X.2018.1549583

de Ridder, D. T. D., Lensvelt-Mulders, G., Finkenauer, C., Stok, F. M., & Baumeister, R. F. (2012). Taking stock of self-control: A meta-analysis of how trait self-control relates to a wide range of behaviors. *Personality and Social Psychology Review*, *16*(1), 76–99. https://doi.org/10.1177/1088868311418749

Desharnais, R., Bouillon, J., & Godin, G. (1986). Self-Efficacy and outcome expectations as determinants of exercise adherence. *Psychological Reports*, *59*(3), 1155–1159. https://doi.org/10.2466/pr0.1986.59.3.1155

Fletcher, D., & Sarkar, M. (2013). Psychological resilience: A review and critique of definitions, concepts, and theory. *European Psychologist*, *18*(1), 12–23. https://doi.org/10.1027/1016-9040/a000124

Gucciardi, D. F. (2017). Mental toughness: Progress and prospects. *Current Opinion in Psychology*, *16*, 17–23. https://doi.org/10.1016/j.copsyc.2017.03.010

Hamilton, R. A., Scott, D., & MacDougall, M. P. (2007). Assessing the effectiveness of self-talk interventions on endurance performance. *Journal of Applied Sport Psychology*, *19*(2), 226–239. https://doi.org/10.1080/10413200701230613

Harrison, D., Sarkar, M., Saward, C., & Sunderland, C. (2021). Exploration of psychological resilience during a 25-day endurance challenge in an extreme environment. *International Journal of Environmental Research and Public Health*, *18*(23), 12707. https://doi.org/10.3390/ijerph182312707

Hatzigeorgiadis, A., Bartura, K., Argiropoulos, C., Comoutos, N., Galanis, E., & D. Flouris, A. (2018). Beat the heat: Effects of a motivational self-talk intervention on endurance performance. *Journal of Applied Sport Psychology*, *30*(4), 388–401. https://doi.org/10.1080/10413200.2017.1395930

Hatzigeorgiadis, A., Zourbanos, N., Galanis, E., & Theodorakis, Y. (2011). Self-talk and sports performance. *Perspectives on Psychological Science*, *6*(4), 348–356. https://doi.org/10.1177/1745691611413136

Howle, T. C., Dimmock, J. A., & Jackson, B. (2016). Relations between self-efficacy beliefs, self-presentation motives, personal task goals, and performance on endurance-based physical activity tasks. *Psychology of Sport and Exercise*, *22*, 149–159. https://doi.org/10.1016/j.psychsport.2015.06.010

Hulleman, M., De Koning, J. J., Hettinga, F. J., & Foster, C. (2007). The effect of extrinsic motivation on cycle time trial performance. *Medicine & Science in Sports & Exercise*, *39*(4), 709–715. https://doi.org/10.1249/mss.0b013e31802eff36

Inzlicht, M., & Marcora, S. M. (2016). The central governor model of exercise regulation teaches us precious little about the nature of mental fatigue and self-control failure. *Frontiers in Psychology*, *7*(May). Frontiers Research Foundation. https://doi.org/10.3389/fpsyg.2016.00656

Kajanus, A. (2018). Mutualistic vs. zero-sum modes of competition – a comparative study of children's competitive motivations and behaviours in China. *Social Anthropology*. https://doi.org/10.1111/1469-8676.12578

Kohn, A. (1992). *No contest: The case against competition*. Houghton Mifflin Harcourt.

Leach, J., & Ansell, L. (2008). Impairment in attentional processing in a field survival environment. *Applied Cognitive Psychology, 22*(5), 643–652. https://doi.org/10.1002/acp.1385

Luthar, S. S., Cicchetti, D., & Becker, B. (2000). The construct of resilience: A critical evaluation and guidelines for future work. *Child Development, 71*(3), 543–562. https://doi.org/10.1111/1467-8624.00164

Maier, H. N., & Taber, K. (2007). Measurement of initiative in high-speed tactical decision making. In Robert R. Hoffman (Ed.), *Expertise Out of Context* (pp. 199–218). Taylor & Francis Group, LLC.

Marcora, S. M., Bosio, A., & de Morree, H. M. (2008). Locomotor muscle fatigue increases cardiorespiratory responses and reduces performance during intense cycling exercise independently from metabolic stress. *American Journal of Physiology-Regulatory Integrative and Comparative Physiology, 294*, 874–883. https://doi.org/10.1152/ajpregu.00678.2007.-Locomotor

Marcora, S. M., & Staiano, W. (2010). The limit to exercise tolerance in humans: Mind over muscle? *European Journal of Applied Physiology, 109*(4), 763–770. https://doi.org/10.1007/s00421-010-1418-6

Martin, J. J., & Gill, D. L. (1991). The relationships among competitive orientation, sport-confidence, self-efficacy, anxiety, and performance. *Journal of Sport and Exercise Psychology, 13*(2), 149–159. https://doi.org/10.1123/jsep.13.2.149

McCormick, A., Meijen, C., & Marcora, S. (2015). Psychological determinants of whole-body endurance performance. *Sports Medicine, 45*(7), 997–1015. https://doi.org/10.1007/s40279-015-0319-6

Mees, A., Toering, T., & Collins, L. (2021). Exploring the development of judgement and decision making in 'competent' outdoor instructors. *Journal of Adventure Education and Outdoor Learning.* https://doi.org/10.1080/14729679.2021.1884105

Molden, D. C., Hui, C. M., & Scholer, A. A. (2016). Understanding self-regulation failure: A motivated effort-allocation account. *Self-regulation and ego control* (pp. 425–459). Elsevier. https://doi.org/10.1016/B978-0-12-801850-7.00020-2

Neal, D. T., Wood, W., & Drolet, A. (2013). How do people adhere to goals when willpower is low? The profits (and pitfalls) of strong habits. *Journal of Personality and Social Psychology, 104*(6), 959–975. https://doi.org/10.1037/a0032626

Oxford English Dictionary. (2022). https://www.oxfordlearnersdictionaries.com/definition/english/endurance

Pageaux, B. (2014). The psychobiological model of endurance performance: An effort-based decision-making theory to explain self-paced endurance performance. *Sports Medicine, 44*(9), 1319–1320. https://doi.org/10.1007/s40279-014-0198-2

Pageaux, B., & Lepers, R. (2016). Fatigue induced by physical and mental exertion increases perception of effort and impairs subsequent endurance performance. *Frontiers in Physiology, 7.* https://doi.org/10.3389/fphys.2016.00587

Rice, V., & Liu, B. (2016). Personal resilience and coping Part II: Identifying resilience and coping among U.S. military service members and veterans with implications for work. *Work, 54*(2), 335–350. https://doi.org/10.3233/WOR-162301

Roelands, B., Hasegawa, H., Watson, P., Piacentini, M. F., Buyse, L., de Schutter, G., & Meeusen, R. R. (2008). The effects of acute dopamine reuptake inhibition on performance. *Medicine and Science in Sports and Exercise, 40*(5), 879–885. https://doi.org/10.1249/MSS.0b013e3181659c4d

Röthlin, P., Wyler, M., Müller, B., Zenger, N., Kellenberger, K., Wehrlin, J. P., Birrer, D., Lorenzetti, S., & Trösch, S. (2022). Body and mind? Exploring physiological and psychological factors to explain endurance performance in cycling. *European Journal of Sport Science*, 1–8. https://doi.org/10.1080/17461391.2021.2018049

Schiphof-Godart, L., Roelands, B., & Hettinga, F. J. (2018). Drive in sports: How mental fatigue affects endurance performance. *Frontiers in Psychology*, *9*. https://doi.org/10.3389/fpsyg.2018.01383

Schmeichel, B. J., & Zell, A. (2007). Trait self-control predicts performance on behavioral tests of self-control. *Journal of Personality*, *75*(4), 743–756. https://doi.org/10.1111/j.1467-6494.2007.00455.x

Shanker, S., & Barker, T. (2017). *Self-reg: How to help your child (and you) break the stress cycle and successfully engage with life.* Penguin books.

Shigihara, Y., Tanaka, M., Ishii, A., Tajima, S., Kanai, E., Funakura, M., & Watanabe, Y. (2013). Two different types of mental fatigue produce different styles of task performance. *Neurology, Psychiatry and Brain Research*, *19*(1), 5–11. https://doi.org/10.1016/j.npbr.2012.07.002

Skorski, S., & Abbiss, C. R. (2017). The manipulation of pace within endurance sport. *Frontiers in Physiology*, *8*. https://doi.org/10.3389/fphys.2017.00102

Sliter, M., Kale, A., & Yuan, Z. (2014). Is humor the best medicine? The buffering effect of coping humor on traumatic stressors in firefighters. *Journal of Organizational Behavior*, *35*(2), 257–272. https://doi.org/10.1002/job.1868

Taylor, I. M., Boat, R., & Murphy, S. L. (2020). Integrating theories of self-control and motivation to advance endurance performance. *International Review of Sport and Exercise Psychology*, *13*(1), 1–20. https://doi.org/10.1080/1750984X.2018.1480050

Tice, D. M., Baumeister, R. F., Shmueli, D., & Muraven, M. (2007). Restoring the self: Positive affect helps improve self-regulation following ego depletion. *Journal of Experimental Social Psychology*, *43*(3), 379–384. https://doi.org/10.1016/j.jesp.2006.05.007

van Cutsem, J., Marcora, S., de Pauw, K., Bailey, S., Meeusen, R., & Roelands, B. (2017). The effects of mental fatigue on physical performance: A systematic review. *Sports Medicine*, *47*(8), 1569–1588. https://doi.org/10.1007/s40279-016-0672-0

Waldvogel, K. J., Nikolaidis, P. T., di Gangi, S., Rosemann, T., & Knechtle, B. (2019). Women reduce the performance difference to men with increasing age in ultramarathon running. *International Journal of Environmental Research and Public Health*, *16*(13), 2377. https://doi.org/10.3390/Ijerph16132377

4
DEALING WITH THE UNKNOWN

Jennifer Pickett and Paula Reid

From an Adventurer's Point of View – Finding my Way

I've been a dog musher for 15 years. That was our only transportation here in McCarthy, Alaska.

Sometimes we'd take all eight together or split them into two teams of four ... Essentially, the more dogs you have the more power you have, and the more power you have the further you can go with them. It was an adventurous feeling and I look back now, and I think how ...? I had a lot of energy – I had so much energy!

I went round the whole Seward peninsula, up through the middle, and just started going further and further ... So essentially, I've done the whole North American continent above the Artic Circle. 5800 miles or something. With a dog team.

You know what the whole thing probably is if you summed it up? Adventure. That's it. I wanted adventure. Literally all my growing up, growing up outside ... always outside doing things. Hunting. Fishing. Playing.

The city is not where my real being wants to be all the time. I like being outside. And being outside for me was living in a place like this. Here in McCarthy. Or in Alaska in general. And I like the adventure.

Anything is an adventure. For me it literally was to the point where ... there was adrenaline. If it's not causing me to have a feeling of... like being a little bit afraid, then it wasn't an adventure, it was a little more tame. But I like that feeling of being lost ... it's so overwhelming, it's almost like a paranormal feeling sometimes, where you get like this feeling, scared, where your hair's standing up ... S★★t I'm lost! And you're going like, where am I lost? You know? Like most of the dog-mushing adventures I had were pre GPS, so they were all by maps if we had them. There was no cell, no

DOI: 10.4324/9781003173601-7

phones, nothing to look at to see where you were. So, every day there was definitely a feeling of, if you're in a whiteout, you can't locate your position. You can't keep saying we'll go this way … and it's a spooky feeling. To be up in the Artic, where everything's flat, and you don't know which way you're going. I mean, you are literally going by compass, that's all. And then you try to get to a place at night and go, "Oh, look there, so that's the highest point … That must be what that is. So, we must be up here." But the adventure levels are such that … there were definitely moments of boredom interspersed with sheer terror. Going across sea ice. Learning … You know, when you look at it, most of adventure is about learning something. These big rivers out here, the Chena, the Nizina, I mean, you got stories of people falling in. Never to be seen again. So, you kinda have to learn at a level that you're not going to kill yourself. And so it takes years. And experience. You don't just blindly …

So essentially, it wasn't, just a haphazard like, oh, I'm just going to go to the Arctic. It was incrementally more and more. And it's like a bad drug. You want more and more.

After a while, when you've mastered your back yard, you might go down the street, and when you've done that, you're like, what's the next town over, after that town, it's the same thing, and then you start reading ice. And it takes so long to do that. Years and years. It wasn't like, I just jumped out on the big rivers right away. But crossing by myself and having the confidence to do that. And find my way. And be able to say, right, I can do this.

Finding my way
Malcolm Vance

Dealing with the Unknown

I started wearing ear plugs just so I didn't hear the roar of these rivers coming up. Just to help keep me calm. Because some of these roars you can hear them forever. And you know it's going to be bad [laughing].

Steve Jordan, White Water Kayaker, McCarthy, Alaska

What makes someone choose to go (knowingly) into the unknown? Knowing that they are likely to be in harm's way, encounter hardship, and potentially fear for life and limb? In this chapter, we explore the motivations, personalities, survival responses, cognitions, and coping skills of those who manage the uncertainty of an adventure willingly and repeatedly. We aim to understand the mindset and skills of the explorers who manage to navigate the unknowns that an adventure presents – the sometimes unpredictable, potentially ambiguous, and often volatile and variable – hazards, risks and obstacles; or even how they navigate the uncertainty of the future. The "advent" (forthcoming) of the "venture" (challenging undertaking). The path yet trodden. The life yet lived.

We delve into the stressors and cognitive loads that are put upon adventurers as they journey in *terra incognita;* reflecting upon the contextual demands which test their ability to make "correct" interpretations and decisions which may be life-enhancing or life-saving.

★ ★ ★ ★

Early explorers quite literally travelled without a map as they sailed, climbed or trekked into "uncharted" territory. In the modern world, adventurers are still travelling into *terra incognita*, dealing with the unknowns of both their inner and outer worlds. They may face immediate, medium- or long-term uncertainty as they encounter ever-changing environments and situations. How do they navigate, make decisions, and cope?

Uncertainty is not a naturally comfortable status for us human beings. We seek and appreciate certainty and we are somewhat intolerant of ambiguity, variability and poor discernibility. We like to know. We like to articulate. Evolution and adaptation requires us to understand our perceptions ("what is that?") and know our actions ("what do we do about it?"). In the Entropy Model of Uncertainty (EMU), Hirsh et al., suggests that "uncertainty is a critical adaptive challenge for organisms, and thus, managing uncertainty is important" (2012). According to Schrödinger, life is "negentropic" in our continuous effort to create order out of chaos, and therefore we are constantly sense-making and meaning-making from the multitude of sensations hitting our brains and nervous system. We have a pre-existing model of the world (going knowingly) with which our current perceptions and sensations (into the unknown) aim to correlate inputs. Hence dealing with – and interpreting – uncertain or ambiguous (chaotic or incoherent) environments and events is effortful and not everyone's choice of experience. Similarly, the "Bayesian brain" theory suggests that our brain serves as a kind of probability machine required to make decisions stemming from the uncertainties of the outside world. We are "wired" to want to know.

Hirsh et al., also suggest that uncertainty can be experienced as anxiety since our perceptions and actions are two evolutionary critical tasks, and uncertainty produces conflict between perceptual and behavioural utility. It takes effort and is slow going for us to fathom answers, or routes, or good decisions, amidst uncertainty and disruption. And yet, adventurers choose to leap – a leap of faith maybe – into the void. For those who claim they are not the adventurous type, it can be difficult to imagine what drives adventurous people – people like Steve Jordan, the kayaker, for instance …

In early April 1974, on a warm, sunny spring day in Fairbanks before the breakup of ice, Steve spent more time portaging his canoe across the ice then he did paddling down the Chena River:

> I was fresh to Alaska and didn't know that just because you put in in clear water, that doesn't mean the water will stay clear. I soon had to try to avoid the water that was running under the ice. Of course, I swamped my canoe. That was my first introduction to the Chena.

Then Steve bought a sixteen-foot raft to check out the haystacks, holes, and thrills of the Nenana River near Denali – a much steeper and faster river with class III and IV rapids. From there, he got into white water kayaking, making many first descents throughout Alaska because: "Finding places to play in the river, behind boulders, getting thrashed around and tossed about is fun! The power of the water made it fun. But that's also one of the things that made it challenging." We could describe this as Steve experiencing psychological flow – where high challenge meets high skill. Or we could describe this is an experiential adventurous state which demands skill, versatility and mindfulness/presence from the adventurer as they tackle the unknown within a challenging context.

Adventurous people put themselves into unknown situations for a variety of reasons. Choices are often shaped by personality, experiences, and opportunities. Most, if not all, adventures contain some degree of risk. Yet, many adventurers will say that they go adventuring not because of the risk involved, but despite it. If this is the case, what is the draw? Is it indeed the unknown itself? And if so, what draws us to "go knowingly into the unknown" (Reid & Kampman, 2020) and more importantly, what psychological processes and skills are needed to navigate the unknown? Are there certain personality profiles that firstly, seek out and secondly, cope better with the hyper-dynamic environment that typically encompasses adventures? Or is it that being in nature produces such positive emotions and states that adventurers are peaking at optimal psychological performance, thus enabling effective decision making? Or that the dynamics of the context – change, challenge and uncertainty to name three – force adventurers to be more fully present/mindful and sharply focused on their adaptability or cognitive flexibility?

In this chapter, we explore these questions with theories by drawing from different areas of psychology such as wilderness therapy, performance psychology, crisis management, survival psychology, working in extreme environments, evolutionary psychology and the like. The main aim is to ascertain how and why some so successfully cope with the unknown, and to create a roadmap for others who may be less comfortable with uncertainty. Our hope is that this will help people deal more capably with the unknown, uncertainty and ambiguity when they occur in everyday or business life.

First, we need to take a step back and briefly dissect what an adventure is. Adventures are typically complex; multifaceted; can be fun and exciting; and can often pose serious challenges. Adventurers are usually self-reliant, agile, confident and possess a certain amount of self-efficacy or self-belief. Adventures take place in the out of doors, in nature or in the wilderness.

Nature Relatedness

Typically, adventures happen in the out of doors, often within a natural setting. As such, it would be remiss to not address that a connection with nature has been imprinted upon us for millions of years. "Biophilia" (Wilson, 1984) is humanity's desire to bond with nature and is culturally universal. Meaning, humans everywhere are attracted to trees, a vista with a view, water, wildlife, and the like. While connecting with nature, people are also reconnecting with themselves which in turn enhances physical health, self-concept, interpersonal relationships and an increase in happiness (Gass et al., 2012). These restorative effects collectively increase psychological functioning which then improves the capacity to cope with uncertainty or a dynamic environment. Not only has the therapeutic value of the natural world been espoused by philosophers, writers, and researchers, (including the influential 19th century Scottish-American wilderness enthusiast John Muir), it has also been documented for centuries and was the basis of wilderness therapy. Wilderness therapy is a mental health treatment strategy in the out of doors for adolescents with behavioural challenges though research shows it is advantageous for adults too.

The healing benefits of nature were documented in 1901 when the New York Asylum for the Insane had issues with overcrowding and placed tubercular psychiatric patients in tents to keep them from infecting other patients. Unexpected beneficial outcomes were discovered as many of the outside patients, previously bed-ridden, showed substantial improvement both physically and mentally (Caplan, 1974; Williams, 2000). Nature tends to affect us both emotionally and psychologically at deep and profound levels as an aspect of self-identity strives to reconnect with nature (Wilson, 1984). The restorative benefits of the natural world have the tendency to reduce negatively valenced emotions while simultaneously bolstering positively valenced emotions, thus combatting mental fatigue (Gass et al., 2012; Kaplan & Kaplan, 1989). Reducing mental fatigue increases, among other positive benefits, psychological wellbeing which increases decision making, coping mechanisms, and managing whatever comes one's way. As most adventures happen in the wilderness or in the very least, out of doors, ergo, they are, in and of themselves, beneficial. On the other hand, if the out of doors is a drastic difference from an individual's accustomed milieu, this could pose a serious challenge to wellbeing and even survival as one grapples with the novel environment and adaptations required, creating even more uncertainty.

Clear Thinking and Cognitive Flexibility

A dynamic or extreme environment can challenge the cognitive and or cognitive/emotional process of an individual. Long-duration adventures typically consist of periods of down time, which can be boring, punctuated with periods of intense or even frantic situations. The down times are when one tends to lose focus on the task at hand or stop paying attention to one's surroundings as thoughts drift elsewhere. Conversely, when intense situations arise, sojourners focus on the goal or task at hand be it concentrating on class VI rapids, negotiating a physical obstacle or weather system, or fixing a broken piece of equipment. Having the cognitive means to tame deep uncertainty includes having an effective approach to recognising new risks in addition to grasping the dynamics of an unfolding situation (Ansell & Boin, 2019).

Some principles that can be applied by adventurers pre-, during, or post-adventure (and challenges involving uncertainty) can be drawn from crisis planning and management. Here individuals or teams are faced with the "unknown unknowns" of crises, and crisis planning techniques provide a way to not only prepare for, but cope with, emerging risks and crises. Crisis management is a challenging task in a hyper-dynamic environment, rife with evolving developments and short decision times that may have huge and lasting impacts on the lives of millions. Research from this area of psychology recognises that contemporary crises are complex and multifaceted, and is dedicated to combatting identified pitfalls of crisis managers. What helps with effective cognitive flexibility, is early detection (recognising a crisis), sense making (grasping the nature of the crisis) and decision making (organising an appropriate response) (Boin & Bynander, 2015). It is crucial to at least partially possess the cognitive means to tame the deep uncertainty or ambiguity that comes with crises (and adventure) and to comprehend the (d)evolution of dynamic events, recognise risks and/or make sense of the situation (Ansell & Boin, 2019).

Managing dangerous events can be a long-term task. A forward-thinking approach is needed when handling the multiple effects of a crisis because poor decisions tend to exacerbate the situation and delay or negate recovery from the incident. Consequently, it is wise that adventurers test themselves in a variety of situations to gain the self-efficacy needed to get themselves out of a variety of potential pitfalls. This may involve skills acquired from past actual adventures and expeditions, or "classroom" techniques such as crisis management, scenario planning, anticipatory thinking and survival training for example, either in the field or pre-departure. Performing at optimal psychological functioning and mental capacity, cultivating situational awareness, and increasing existing skills, knowledge and resources when dealing with the unknown, are all essential for a successful trip and return.

Moreover, managing stressors and cognitive load is necessary for finding the maximum psychological functioning needed for demanding tasks. Stressors bring extra pressure to the systems: to neuro functioning; emotion regulation; and physical ability for instance. High stressors can dramatically impair functioning and decision making, making it even harder – and even more stressful – to mentally and physically cope with uncertainty. Stressor analysis and appraisal may be especially difficult within ambiguous contexts when clarity of information is a rarity.

Cognitive load is the processing of information needed for task performance. When there is a high volume or/and highly intense sensory inputs – as is likely while on an adventure – plus other data inputs requiring attention within the broad context of uncertainty, then cognitive load is likely elevated. The adventurer may struggle to think clearly or generate strategies or creative solutions. Essentially, decision making becomes hindered when the mental load is high. Other types of fatigue – such as physical or emotional, can also hinder or slow down decision making (Keller et al., 2019) and factors such as sleep, fluid or food deprivation will also negatively impact the ability to make sound decisions especially in uncertain contexts (Caldwell et al., 2009). All of which are of course likely scenarios on expeditions.

Repeated or complex sense making and decision making utilises cognitive resources leading to decision fatigue, which in turn effects the ability to balance information by depleting self-regulatory resources. However, self-regulation is akin to a muscle and can be trained. This can be exercised by, for example, the Professional Judgement Decision-Making Model (PJDM; Collins & Collins, 2020). The PJDM addresses the procedures or "the what, why and how" of making sense and decisions in stressful situations. Specifically, the PJDM can be employed to manage demanding task complexities and once established, the PJDM is transferable and can be employed in new settings or situations. Other methodologies are taught or applied in associated contexts such as survival, military or pilot training in which the cognitive load is reduced by introducing procedural habits or drills. Teaching coping mechanisms to manage stressors and pressure enhances an adventurer's detection, sense making and effective decision making in the unknown.

Another methodology useful for the pre-emptive handling of uncertainty is "Anticipatory Thinking" (AT). Whereas in Sport Psychology a performer may utilise visualisation techniques to picture a successful future, an adventurer may find it more beneficial to use AT techniques to rehearse a challenging or ambiguous future – to visualise a "bad day on the mountain" instead of a "perfect day on the mountain." Klein describes this as "not trying to guess the future, … [but] trying to adapt to possible futures" (Klein, 2017). This realistic or feasible psychological preparation is more pertinent to adventuring and survival or crisis management, than for instance, preparing to win in a team sport within fairly predictable conditions. By imagining or anticipating the "unexpected" we begin the process of responding more quickly and decisively to what may occur. We may go knowingly on our adventures by using hindsight, insight, and foresight, to scenario plan, crisis plan, anticipate or mentally rehearse, so that future unknowns are at least more psychologically known to us before we get into trouble. We can therefore adapt quicker, and survival is more likely.

Moreover, research by Bloom and colleagues (2014) found that recreational travel increases cognitive flexibility, creativity and increases positive emotions – all of which help manage uncertainty. Recreational travel can relieve individuals from stress, while also provide diverse experiences for them to respond to or adapt toward and thus equip them to go "more knowingly into the unknown" next time. All three elements – cognitive flexibility, creativity and positive emotions – are beneficial for not only surviving but thriving in dynamic environments. Positive emotions lead to more creativity, which in turn leads to more agile decisions in situ (Csikszentmihalyi, 1996). This is supported by Fredrickson's *broaden-and-build theory* (2004). According to Fredrickson, positive emotions such as joy, curiosity, hope and awe – all of which are often reported in the wilderness – help accrue essential resources, broadening awareness and repertoire. For instance, the thought-action tendency surrounding joy is play, which leads to skills gained from experiential learning. Hope brings resilience and optimism, while awe leads to new world views. Collectively, these emotions lead to a broadened mindset which engenders discovery, entrepreneurship, and the acquisition of new knowledge and skills.

Having a momentarily broadened mindset is not a key ingredient in the recipe for any quick survival manoeuvre. It is, however, in the recipe for discovery, discovery of new knowledge, new alliances, and new skills. In short, broadened awareness leads to the accrual of new resources that might later make the difference between survival and succumbing to various threats.

In other words, positive emotions broaden novel thoughts, relationships, and activities, which in turn builds personal resources (e.g., resilience, skills, social support), which in turn enhances fulfilment, health, and survival. Collectively, these positive emotions are key to unlocking the optimal psychological functioning needed to: maintain cognitive and emotional regulation; employ coping mechanisms; and engage high-stakes decision making in hyper dynamic (i.e., unknown) environments.

Dealing with the unknown on adventures requires mental dexterity. The more flexible an individual is, the quicker they may respond to their situational awareness, and potentially realise that a situation is shifting and requires the adventurer to adapt. Sometimes adaptation is key to survival. The sooner an adventurer understands the dynamics of a situation, the quicker an appropriate reaction can be formulated. This is also found in survival psychology when understanding the most effective psychological responses to disaster.

Survival Psychology

One description of disaster (see Leach, 1994, for a full review) details overlapping stages unfolding from pre-impact to post-trauma. These stages comprise: pre-impact (both the threat and the warning), impact, recoil, rescue, and finally post-trauma. This dynamic model is used as a framework to study human behaviour and psychology in hostile or hyper-dynamic conditions. The pre-impact phase is when the signs of danger are noticed and the individual is alerted that a calamitous situation or event is highly likely. This is subdivided into two phases: threat and warning. At the threat phase (encompassing the likelihood of a real danger to life or limb), the threat is acknowledged psychologically. At the warning phase the individual is alerted to the fact that danger is imminent and will strike. A common psychological reaction to this is denial which leads to inactivity. When an individual is faced with information that cannot be satisfactorily resolved or is conflicting with one's self-preservation – such as an alarm going off – cognitive dissonance occurs. Here an individual may reduce or remove information to a level which they are cognitively comfortable with so that information fits with one's self-preservation.

Moreover, in times of uncertainty, people tend to conform to the behaviour of the group. Individuals with training or experience are more psychologically prepared and a warning phase allows them time to gather their wits, assimilate and assess information, and take action (Leach, 1994).

The period of impact typically, but not always, is preceded by the pre-impact phase (unless a disaster strikes so suddenly, there is no time). The typical psychological reaction is that of a deer in headlights – incomprehension and confusion – or "freezing." No amount of training or experience will entirely prepare an individual for the impact or remove this psychological response (Leach, 1994). This initial impulsive reaction will then be proceeded by either relative calm and clear headedness; shock and awe; or panic: typically 20%, 75% and 5% of the population, respectively (Leach, 1994). Recoil begins as soon as the initial dangers are over, be that naturally or by survivors escaping. Recoil is typically met with confusion as the realisation of the extent of the disaster or damage is revealed. The final phase of post-trauma is experienced after the disaster when individuals endeavour to rebuild their lives. This can be when post-traumatic stress (PTSD) is experienced, namely anxiety, depression, or psychosomatic issues (lack of sleep), or post-traumatic growth (PTG) can occur (characterised for instance, by newfound compassion and altruism, strengthening of close relationships, spiritual change, and appreciation for life).

These human behaviours or reactions to a disaster tend to follow a pattern and are remarkably consistent (Leach, 1994). Being armed with this information helps us to understand how some cope better with uncertainty and deal with the unknown, or respond effectively to dynamic and evolving conditions.

Personality and Context

Broadly defined, personality is an individual's characteristic traits of cognition, affect and actions. Personality is key when studying human behaviour because it reflects individual differences in a person's distinctive patterns of thinking, feeling, and behaving. We may now look at adventure through the lens of personality when exploring the motivation of people who seek adventure or choose to enter extreme environments, and specifically in this chapter, to answer the question posed at the very beginning: "Are there certain personality profiles that firstly, seek out and secondly, cope better with the hyper-dynamic environment that typically encompasses adventures?" Three personality dimensions that seem interesting for this exploration are extraversion, conscientiousness, and openness. Individuals who score highly on the measures of trait extraversion tend to bore easily, seek stimulation and experiences. Conscientious individuals are reliable, dependable and goal oriented. People who score high on openness are imaginative, curious, flexible, and good at absorbing information and combining new information. The combination of these traits and a preference for adventure makes intuitive sense and research has explored "the right stuff" required in a person to thrive in adventurous and extreme environments (see Kjærgaard et al., 2015). When it comes to studying people's thoughts, feelings, and behaviours in the unknown, personality impacts our selection or avoidance of situations, our reactions to those situations, the coping mechanisms we use, our resilience and subjective wellbeing or adaptability.

Another trait worth considering here is that of curiosity and how curiosity plays a part in exploration and the tolerance of ambiguity, inference, and decision making. Todd Kashdan et al. developed a five-dimension (5D) model of curiosity (Kashdan et al., 2018) which included curiosity motivated from the need for information (to fill a gap in knowledge), and a tolerance of the stress associated with accepting the anxiety of novelty. Thrill seeking and joyous exploration were other factors which would suggest an "adventurous" type more open to dealing with unknowns.

Our behaviours, feelings and thoughts are not only influenced by internal factors, such as personality, but also external factors, such as the situation one finds oneself in (Ziegler et al., 2019). As an individual navigates situations, they encounter various situational cues, and these different situational cues will activate different personality traits, which in turn leads to different behaviours, feelings, and thoughts (Tett & Fisher, 2020). For example, a social situation will likely activate extraversion, while stressful tasks will activate conscientiousness.

When adventurers face such stressors, particularly over an extended period of time, it can parlay into psychological stress. It is important to mention, however, that "stressors" do not necessarily result in negative stress, they can also result in a positive interaction or eustress. Moreover, research shows that optimism, or focusing on the positive even in a negatively valenced situation, can play an important role when employing mechanisms to cope or adapt (Sandal et al., 2006). Eustress, salutogenesis (Antonovsky, 1987) or positive experience generates healthy and favourable conditions where states such as resilience, self-efficacy, improved crew relations and increased self-awareness can occur (Pickett & Hofmans, 2019). All of this implies that positive and negative effects are not mutually exclusive, they can and do simultaneously occur as a person can enjoy an experience even though they are subjected to a psychological or environmental stressor.

Improving adventurers' mental capacities, cultivating awareness, and increasing existing skills, knowledge and resources when dealing with the unknown are all essential for obtaining maximum psychological functioning needed for demanding tasks such as high-stakes decision making in hyper-dynamic environments. Improving cognitive assets through the transfer of skills to improve detection, sense making, and high-stakes decision making under pressure, along with successfully maintaining optimal psychology functioning and sustaining (long-term) subjective wellbeing necessary to manage the stressful situations and other adventure demands. To do so, we may look to the Psychological Capitol Model (PsyCap) to enhance the necessary resources to navigate a crisis. Building on the personality traits of hope, self-efficacy, optimism, and resiliency has been shown to be effective (Luthans et al., 2010; Milosevic et al., 2017; Pickett et al., 2019). PsyCap builds resources needed to navigate, prepare, persevere and deal with the unknown.

Concluding Thoughts

There are many psychological, physical, social and emotional trials associated with experiencing uncertainty. It is not a condition we are generally designed to be comfortable with. Challenges include: the stress of not-knowing; the anxiety of novelty or change; decision making in ambiguity; dealing with dynamic crises as they unfold; cognitive load; mental fatigue; disaster or survival response-ability; necessity for flexibility and adaptability; and so on.

However, the ability to cope with uncertainty seems to also be a human skill that can indeed be developed and strengthened (albeit also associated with certain personality traits). Benefits may include the positive state found inside biophilia and the mental alertness and presence facilitated by exploring in the out of doors. The ability to deal with uncertainty is a key life-skill which would be useful in everyday living, running a business, and experiencing an adventurous challenge. The ability to be agile, adaptive, and make decent decisions during Volatile, Uncertain, Complex and Ambiguous (VUCA) contexts is a useful one. Adventure Psychology harnesses our abilities to deal with uncertainty and enable people to go knowingly into the unknown. As white water kayaker Steve Jordans puts it: "My adventurous spirit has always been there. The outdoors, challenging myself, the personal satisfaction and accomplishment. Not for the numbers, the books, or notoriety, but I do it for the memories that only I can fully appreciate."

References

Ansell, C., & Boin, A. (2019). Taming deep uncertainty: The potential of pragmatist principles for understanding and improving strategic crisis management. *Administration & Society*, *51*(7), 1079–1112. https://doi.org.10.1177/0095399717747655

Antonovsky, A. (1987). *Unraveling the mystery of health: How people manage stress and stay well.* San Francisco, CA: Jossey-Bass.

Boin, A., & Bynander, F. (2015). Explaining success and failure in crisis coordination. *Geografiska Annaler: Series A, Physical Geography*, *97*(1), 123–135.

Caldwell, J. A., Mallis, M. M., Caldwell, J. L., Miller, J., Paul, M., & Neri, D. (2009). Fatigue countermeasures in aviation. *Aviation, Space, and Environmental Medicine*, *80*(1), 28–59.

Caplan, R. (1974). Early forms of camping in American mental hospitals. In T. P. Lowry (Ed.), *Camping therapy: Its uses in psychiatry and rehabilitation* (pp. 8–12). Springfield, IL: Charles C. Thomas.

Collins, D., & Collins, L. (2020). Developing coaches' professional judgement and decision making: Using the 'Big 5'. *Journal of Sports Sciences*, 115–119.

Csikszentmihalyi, M. (1996). *Creativity: Flow and the psychology of discovery and invention.* New York: Harper Perennial.

Gass, M. A., Gillis, H. L., & Russell, K. C. (2012). *Adventure therapy: Theory, research, and practice.* New York, NY: Routledge.

Hirsh, J. B., Mar, R. A., and Peterson, J. B. (2012). Psychological entropy: A framework for understanding uncertainty-related anxiety. *Psychological Review*, *119*, 304–320. https://doi.org/10.1037/a0026767

Kaplan, R., & Kaplan, S. (1989). *Experience of nature.* New York: Cambridge University Press.

Kashdan, T. B., Disabato, D. J., Goodman, F. R., & Naughton, C. (2018, September–October), The five dimensions of curiosity. *Harvard Business Review.* Available from https://hbr.org/2018/09/curiosity

Keller, J., Mendonca, F. C., & Cutter, J. E. (2019). Collegiate aviation pilots: Analyses of fatigue related decision-making scenarios. *International Journals*

Kjærgaard, A., Leon, G. R., & Venables, N. C. (2015). The "right stuff" for a solo sailboat circumnavigation of the globe. *Environment and Behavior, 47*(10), 1147–1171. https://doi.org/10.1177/0013916514535086

Klein, G. (2017, February 8). *Anticipation: How do we prepare ourselves for the unexpected?* Psychology Today. https://www.psychologytoday.com/gb/blog/seeing-what-others-dont/201702/anticipation

Leach, J. (1994). *Survival psychology.* Basingstoke: Palgrave Macmillan.

Luthans, F., Avey, J. B., Avolio, B. J., & Peterson, S. J. (2010). The development and resulting performance impact of positive psychological capital. *Human Resource Development Quarterly, 21*(1), 41–67. https://doi.org/10.1002/hrdq.20034

Milosevic, I., Bass, A. E., & Milosevic, D. (2017). Leveraging positive psychological capital (PsyCap) in crisis: A multiphase framework. *Organization Management Journal, 14*(3), 127–146. https://doi.org/10.1080/15416518.2017.1353898

Pickett, J., & Hofmans, J. (2019). Stressors, coping mechanisms, and uplifts of commercial fishing in Alaska: A qualitative approach to factors affecting human performance in extreme environments. *Journal of Human Performance in Extreme Environments, 15*(1), 8.

Pickett, J., Hofmans, J., & De Fruyt, F. (2019). Extraversion and performance approach goal orientation: An integrative approach to personality. *Journal of Research in Personality, 82*, 103846. https://doi.org/10.1016/j.jrp.2019.103486

Reid, P., & Kampman, H. (2020). Exploring the psychology of extended-period expeditionary adventurers: Going knowingly into the unknown. *Psychology of Sport and Exercise, 46*, 101608. https://doi.org/10.1016/j.psychsport.2019.101608

Sandal, G. M., Leon, G. R., & Palinkas, L. (2006). Human challenges in polar and space environments. *Reviews in Environmental Science and Bio/Technology, 5*(2–3), 281–296.

Tett, R., & Fisher, D. (2020). Personality dynamics in the workplace: An overview of emerging literatures and future research needs. In J. F. Rauthmann (Ed.) *The Handbook of Personality Dynamics and Processes* (pp. 1061–1086). Academic Press, 2021. https://doi.org/10.1016/B978-0-12-813995-0.00041-8.

Williams, B. (2000). The treatment of adolescent populations: An institutional vs. a wilderness setting. *Journal of Child and Adolescent Group Therapy, 10*(1), 47–56.

Wilson, E. O. (1984). *Biophilia.* Cambridge, MA: Harvard University Press.

Ziegler, M., Horstmann, K. T., & Ziegler, J. (2019). Personality in situations: Going beyond the OCEAN and introducing the Situation Five. *Psychological Assessment, 31*, 567–580. https://doi.org/10.1037/pas0000654

5

ADVENTURE, POSITIVE PSYCHOLOGY, AND NARRATIVE

The Wellbeing Impacts of Answering the Call to Adventure

Kitrina Douglas, David Carless, Paula Reid and Ruth Hughes

An Adventurer's Point of View: Becoming Someone Else

As soon as you start, you're there. You're - you're almost mentally someone else. You become the adventurer person. You cast off all your inhibitions and normalness and just, um, restrictions that come with middleaged person living in middle-England and there's less – it's hard to describe. You're expected to be a certain type of person when you're not adventuring and there's limitations to that almost, like you're not expected to go up a ladder and paint the front of your house because society assumes you shouldn't or it's dangerous or it's not safe so that feels quite restrictive. So, you become a shadow of … or you become, I think, less a person because of society's expectations and norms and worries and fears and all that. But then when you're on an adventure, you can just really, really be yourself and you can become stronger again and more natural perhaps, more capable. You can wear what you want, kind of do what you want, but you haven't got that peer pressure of not climbing that tree or caution that comes with the health and safety age of living in modern Britain. So, during [adventure] – lovely; freedom, liberation, be who you want to be, stronger, more decisive, more capable. I can navigate when I'm an adventurer. I can't navigate when I'm not an adventurer. I can do scarier stuff when I'm adventurer. I'm not allowed to do scary stuff when I'm not an adventurer. I can be fit and healthy and muscly and work hard and sweat and cry and bleed when I'm an adventurer, but I'm not supposed to be when I'm not an adventurer. It's so … it's a hugely … it feels more authentic, uh, there's another word like authentic, um, compatible or something. Coherent, I think. So, and then your head is in the right zone, so although it's the same worries and the situation that you've prethought about, once you're in it, you just deal with it. You just calculate everything

DOI: 10.4324/9781003173601-8

and make decisions and when you're in country, if you're in another country, the attitude is so much more, you know, we can and we can solve it and don't worry or no worries. And even when the going gets tough if you're in adventure mode. So, sometimes I liken myself to becoming Lara Croft when I'm adventuring because I just become her. I'm tougher and wiser and more capable without the cotton-wool stuff that I get at home.

'Lara'

Adventure, Positive Psychology, and Narrative: the Wellbeing Impacts of Answering the Call to Adventure

Adventures and Positive Psychology

This chapter aims to explore the role of positive psychology and narrative theory in informing our understanding of adventures, adventurers, and the adventure story. We will consider factors which motivate and reward the adventurer, including inspiring narratives where adventurers leave behind the ordinary world and push beyond pre-existing boundaries. Whilst recognising that not all adventures result in positive or positively transformative outcomes, this chapter seeks to use the lens of evidence-based positive psychology to better understand how adventure stories might promote flourishing in both the adventurers recounting them, and the audiences receiving them.

Answering the call to adventure can result in multiple and diverse experiences which may be "positive" or "negative". In the heart of an adventure, we can be enduring, surviving, coping, or flourishing; often stretching our understanding of who we are and of what we are capable. As Reid and Kampman propose, "to 'go on an adventure' is to choose to have a natural peak experience that is good for our eudaemonic happiness and psychological wellbeing" (2020, p. 8). Positive Psychology (PP) is described as "the study of the conditions and processes that contribute to the flourishing or optimal functioning of people, groups and institutions" (Gable & Haidt, 2005, p. 103). Although there are other frameworks through which to consider the adventure experience, an understanding of evidenced positive psychology offers us insight into how and why adventures, adventure stories and the use of adventurous language, metaphors and words, might result in positive affect both for the adventurer and the listener or reader.

The origin of positive psychology owes much to ancient Greek philosophers, to the Humanistic psychology movement and to therapeutic psychology, among others, and still this evolving field continues to develop and redefine itself, embracing all that contributes to optimal human functioning and flourishing, including so-called "negative" emotions (Lomas, 2016) or negative inputs (Wong, 2011). At the 1999 American Psychological Association annual conference, Seligman reminded his audience of their responsibility to nurture "what is best in ourselves" (Seligman, 1999, p. 560) and as Rona Hart puts it, to "draw on what is right with people – their strengths, courage, optimism, resilience and many other capacities" (2020, p.2) all of which undoubtedly contribute to the positive experiences – or mindsets – of many adventurers.

Let's take a brief look at three of the more well-established PP models and how they may relate to adventuring. The five elements of Martin Seligman's positive psychology PERMA model (Seligman, 2018) are commonly reported as being experienced on adventures: Positive emotions (Fredrickson, 2013), Engagement (Youssef-Morgan & Bockorny, 2014), Relationships with others (Reis & Gable, 2003), finding Meaning (Peterson & Park, 2014), and a sense of Achievement (Howell, 2009). Adventurers may also experience the positive aspects described in Ryff's Psychological Wellbeing model (1989) including: Life-Purpose; Autonomy; Personal Growth; Environmental Mastery; Positive Relationships and Self-Acceptance – six categories central to the facilitation of optimal wellbeing. Finally, within the concept of Psychological Capital, can be found "HERO" with its four tenets of Hope, Efficacy, Resilience, and Optimism; all linking to life satisfaction and adventure experiences (Luthans & Youssef-Morgan, 2017).

Clearly there are many Positive Psychology concepts that underpin the purpose and benefits of "going on an adventure" or participating in adventurous activities, including the "dark side" of the journey. Experiencing "negative" emotions during times of difficulty and challenge can arguably have positive outcomes, as adventurers experience stressors, challenge and adversity, potentially resulting in resilience and coping skills (Lazarus & Folkman 1984), and harnessing flow, optimism, self-efficacy and grit, to name a few.

Adventure itself could be described – or prescribed – as a Positive Psychology Intervention (PPI) which demands a state of mindfulness or flow from the adventurer, both of which are deemed to be positive states of wellbeing. Additionally, the language and narratives associated with adventuring (such as *rising to the challenge, weathering the storm, getting to the summit,* or *turning the corner*), may incorporate a similar explanatory style to second wave positive psychology (Ivtzan et al., 2015) and heroic or relational narratives, which will be reviewed further in this chapter.

Adventure Storytelling

Adventure stories call us into the elsewhere, transporting us beyond our ordinary lives and across time. From *once upon a time* to "a galaxy far, far away" (Lucas, 1977) we may "boldly go where no man has gone before" (Delahunty, 2010, p. 52). It is the stuff of Legends. Some of the oldest and most enduring stories are great adventure tales: The Epic of Gilgamesh (Kovacs, 1989); The Odyssey (Homer, 2015); The Mahabharata (Rajagopalachari, 1970) and Beowulf (Klaeber, 1936), for example. These epic stories, and the influence they have on other stories, seep into our understanding of reality, socially constructing what is possible, who we think we are, and, indeed, who we have the potential to become.

We, and our identities – and our potentiality – are influenced by stories. In every culture we use stories to build and shape our understanding of the world, how it works and how we work within it. This influences our mindsets and feeds our wisdom. The recounting of an adventure story involves reflection, sense-making and awareness (whether conscious or unconscious) of narrative form.

Many of us, as readers or as audience, are entertained and inspired by stories of adventure, creating meaning in a world where story form has been inundated by bite-sized social media and messages of consumerist materialism. Stories of perseverance, grit, determination, success, failure and achievement over the odds can play a role in boosting, rather than reducing, positive affect (Mager & Stevens, 2015).

Evidence suggests that both the recounting and receiving of a story could be a positive psychology intervention (Rutledge, 2016). The recounting of the adventure story may prove to be of benefit to the wellbeing of the adventurer reflecting on their reality, narrating (and perhaps reauthoring) selected events, but also to the recipient as a form of Aristotelian catharsis (Kruse, 1979), in the experiencing of which they can safely process unsafe emotions; or to reveal possibilities, inform and inspire. As Parker and Wampler explain (albeit when talking about the use of story in therapy):

> It is common to experience emotional changes while engaged in a book, television program, or movie. Feelings of excitement, sadness, and other emotions are experienced while following the storyline. *[If the recipient of the story]* is able to identify with the protagonist of this story and experience the emotional changes, having these feelings can be useful… shifting the emotion from discouragement to success can begin to open up possibilities …
> *(2006, p. 155)*

Adventure stories recount the capacity of humans to overcome adversity and transform themselves and their life's purpose through suffering, struggle and privation, giving us hope we can ourselves do something never done before. This harnessing of meaning (such as can be found in Viktor Frankl's *Man's Search for Meaning*, 2004), can be utilised for overall positive effect; acknowledging and accepting the power of negative emotions we experience when enduring difficulties and providing coping or performance enhancing strategies (Lomas, 2016). Essentially, the adventure creates opportunities for the adventurer to be broken and remade, and thus to grow and transcend (Dabrowski, 1966). Emotionally, the adventure story can do likewise for its recipient.

As Crites writes in his seminal paper *The Narrative Quality of Experience*, "we live our lives from day to day, but we understand our life as if it were a story" (1971). The paper lists the benefits of journaling for adults, including: personal growth and development; intuition and self-expression; problem-solving; stress-reduction and health benefits; and reflection/critical thinking. Thus, journaling may be regarded as another form of storytelling (or processing) – an activity that many adventurers undertake to capture their lived experience whilst on adventure. Journaling, or writing down the adventure story, may also prove to be a useful tool for reviewing or debriefing, thus potentially decreasing risk whilst on adventure, or reducing mental or physical distress.

The processing and telling of the adventure story itself could be considered as related to the epochs of adventuring: pre-, during and post-experience for both the participant(s) and the listeners. Preparing for and anticipating the adventure, engaging in the adventure, and savouring memories through recounting the experience can boost positive affect as we mentally time travel (Suddendorf & Corballis, 2007). Reid & Kampman (2020) also discerned the significance of the adventure epochs in their research on the purpose and benefits of expeditionary adventuring. The experience – and the story – starts at the very first thought of adventure and has the potential to continue to journey's end.

Adventure Narratives

Introduction

Across the centuries a variety of scholars from different traditions and disciplines have contributed to our current understanding of Narrative Theory (see for example Mikhail Bakhtin, David Epstom and Michael White). For us, the insights of John Mcloud, Dan McAdams, Arthur Frank and Hilde Lindeman Neilson have richly infused our research. Below, we outline some of the theoretical tenets of narrative theory which will be followed by some practical implications.

Narrative Theory

Before looking at what the theory means in practice there is an element to clarify. Some scholars use the terms "story" and "narrative" interchangeably, others believe there are subtle differences worth maintaining. When we use the term *story* it usually relates to a tale about a character or event and what happens, there is a plot, and an arc to what is being described as well as consequences. In contrast *narrative*, takes on a more symbolic, overarching framework. Arthur Frank (2010) suggests a narrative type is the most general storyline that can be recognised underlying the plot and tensions of particular stories. When we listen to people's stories, *narrative* becomes a listening device to unpick and understand cultural expectations, the types of actions that will be validated and the types of actions that will cause trouble for the teller including silencing, exclusion, stigmatisation, or loss of mental health.

While there are many insights that might be gleaned from studying narrative the following are some of the most important to keep in mind:

- Humans are storytelling animals who make sense of their experience, of time, relationships, events, and so on, through creating and sharing stories.

- An individual begins to shape a particular identity through talking about their motivations, experiences, and what they mean; and by sharing stories. In other words, they begin to understand themselves as a 'person' who will do A but not B. From observing the actions and behaviour of the individual, others – such as family, friends, the media – also begin to shape the individual's identity, by telling their own stories about them. Thus, our identities are both personally and culturally shaped and validated.
- A storyteller uses the building blocks available within their environment to create and share their stories. That is the words, metaphors, similes, adjectives, the way the story is put together, along with how the story is narrated, is learned from what is accessible. Thus, from an individual story we also learn about the storyteller's community, and the conventions of that culture or sub-culture.
- Over time, stories tend to cluster in ways that give rise to recognisable types of plot. The one we often use is the hero narrative, which is where the protagonist takes on a series of daring acts to achieve a super-human feat.
- The process whereby some story plots gain greater recognition leads to master or dominant narratives. These are stories that either carry a moral force such that certain actions and behaviours are justified over others, or leads to some behaviours becoming devalued, silenced and / or tabooed.
- A problematic aspect of dominant narratives is they can misrepresent, oppress, finalise and silence people whose lives and stories fail to align or conform with the dominant story plot. They might also silence those who have evidence that challenges the truth of the dominant story. For example, most of us will recognise the American Dream, but also know it is not working for many ethnic and minority groups in the USA. Reports about adventurers such as Captain Preet Chandi and Nirmal 'Nims' Purja also help reduce the dominant narrative of white, western male conquerors.
- Counter narratives, in contrast, are plots that identify, resist and undermine the authority of dominant narratives by bringing to light morally relevant details that are missing or misrepresented (Douglas & Carless, 2015).
- The stories we tell (and those that we are fearful of telling), and the identity that is shaped in the process, are linked in very powerful ways to our mental health; to being accepted and validated within the cultures we live and work. The opposite is also the case.

Identifying Narrative Types

In considering narrative types, we might want to reflect on how different kinds of narratives act as listening devices around stories and thus how they impact upon us.

For example, Arthur Frank identified three different types of stories that cancer patients shared regarding their cancer journey. The first, he called the *restitution narrative*, a story plot which focussed on getting back to health. In its most succinct form, the story plot was "yesterday I was healthy, today I am sick, and tomorrow I will be healthy again". Such story plots act like a map for the ill person's journey influencing the types of treatments doctors offered, the expectancy of the patient and how they (and family) describe their experiences. A parallel for this in adventure might be of an adventurer overcoming significant hurdles to achieve their adventure objectives and return safely home.

The second type of illness story – a *chaos narrative* – reported by Frank was largely incommunicable; the individual lived in trauma or fear, was unable to express what they were experiencing and had no map for how to escape, in short, life was in chaos. On an adventure, the protagonist may be physically or psychologically lost, meandering on their journey of ups and downs with no real sense of direction or conclusion.

The third type of narrative was the *quest narrative*. Here the ill person is on a journey where a return to health was not the only or most important destination. These storytellers talked about being transformed by their experiences such that they had learned something important or become something they wouldn't have expected but now value. Whether surviving cancer, or in death, the transformation of this *journey* was key, as opposed to getting back to health. Additionally, often these storytellers storied their cancer as a positive step on this transformational journey. Transformative quests for adventurers are referred to later in the hero's journey section (or see Chapter 12).

Frank suggested one issue with the restitution narrative with a 'return to health' story being the only outcome, led to there being few conversations about death, and no room for cancer to be storied positively. Without considering death and the type of death that might be best, there was little option for refusing treatment and it sometimes led to sick patients trying new medicines and treatments with no hope of success, often encouraged to do so by loving caring relatives desperate for them to live. If getting better was the only goal with everything invested in this outcome, its unsurprising that the types of stories that were developed were about "fighting" and "beating cancer" as the patient became the battle ground. In this context "fighting to the end" was storied as a positive result.

Similarly, if adventure narratives focus solely on achieving the end objective of the adventurer, such as reaching the summit, there may be less room for transformation, connection, achievement, purpose and growth in the upwards climb.

Narrative Types in Sport

In analysing the life stories of multiple tournament winners in sport we discovered three core narrative types (see Carless & Douglas, 2009; Douglas & Carless, 2006; Douglas & Carless, 2009). These may also be applied to the adventurer story (especially those that involve elements of competition, or specific goal attainment). The first we called the *performance narrative;* a story plot where the individual is expected to dedicate their life to winning, and tends to story a need to sacrifice all other activities, interests or relationships to win. For these individuals winning increases self-worth and esteem, while losing has the opposite effect, reducing self-confidence and worth. The results for tellers of performance narratives is that life often becomes an emotional yoyo, dependent on the next win or what was happening on the course.

The *discovery narrative*, in contrast, is the antithesis to what we have just described. The discovery storyteller recounts achieving success without prioritising winning ahead of relationships, education, self-development, and other interests. As such these individuals develop a multidimensional identity and sense of self and these provide additional sources of self-worth not related to sport success.

The third type of narrative we called a *relational narrative*. These storytellers talked about the journey as being important rather than the destination, and other travellers on this journey as being important, as opposed to the trophy, cup or medal. Though it should also be said, these individuals were no less successful to those in the performance narrative group.

By presenting three different narratives in sport, these counter narratives provide an important resource and new options for narrating life experiences. In 2015, after reading the three different types of story at the Recreation Alliance Conference "Sporting Minds" at Wembley Stadium, a mountain climber introduced himself to us and we chatted about what he took from the stories. He mentioned that the narrative types were similar to what he was experiencing in climbing where some people wanted to "conquer" the mountain and would let nothing get in their way to the summit. Others, like him he said, aligned more with the discovery narrative and viewed the experiences as an opportunity to learn and discover something about themselves, their climbing partners or their technique. What was validating to this individual was that his way of experiencing climbing had in some way been validated, he didn't have to focus on beating the mountain or sacrifice his love of discovery.

The Hero's Journey Explored through a Positive Psychology Lens

Although there are many forms of plot, the universal story of "The Hero's Journey" (Campbell, 1949) is a useful lens to connect real and fictional adventure stories with positive psychology theory, thus further exploring potential psychological benefits within the adventures we experience and narrate. The basic premise of "The Hero's Journey" (a global monomyth) is that a story's protagonist goes on a journey comprising trials, allies and enemies, and returns a hero. It provides a rite of passage narrative, depicting a departure from the known world, a journey of tests, initiation and transformation, and a returning back to home. This classic structure is found in many iconic films, books and games, such as Star Wars, The Hobbit, Alice in Wonderland, The Matrix, Frozen, The Lion King, Harry Potter, Lost, The Legend of Zelda, and so on. Campbell describes it thus:

> A hero ventures forth from the world of common day into a region of supernatural wonder: fabulous forces are there encountered and a decisive

victory is won: The hero comes back from this mysterious adventure with the power to bestow boons on his fellow man.

(2014, p. 23)

Campbell divided the whole journey into specific stages of story, which we can further explore in terms of wellbeing and specific positive psychology concepts relating to these stages. Each stage is listed below with potential psychological associations. This is a suggested relationship with examples below:

Hero's Journey Stages	*Positive Psychology Concepts*
1. the ordinary known world	
2. the call to adventure	Optimism & hope
	Self-determination
	Motivation towards / away from
	Psychology of Possibility
	Growth mindset
3. crossing the threshold	Goal pursuit
	Shattering of the assumptive world
	Commitment
	Fear, Courage
	Liberation
4. the journey	Goal Agency and Pathways
	Hedonism & eudaemonia
	Flow, mindfulness, presence
	Psychophysiological movement
	Motivation, Drive
	Savouring
	Awe
5. trials, challenges and tests	Resilience, grit, hardiness
	Mental toughness (not mental fragility)
	Sisu
	Self-efficacy
	Coping
	Character strengths & virtues
	Positive power of negative emotions
6. mentors and allies	Positive relationships, social support
	Gratitude
	Compassion
	Empathy
7. enemies, temptations and distractors	Self-regulation
	Forgiveness
8. the ultimate ordeal	See (5) above
	Mortality awareness
	Peak & Plateau experiences

9. reward (achievement, positive emotions)	Eudaemonic wellbeing Meaning Accomplishment Self-awareness Identity Atonement
10. transformation and resurrection	Post-Traumatic Growth Post Adventure Growth Cross-cultural growth Identity integration Transformation Transcendence
11. return & adjustment, returning with the boon	Gratitude Wisdom Growth Positive ageing

The Hero's Journey and the Call to Adventure

In this section we will follow the different stages of the hero's journey and link them to adventure experiences. Some of these concepts particularly resonate with "extended-period expeditionary adventuring" (Reid & Kampman, 2020) – enduring, "heroic" journeys involving pre-, during and post-adventure epochs. In the original qualitative research, Reid interviewed seven expeditionary adventurers with multiple, extended adventures under their belts. Between them they cycled, walked, sailed, run, skied and climbed around the world several times, including both Poles and the tallest peaks. In their phenomenological storytelling (and as seen in the selected quotes below), we can begin to understand the external and internal journeys these adventurers experienced. Starting from a place of dissatisfaction in their known, ordinary world; through to their return as "heroic" figures; resurrected, transformed, self-actualised – or at the very least, psychologically stronger and wiser.

Here Ted – one of the seven expeditionary adventurers interviewed – begins his "hero's journey" at Stage One in his known and ordinary world as a discontented tennis teacher:

> … I could feel inside I didn't feel like I was fulfilling my potential. And so I had my big massive dream to be like, you know, the next big Tim Henman and there I was teaching tennis to children just thinking, "I'm a waste, I'm useless." … and then I started to reflect a little bit on my life and I took time out of my life, which I've never done before, you know, to actually think.

Other adventurers did not always feel happy or fulfilled in their ordinary worlds, like Jack, a round-the-world sailor: "It's not about just ticking along and then you die. What a waste". He felt there was more to life, as did multi-expeditioner Lara: "... not sitting at home and doing tapestry or something. I would have gone mad if I'd have grown up in the Victorian era". Sitting at home, adventurers may want more, as they strain against perceived mundanity. For these individuals, their known world may not provide them with sufficient growth, challenge and newness to extend their potential and drive for self-development. In Seligman's PERMA model engagement is key to wellbeing, and for adventurers, engagement with the unknown may be more appealing than residing in the ordinary world.

The second – and critical – stage of the hero's journey: the *call to adventure*, may be subtle: "It sat there like a seed ... I didn't even know it was there ..." (Ted); a call that shines: "... it was like a light that came on" (Dora) or an actual call such as the one Joanna received:

> ... the chance happening, if you like, was a phone call in the office. I was working as a journalist in London and I had a friend ... asking if I would like to report on an expedition on Everest and, um, I said yes.

Campbell provocatively suggested: "We must let go of the life we have planned, so as to accept the one that is waiting for us. The old skin has to be shed before the new one can come" (Osbon, 1991, p.8). Referencing the snake reminds us of a Harry Potter symbol: Voldemort's archetype and the symbol of the Slytherin in Hogwarts, whose headmaster suggests: "It is our choices, Harry, that show what we truly are, far more than our abilities" (Rowling, 1998). One choice we make is how we respond to the call to adventure.

The choice to answer the call is an intriguing and life-hanging moment of decision-making. The "Yes Tribe" founded by adventurer Dave Cornthwaite embodies just that point – to say yes more (www.sayyesmore.com) and thus prevent life passing by. Assuming the call to adventure is answered with an affirmative, the adventurer then *crosses the threshold* and departs their known (safe, secure, comfort zone) world taking a leap of faith into the unknown. The adventurer Lara describes it thus:

> I think the day before you start is possibly the hardest day because it's all built up into a big tidal wave of anticipation and all your energy is in check because you haven't started and you haven't set foot out there and, um, it's kind of worry about the unknown, I suppose.

At this point of departure, Jack describes the new world as a "bubble world" when "your focus is on your adventure" and you perhaps change your narrative or identity becoming "Lara Croft". This is an early stage of transformation, where both the landscape, and the inner world of the hero, changes from *terra firma* to *terra incognita*. We go from the known world into the unknown; from our comfort zone to our stretch. *Crossing the threshold* into the realm of adventure, necessitates the adventurer engaging with a goal. The reality of the new endeavour can cause the pre-existing assumptive world to shatter (Janoff-Bulman, 1989) opening new perspectives and possibilities.

It is now time for the journey itself "getting further and further away from home" (Emma). Ted, our frustrated children's tennis coach, is now off on an epic adventure, cycling 40,000 miles:

> And I felt the transition from the beginning more kind of like just scrambling and just trying to fight through every day because it was all a bit too much, but then as I started to progress in the journey, I was like, "Okay. Now I know what this is all about … I've just got to get to the end of every day."
>
> … it's like the journey just became bigger than me, just totally and utterly like this wasn't to do with me anymore.

The adventurous, heroic journey is not an easy one, and we posit that it is sometimes purposefully chosen by adventurers to strengthen or test themselves. Sean, a *Grand Slam Adventurer* describes it as: "testing myself, you know, pushing the boundaries". Sean goes on to describe a very challenging time when he was stuck up Denali (mountain) in a storm:

> … that was physically horrible. It was painful. I was hallucinating after a couple of days on the mountain, just lying there on the ice. It was not enjoyable and I do remember saying, "I'm never going to do this again."

Perhaps for Sean, this was also a point of utmost despair and the nadir of that particular expedition.

Adventurers face *trials, challenges and tests* inherent in the journey, and if we include the Hero's Journey structural elements of *enemies, temptation and distractors*, and the concept of *the ultimate ordeal*, the positive psychology concepts of coping, resilience and post-traumatic growth may be of particular relevance in supporting adventurers. Second wave positive psychology (Ivtzan et al., 2015) suggests that through adversity the characteristics of resilience and recovery result in transformational growth. Duckworth and Gross (2014) advocate the employment of self-control and grit as determinants of success, especially when performing in extremes and beyond self-perceived limits (Lahti, 2019). Evidence from stories told by adventurers suggest these factors surely contribute to mental toughness and endurance under pressure (Crust & Clough, 2005).

En-route, challenges include *enemies, distractions and detractors* such as the dementors in Harry Potter described thus: "Dementors … drain peace, hope, and happiness out of the air around them … Get too near a Dementor and every good feeling, every happy memory will be sucked out of you" (Rowling, 1999). Ordinary people also can drain the hero, (or anyone anytime in life), as our adventurers describe: "they'd just try and scare me and, … one guy it's like said, 'Oh, you'll never make that' " (Ted); or "… of course people are going to tell you that you're stupid and you're foolish and, you know, you're silly for even thinking that, you know, that you can accomplish that thing" (Emma). The detractor or enemy can even be yourself: "It's proving to me that I can do it. Proving to me that I'm not as bad as I think I am" (Sean).

There are also positive forces who aid the adventurer on their journey; *allies, mentors and supporters* who facilitate progress, who encourage, motivate and strengthen with their kindness. Ted, at a time of loneliness as he ran 5,000 miles solo across Canada, came to a point where: "I finally cracked and I thought, I just need people, just need human contact … eventually I got invited into her house for tea and biscuits"; and Emma: "going into a bread shop bursting into tears and being so thankful that he'd just given me a bag of stale bread". Sometimes the friendly ally is more significantly helpful such as a guide or Sherpa as Joanna recounts from her Everest climb: "I mean, but for Tran, I probably wouldn't have done it … he kind of just allowed my confidence to fall to the right side of the line".

It is unsurprising that good relationships support positive psychology concepts of subjective wellbeing, (Lucas & Dyrenforth, 2006). For the adventurer, especially for those in extreme situations, support from fellow travellers and those they encounter, can be the difference between life and death. Although definitions of support are debatable (Veiel & Baumann, 2014), research suggests that those in receipt of support do better in adverse conditions than those who do not have access to it.

At the darkest hour, there is an *ultimate ordeal* or nadir of the journey; the fundamental test (and thus strengthening of the spirit or *psyche*). Described as the "belly of the whale" this place is dark and deep, often portrayed in film as a tunnel, cave or dungeon – or even garbage disposal pits such as in *Star Wars: A New Hope* and *Toy Story 3* – and may represent our subconscious: "On an expedition when, you know, you don't think you could get any lower and all you want to do is find a dark hole and live in it", Emma appreciates however that it may be the contrast with the darkness – the struggle or suffering – that provides the enlightenment; the post-traumatic growth:

> I try and embrace that feeling because I know that when I come out of that bad place, the - the happiness after is going to be so amazing and intense and I'm going to be so much stronger from the pain that I felt that's it's - that I think it's something to be embraced and appreciated, I think.

The *reward* is the boon. The elixir of life; the *transformation and resurrection* of the spirit, soul or heart: "I know that adventure saved my life", says Dora; "my heart is fixed" claims Emma; "I ultimately felt, um, accepted and it was almost like I was an onion and I just peeled back loads of layers of myself and – and it was okay. People actually liked me and it was okay" says Ted.

On returning home – and "there's no place like home" according to Dorothy (Vidor et al., 1939) – the hero needs to adapt back to the ordinary world and the adventurer needs to adjust too, while perhaps grappling with "post-adventure blues" (Smith & Barrett, 2016). After such peak experiences, adventurers and heroes return home transformed and resurrected (Hopkins & Putnam, 2013), bearing gifts potentially including wisdom, gratitude and altruism as, through story, they support would-be adventurers and inspire the next generation.

In conclusion the journey itself may promote physical and psychological wellbeing. Quite aside from the effects of being outdoors in green or blue spaces (Gascon et al., 2015, Gascon et al., 2017), there are well-evidenced mental wellbeing impacts from the physical engagement of moving and using one's body. As a wellbeing intervention, physical activity operates on many levels, improving positive emotions (Ekkekakis et al., 2005), encouraging autotelic engagement and flow (Nakamura & Csikzentmihalyi, 2014) and facilitating a number of human needs inherent in goal pursuits (Deci & Ryan, 2000). Adventurers report joy and awe in savouring the environment around them (Buckley, 2020; Reid & Kampman, 2020) – the process and the journey mattering as much as the destination. This savouring in the present time, recalled through the adventure story, can also create wellbeing and, arguably, further aspects of optimism and hope towards future adventures to come (Biskas et al., 2019).

Let's leave the last words of our narrative with Ted the disillusioned tennis coach, who finally concluded that adventure: "… fills your soul, there and then, you move on with life".

References

Biskas, M., Cheung, W. Y., Juhl, J., Sedikides, C., Wildschut, T., & Hepper, E. (2019). A prologue to nostalgia: savouring creates nostalgic memories that foster optimism. *Cognition and Emotion, 33*(3), 417–427.

Buckley, R. (2020). Nature sports, health and ageing: The value of euphoria, *Annals of Leisure Research, 23*(1), 92–109. DOI: 10.1080/11745398.2018.1483734

Campbell, J. (1949). *Joseph Campbell's the hero with a thousand faces.* Princeton University Press.

Carless, D., & Douglas, K. (2009). "We haven't got a seat on the bus for you" or "All the seats are mine": Narratives and career transition in professional golf. *Qualitative Research in Sport and Exercise, 1*(1), 51–66.

Crites, S. (1971). The narrative quality of experience. *Journal of the American Academy of Religion, 39*(3), 291–311.

Crust, L., & Clough, P. J. (2005). Relationship between mental toughness and physical endurance. *Perceptual and Motor Skills, 100*(1), 192–194.

Dabrowski, K. (1966). The theory of positive disintegration. *International Journal of Psychiatry, 2*(2), 229–249.

Deci, E. L., & Ryan, R. M. (2000). The "what" and "why" of goal pursuits: Human needs and the self-determination of behavior. *Psychological Inquiry, 11*, 227–268.

Delahunty, A. (2010). *Adonis to Zorro: Oxford dictionary of reference and allusion.* Oxford University Press.

Douglas, K., & Carless, D. (2006). Performance, discovery, and relational narratives among women professional tournament golfers. *Women in Sport and Physical Activity Journal, 15*, 14–27. 10.1123/wspaj.15.2.14

Douglas, K., & Carless, D. (2009). Abandoning the performance narrative: Two women's stories of transition from professional golf. *Journal of Applied Sport Psychology, 21*(2), 213–230.

Douglas, K., & Carless, D. (2015). *Life story research in sport: A narrative approach to understanding the experiences of elite and professional athletes.* Routledge.

Duckworth, A., & Gross, J. J. (2014). Self-control and grit: Related but separable determinants of success. *Current Directions in Psychological Science, 23*(5), 319–325.

Ekkekakis, P., Hall, E., & Petruzzello, S. (2005) Variation and homogeneity in affective responses to physical activity of varying intensities: An alternative perspective on dose–response based on evolutionary considerations, *Journal of Sports Sciences, 23*(5), 477–500.

Frank, A. W. (2010). *Letting stories breathe: A socio-narratology.* University of Chicago Press.

Frankl, V. (2004). *Man's Search for Meaning.* Rider.

Fredrickson, B. L. (2013). Positive Emotions Broaden and Build. In P. Devine, & A. Plant (Eds.), *Advances in Experimental Social Psychology* (Vol. 47, pp. 1–53). Burlington: Academic Press.https://doi.org/10.1016/B978-0-12-407236-7.00001-2

Gable, S. L., & Haidt, J. (2005). What (and why) is positive psychology? *Review of General Psychology, 9*(2), 103–110.

Gascon, M., Triguero-Mas, M., Martínez, D., Dadvand, P., Forns, J., Plasència, A., et al. (2015). Mental health benefits of long-term exposure to residential green and blue spaces: A systematic review. *International Journal of Environmental Research and Public Health, 12*(4), 4354–4379. DOI: 10.3390/ijerph120404354

Gascon, M., Zijlema, W., Vert, C., White, M. P., Nieuwenhuijsen, M. J. (2017). Outdoor blue spaces, human health and well-being: A systematic review of quantitative studies. *International Journal of Hygiene and Environmental Health, 220*(8), 1207–1221. https://doi.org/10.1016/j.ijheh.2017.08.004

Hart, R. (2020). *Positive psychology: The basics.* Routledge.

Homer, H. (2015). *The Odyssey.* Xist Publishing.

Hopkins, D., & Putnam, R. (2013). *Personal growth through adventure.* Routledge.

Howell, A. J. (2009). Flourishing: Achievement-related correlates of students' well-being. *The Journal of Positive Psychology, 4*(1), 1–13.

Ivtzan, I., Lomas, T., Hefferon, K., & Worth, P. (2015). *Second wave positive psychology: Embracing the dark side of life.* Routledge.

Janoff-Bulman, R. (1989). Assumptive worlds and the stress of traumatic events: Applications of the schema construct. *Social cognition, 7*(2), 113–136.

Klaeber, F. (1936) *Beowulf and the Fight at Finnsburg.* Рипол Классик.

Kovacs, M. G. (1989). *The epic of Gilgamesh.* Stanford, CA: Stanford University Press.

Kruse, N. W. (1979). The process of Aristotelian Catharsis: A reidentification. *Theatre Journal, 31*(2), 162–171.

Lahti, E. (2019). Embodied fortitude: An introduction to the Finnish construct of sisu. *International Journal of Wellbeing, 9*(1), 61–82. https://doi.org/10.5502/ijw.v9i1.672

Lazarus, R. S., & Folkman, S. (1984). *Stress, appraisal, and coping.* Springer Publishing Company.

Lomas, T. (2016). *The positive power of negative emotions: How harnessing your darker feelings can help you see a brighter dawn.* Hachette UK.

Lucas, R. E., & Dyrenforth, P. S. (2006). Does the existence of social relationships matter for subjective well-being? In K. D. Vohs & E. J. Finkel (Eds.), *Self and relationships: Connecting intrapersonal and interpersonal processes* (pp. 254–273). The Guilford Press.

Lucas, G., dir. (1977). *Star wars episode IV: A new hope.* Twentieth Century Fox. Film.

Luthans, F., & Youssef-Morgan, C. M. (2017). Psychological capital: An evidence-based positive approach. *Management Department Faculty Publications* 165. https://digitalcommons.unl.edu/managementfacpub/165

Mager, B. J., & Stevens, L. A. M. (2015). The effects of storytelling on happiness and resilience in older adults. Sophia, the St. Catherine University repository. Accessed from https://sophia.stkate.edu/ma_hhs/3

Nakamura, J., & Csikszentmihalyi, M. (2014). The concept of flow. In *Flow and the foundations of positive psychology* (pp. 239–263). Dordrecht: Springer. https://doi.org/10.1007/978-94-017-9088-8_16

Parker, T. S., & Wampler, K. S. (2006). Changing emotion: The use of therapeutic storytelling. *Journal of Marital and Family Therapy, 32*(2), 155–166.

Peterson, C., & Park, N. (2014). Meaning and positive psychology. *International Journal of Existential Psychology and Psychotherapy, 5*(1), 2–8.

Osbon, D. K. (1991). *Reflections on the art of living: A Joseph Campbell companion*. HarperCollins.

Rajagopalachari, C. (1970). *Mahabharata* (Vol. 1). Diamond Pocket Books (P) Ltd.

Reid, P., & Kampman, H. (2020). Exploring the psychology of extended-period expeditionary adventurers: Going knowingly into the unknown. *Psychology of Sport and Exercise, 46*, 101608.

Reis, H. T., & Gable, S. L. (2003). Toward a positive psychology of relationships. In C. L. M. Keyes & J. Haidt (Eds.), *Flourishing: Positive psychology and the life well-lived* (pp. 129–159). American Psychological Association. https://doi.org/10.1037/10594-006.

Rowling, J. K. (1998). *Harry Potter and the Chamber of Secrets*. Bloomsbury.

Rowling, J. K. (1999). *Harry Potter and the prisoner of Azkaban*. Arthur A. Levine Books.

Rutledge, P. B. (2016). Everything is story. In E. M. Gregory & P. B. Rutledge (Eds.), *Exploring positive psychology: The science of happiness and well-being: The science of happiness and well-being*. ABC-CLIO.

Ryff, C. D. (1989). Happiness is everything, or is it? Explorations on the meaning of psychological well-being. *Journal of Personality and Social Psychology, 57*(6), 1069.

Seligman, M. E. P. (1999). Positive Social Science. *Journal of Positive Behavior Interventions, 1*(3), 181–182. https://doi.org/10.1177/109830079900100306

Seligman, M. (2018). PERMA and the building blocks of well-being. *The Journal of Positive Psychology, 13*(4), 333–335.

Smith, N., & Barrett, E. (2016). The transition-reintegration of personnel working in fragile states: Lessons from extreme environments. Conference paper. Conference: 5th British Psychological Society Military Psychology Conference.

Suddendorf, T., & Corballis, M. C. (2007). Mental time travel across the disciplines: The future looks bright. *Behavioral and Brain Sciences, 30*(3), 335–345.

Veiel, H. O., & Baumann, U. (Eds.) (2014). *The meaning and measurement of support*. Taylor & Francis.

Vidor, K., Fleming, V., Cukor, G., Thorpe, R., Taurog, N., & LeRoy, M. (1939). *The Wizard of Oz*. Metro-Goldwyn-Mayer (MGM).

Wong, P. T. P. (2011). Positive psychology 2.0: Towards a balanced interactive model of the good life. *Canadian Psychology, 52*(2), 69–81.

Youssef-Morgan, C., & Bockorny, K.M. (2014). Engagement in the context of positive psychology. In C. Truss, R. Delbridge, E. Soane, K. Alfes, & A. Shantz (Eds.), *Employee engagement in theory and practice* (pp. 36–56). Routledge.

6

THE HUMAN–ENVIRONMENT DYNAMIC

An Ecological Dynamics Approach to Understanding Human–Environment Interactions in the Context of Adventure Psychology

Tuomas Immonen, Eric Brymer, Timo Jaakkola, and Keith Davids

From the Point of View of an Adventurer: Senses

> There it was again, that feeling. This time I was driving hard to leave the safety of the eddy with a route down a Himalayan Grade 4 rapid stuck in my mind. I had been on the water for a few days so my body was attuned to the information required for a successful descent. I knew what I needed to do, not each move so much as where I needed to be and what the features of the water offered in terms of making the journey straight forward. The feeling of being in the right place, of being physically stretched but comfortable, of being wholly aware of my surroundings and where every one of my senses were fully engaged and awake. I could see better, hear more and sense my surroundings far more clearly than normal. I was alive …
>
> Eric

Introduction

From an Ecological perspective the traditional understanding of adventure is limited. Adventure is not a thing done as captured by the idea of going on an adventure, or a thing done to us as might be presumed from reading some of the literature on adventure therapy. Adventure is not even an activity that might be encapsulated by specific task types (e.g., kayaking, mountaineering), duration or intensity. Instead, adventure is an experience in the same way that flow or love is an experience. From an ecological perspective this experience is best understood by referring to the human–environment–activity relationship. To understand the implications of this perspective this chapter first briefly contrasts the ecological approach with the traditional approach before outlining the ecological framework. The notion of adventure sport is sometimes used to frame the examination of adventure.

Traditional theoretical approaches have focused on participation in activities described as *dangerous, reckless, unhealthy,* or *harmful* to participants (Brymer & Schweitzer, 2017; Immonen et al., 2017., 2018). Approaches to understanding psychology in adventure contexts have revealed a classic 'organismic asymmetry' or bias towards seeking internalised explanation within an individual (see Dunwoody, 2007 and Davids & Araújo, 2010 for examples in psychology and sport science). An organismic asymmetry may emphasise individual and cognitive structures, as exemplified by the excessive focus on personality traits (Self et al., 2007), thrill-seeking (Breivik, 2011; Rossi & Cereatti, 1993) and risk-taking (Laurendeau, 2006, 2008) tendencies to explain behaviour, decision-making, or performance regulation of individuals. This somewhat narrow focus has led to definitions and views, where participation is often seen as pathological and a platform for taking socially unacceptable risks. However, a growing body of research has revealed numerous physical, psychological, and social health and wellbeing benefits of adventure (Appelqvist-Schmidlechner et al., 2021; Immonen et al., 2017). Conceptualising adventure as solely dangerous, pathological, highly risky, unhealthy, or practiced by individuals with deviant personalities is based on over-simplified conclusions about the putative motives and psychological aspects of participants that stem from a weak theoretical approach and a reductionist research paradigm.

First, in contemporary research, activities requiring high levels of self-knowledge, personal skills, training, commitment, environmental knowledge, and task knowledge, such as big mountain snowboarding or skiing, are consistently confused with activities that require no previous experience or knowledge of the activity or environment, such as commodified white-water rafting or bungee jumping. The difference between the two types of activities is framed by more and less opportunity for participant *self-regulation* (relying on perception, action, cognition in the form of problem solving and decision-making). Findings from studies (for instance on motivations or risk-perceptions) of individual participants in instructor-led, commodified activities, may not generalise to understanding participation in activities such as high-altitude mountaineering, off-piste ski journeys or self-regulated sea kayaking expeditions. Differences in self-regulation opportunities by individuals is an important notion to consider when recruiting research participants from several sports or activity categories into the same study of adventure experiences.

Second, a wide spectrum of (positive) outcomes and motives for participation have been reported by participants. These include: increased positive psychological outcomes, such as resilience and self-efficacy (Brymer & Schweitzer, 2013; Mackenzie et al., 2011), experiences of connection with nature (Brymer & Oades, 2009; Varley, 2011), increased physical activity levels (Clough et al., 2016), relieving boredom and social relationships (Kerr & Mackenzie, 2012), pushing personal boundaries and overcoming fear (Allman et al., 2009; Brymer & Oades, 2009), enjoyable kinaesthetic sensations (Varley, 2011), control, mastery and skill (Allman et al., 2009), specific goal achievement (Willig, 2008), contribution to deep friendships (Frühauf et al., 2017; Wiersma, 2014), overcoming challenge (Frühauf et al., 2017; Kerr & Mackenzie, 2012), positive transformational experiences (Brymer & Schweitzer, 2017; Holmbom et al., 2017) and opportunities to fulfil basic psychological needs of autonomy, relatedness and competence (Clough et al., 2016). This diversity of effects indicates that attempts to describe all forms and participation styles of adventure under the umbrella of definitions such as "high-risk" or "lifestyle-sports" are fundamentally misleading. In addition, as this diversity exemplifies, outcomes cannot be understood solely as pathological or unhealthy for participants.

Third, adventure activities differ in terms of activity duration and intensity, and it is important to note that this can lead to different interaction effects on behaviour or experiences. For example, an expedition to Everest might take weeks (and months of planning), which exposes individuals to prolonged periods of environmental, social, and psychological uncertainty, whereas the performance window in some organisational- or instructor-led activities might only last a few seconds or minutes. This notion sets specific requirements for methodological approaches and eligibility criteria of research participants. Fourth, in contrast to previous assumptions, participants represent a broad demographic, including males and females of various age ranges and education and income levels (Creyer et al., 2003), suggesting that characterisations of groupings for data interpretation, such as "youth sports", need to be seriously reconsidered as encompassing descriptions.

In relation to a sporting context, adventure can be defined as "constantly evolving forms of activities" that are not usually limited by organisational structures, externally codified rules and regulations or regulated performance environments (social and physical). Adventure entails "activities which flourish through creative exploration of novel movement experiences, continuously expanding and evolving beyond predetermined environmental, physical, psychological or sociocultural boundaries" (Immonen et al., 2017, p.1). The most important defining feature of adventure is that the environment is unconstrained by externally pretrained boundaries. This means that participants need to be highly attuned to information in the environment to make effective decisions, to self-regulate to achieve the performance goals they set, or even just to avoid injury (Immonen et al., 2018).

From psychological and existential points of view, what makes the difference is the exquisite, emerging experiences achieved through these specific participation styles, and the ensuing changes in ways individuals explore, experience, and perceive the world, their everyday life, and fundamental human values (Brymer & Schweitzer, 2017; Holmbom et al., 2017; Immonen et al., 2018). Research has shown that the profound person-environment relationship developed through adventure can act as a facilitator to a deep, positive understanding of *self* and its place in relation to the environment (Albrecht, 2012; Brymer & Gray, 2009). For example, experiencing extreme elation or intense fear can be a potentially meaningful and constructive event in the lives of participants, having implications as a potentially developmental and transformative process (Brymer & Schweitzer, 2013). Importantly, these changes are most likely to occur when specific performances, often by facing danger, injury or potential death, make deep existential structures visible and available to be experienced.

According to insights from contemporary phenomenological research, these changes are not as readily available within traditional, highly regulated activities. Adopting a phenomenological account and an ecological dynamics rationale, adventure consists of an "inimitable person-environment relationship with exquisite affordances for ultimate perception and movement experiences, leading to existential reflection and self-actualisation as framed by the human form of life" (Immonen et al., 2018, p. 1274). This kind of demarcation between activity categories might be useful, for example in research, when considering eligibility criteria from which to include participants. For instance, in a sporting context BASE jumping or Free Solo climbing might align well together due to their similar historical, psychological, or socio-cultural distinctions within their own specific socio-cultural frames of references, whereas bungee jumping or drag racing are probably representative of different characteristics. To emphasise, adventure, including sports in extreme and non-extreme ways of participation, clearly requires specific skills, and personal devotion and commitment to develop necessary skills. This is not the case when individuals participate in commodified activities such as bungee jumping, where preparation and specific skills are unnecessary. Understanding these nuances is crucial for recognising how a variety of socio-cultural values have constrained emerging participation (Immonen et al., 2017).

Constraints, Affordances, and Form of Life in the Adventure Context

Previous psychological research of human behaviour in adventure has emphasised the dualistic view that the individual and their surrounding environment are fundamentally considered as two separate systems. This perspective stands in stark contrast with the ecological approach to human behaviour. In this section, we will explain how our understanding of adventure can be enhanced through *the ecological dynamics* framework. The most fundamental difference to traditional approaches to understanding human behaviour is that the ecological approach advocates the relevance of adopting an individual–environment scale of analysis (Button et al., 2020). Ecological dynamics conceptually recognises humans as dynamic, complex systems constantly interacting with other systems (Button et al., 2020; Komar et al., 2021). As opposed to traditional approaches, the individual and their social, physical, and cultural environments are fundamentally seen as intrinsically and deeply linked, nested systems, where behaviours of individuals self-organise over time under interacting *constraints* (Button et al., 2020; Hristovski et al., 2011; Vaughan et al., 2019). Instead of being imposed by a pre-existing, inherent structure such as a specific personality trait or an individual's inherent risk-taking tendency, behaviour emerges from this confluence of interacting constraints. Inherent tendencies and environmental and task constraints continually provide the boundary conditions over different timescales that shape emerging behaviours on an individual's path towards achieving specific tasks or goals (Button et al., 2020). In an ecological dynamics rationale, perceptions, cognitions and actions are conceptualised as self-organised, interacting phenomena, emerging from the continuously dynamic interplay of a performer's action capabilities (*effectivities*) and opportunities for action (*affordances*) (Gibson, 1979) available in a specific performance environment (*ecological niche*) (Araujo et al., 2006; Ross, Gupta, & Sanders, 2018; Woods, Rothwell, Rudd, Robertson, & Davids, 2021).

Constraints

Newell (1986) defined *constraints* as boundaries or features that shape the emergence of each individuals' cognitions, actions, and decision-making processes. Three key categories of constraints include *individual constraints*, which can be structural (e.g., height, weight, body shape, technical abilities, connectivity of synapses in the brain), functional (e.g., motivations, attitudes, emotions, cognitions, perceptions) and historical (e.g., development to tolerate lack of comfort, experiential knowledge through past experiences of accidents) characteristics of an individual (Button et al., 2020). Individuals are described as active agents with different personal characteristics or features which may shape the distinct strategies used to coordinate actions and solve problems in uncertain environments (Dashper & Brymer, 2019).

Task constraints include specific 'rules' associated with activities, including task goals, objects, equipment, surfaces, boundary areas such as nets or posts or instructional features (Seifert et al., 2017). Different to traditional activities, adventure is predominantly free of organisational frameworks, regulated competitive structures or rule-bound task constraints (Immonen et al., 2017; Immonen et al., 2018). Indeed, as discussed earlier, the freedom from regulatory environmental constraints can be seen as the most fundamental definitive characteristic of adventure (Collins & Carson, 2021; Immonen et al., 2017). However, adventure often involves the participant interfacing with a challenging environment using technology and equipment in their interactions, exemplified in snowboarding, backcountry skiing, canoeing and mountaineering.

Environmental constraints can be physical (e.g., weather, ambient light, temperature, gravity, the shape and size of stopper wave in expedition canoeing), or socio-cultural (e.g., values, family or peer support, (sub)cultural norms or expectations) (Button et al., 2020; Immonen et al., 2017). In adventure, a definitive feature is that physical constraints are not restricted by predetermined environmental boundaries (such as courts or arenas in invasion sports), but can involve surrounding natural conditions, such as characteristics of mountain terrain, river rapids, a track or trail, weather, visibility and snowpack features and stability. For example, in an adventure sports context delineations between traditional sports and adventure sports go well beyond the competitive vs. non-competitive dichotomy (Collins & Carson, 2021). From the ecological point of view, the inherent uncertainty of natural adventure environments (as opposed to stable manicured environments, such as indoor arenas in tennis and gymnastics), inevitably stands for the instability or dynamicity of information sources that surround the performing individual at all times, available for use to functionally adapt and regulate their actions and behaviours.

Affordances

One of the fundamental building blocks of ecological dynamics is the theory of *affordances*, originating in the work of James Gibson (1979). The concept *affordance* refers to opportunities or invitations for actions that emerge as individuals interact with critical information from the environment (Withagen et al., 2012; Withagen et al., 2017). For instance, different surfaces, substances, objects, or other individuals in the environment can *afford* different possibilities for actions in different people relative to their individual capacities, needs, values and motivations acting as constraints. *Effectivities* are complementary action capabilities that can help each individual realise affordances in coherent forms of behaviour (Davids et al., 2016), i.e., the skills, capacities and capabilities an individual can possess within a specific form of life (Peacock et al., 2017). Such coherent behaviour is exemplified by a skilled big mountain skier (attuned to a specific *field of affordances* in a snowy environment through experience and learning). Such an individual might choose a steeper and more exposed line to descend the mountain face, controlling the speed with line choices of carving turns instead of slowing the speed down with skidded turns. Or they may prefer organising a more technical action when jumping off a cliff, compared to a novice (for whom the same *landscape of affordances* is available) (Rietveld & Kiverstein, 2014). Importantly, effectivities might be limited or enabled by environmental constraints, such as natural characteristics of a performance environment or values, social habits and attitudes (Peacock et al., 2017). When the description of the environment is founded in affordances, it changes the description from physical to functional. That is, the environment is described in terms of what it offers a performer, "for good or ill" (Gibson, 1979). In ecological psychology, this idea signifies that when perceiving possibilities for action (such as safe or unsafe passages of travel in the mountains, rivers or trails), one would directly perceive their "goodness" or "badness" in relation to one's skills, values, needs, intentions, motives, emotions, interests, and goals.

Adventure Psychology and a Form of Life

Wittgensteinian's (1953) concept, *form of life,* refers to the potential and common behaviours available to a specific group of organisms (such as a group of humans or a species of fish), influencing how the group interacts with and within the world around them (Peacock et al., 2017; Rietveld & Kiverstein, 2014). For humans, effectivities are not only relative to a particular individual perceiving or detecting affordances, but they have an existence relative to a set of skills and capacities available in specific practice, such as within a particular adventure niche, and, to the abilities available in a human form of life as a whole. Therefore, a form of life implies that socio-cultural practices of humans (constituted by skills, values, beliefs, habits, customs, attitudes and so forth) constrain the emergence of specific behavioural patterns (Ingold, 2002; Wittgenstein, 1953), such as preferred or established ways of acting physically, intentions, or attitudes towards risk-taking within the socio-cultural frame of reference of a specific adventure niche. When individuals perceive affordances of an ecological niche as feasible possibilities for actions, they will effectively orient to, and potentially start regulating their behaviour in relation to, the situationally salient affordances (Chemero, 2018; Pyysiäinen, 2021; Withagen et al., 2012).

Considering the crucial role of socio-cultural constraints on behaviours, the individual–environment system can be characterised as an ecological niche that arises from, and mutually co-creates, a form of life (Immonen et al., 2018; Vaughan et al., 2019). In this line of thinking, each individual–environment system co-exists as an open, dynamic system, meaning it is nested within, and capable of exchanging energy and information with the surrounding ecology at micro and macro scales (Bronfenbrenner, 2005; Vaughan et al., 2019). The nestedness of affordances is understood as multiple affordances that exist in any given situation, and the consequential possibilities of humans to choose among them. Given that affordances reflect the relational nature of multiple properties of individuals as well as the multiple properties of (physical, social and cultural) environments, affordances are considered to be nested in the context of other affordances. This implies that an individual affordance may be superordinate or subordinate to other affordances (Seifert et al.; Wagman & Stoffregen, 2020). For example, a mountaineer ascending a mountain face, might be able to find a route up towards the summit (i.e., subordinate affordance), but fail to pass the "crux", such as a steep and unstable icefall (i.e., superordinate affordance), as they may not have the required skills to do so.

The notion of affordances offers a valuable perspective, especially when examining performance or learning, as it changes the perspective away from a strictly biomechanical, cognitive or physical lens, towards a more relational focus of attunement to information available in the psycho-socio-material environment, specifically highlighting the uncertainty of typical environments in adventure contexts. From an ecological perspective, expertise in adventure can thus be understood as a skilled engagement with the specific banks of available environmental information. This is an important notion from the point of view of practical implications since training outside of the specific context (such as in a stable practice environment which is non-representative of the unstable informational properties of the actual performance environment) has been shown to be ineffective from the perspective of development of skilled actions in multiple traditional domains (Komar et al., 2021). In other words: context is everything. For instance, learning to swim in a swimming pool might not prepare individuals' water competence sufficiently for negotiating different aquatic environments such as a river or ocean surf (Button, Button, Jackson, Cotter, & Maraj, 2020).

Deriving from the work of Vaughan et al. (2019) on football, the dominant form of life (specific way of doing things) in (national, regional, or trending) adventure niches might be conceptualised as deeply acculturated, socially accepted, and often taken for granted. This idea is exemplified in the frequency on the use of helmets and other safety gear in adventure sports or a social push against or towards attending to structured safety or rescue training in whitewater kayaking communities. In this line of thinking individuals' or groups' ways of acting and making decisions are seen as socio-cultural artefacts (Rossing et al., 2019), embodying the manifestation of the relational environment. Ignoring the role of socio-cultural constraints as an inherent feature of participation style limits capacity to comprehend adventure. It fails to understand the importance of nuanced experiences and actions of participants emerging from the interaction of constraints in specific situations and contexts. Thus, researchers and practitioners, trained within the traditional positivist, reductionist research paradigms, might gain an ontologically limited picture of the complexity of human behaviour, experiences, and development of skills and expertise (Vaughan et al., 2019) in adventure. This is arguably a serious limitation on the evaluation and interpretation of data, syntheses of study findings or general study designs.

Tim Ingold's (2002) views of embodied skills of humans as fundamental attributes of cultural variation can help us to distinguish several useful levels of analysis when examining adventure and drawing demarcations between niches. Three levels of analysis are exemplified through the evolution of niches with a basis in an environment which affords gliding and sliding possibilities for people with an adequate behavioural repertoire (Orth et al., 2018). These are: (1) Human forms of life have general action and movement capabilities due to phylogenetic and ontogenetic development processes over millions of years (contrasting with development of, for instance, birds or fish). Also, there has been the potential to collectively manufacture and utilise equipment and tools, which afford gliding on different surfaces in different contexts (such as white-water kayaking as recreation, canoeing as transporting food, locomotion or locomotion-aid in fishing and hunting). (2) There exist specific and distinguishing socio-cultural practices i.e., regularities in the performances, behaviours and experiences of groups of people who utilise gliding and sliding movements recreationally or competitively on specific contexts, situations and geological locations (such as adventurous sea kayaking in open ocean space or kayak expeditions utilising specific features of white water, such as stopper waves to perform creative movements). (3) A more detailed analysis indicates that skilled engagement with affordances is highly individualised, diverse, and multi-dimensional within a specific socio-cultural frame of reference.

Researchers and practitioners need to be clear on the contexts framing each kind of activity being studied and how the results may be generalised, transferred or utilised through this kind of comprehensive background analysis. From an ecological perspective, the important point is that the development of skills is a fundamental component in how niches are mutually formed and evolved through person-environment interactions. Additionally, the evolution of a niche mutually affords a physical, psychological, and socio-cultural environment for individuals and groups to become attuned to and, therefore, to utilise available affordances and develop skills even further.

Bronfenbrenner's (2005) bio-ecological model provides a reference framework to zoom in on different levels of an inherently interconnected and dynamic, complex system (see Figure 6.1). For example, neurobiological, psycho-social, and socio-cognitive subsystems of an individual adventurer, perceiving and

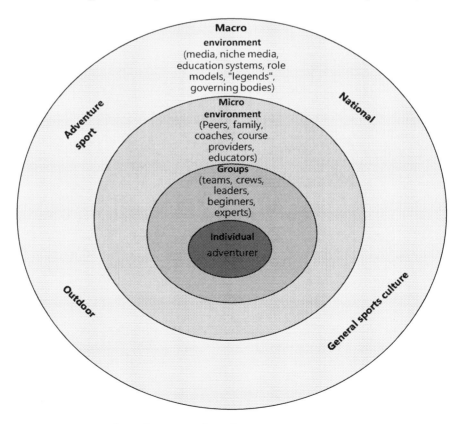

FIGURE 6.1 An ecological context of an adventurer.

acting within the contexts of local / global adventure niches are enclosed by the ecologies of: (i) broader action, adventure, and extreme sport cultures, (ii) (local and global) outdoor culture(s), (iii) national and global (sub)culture(s), (iv) human forms of life as a whole, local, and global political-, economic-, geological-, (v), weather systems and so on.

Characterisation of Skill and Skill Transfer in Adventure Contexts

In traditional terms, skilled performances can be defined and measured quantitively, e.g., in units of time, distance or score or in comparison to other participants. However, this kind of assessment makes it difficult to comprehensively understand skill in adventure. Specifically, the meaning of concepts such as "success", "winning" or "losing" are challenging to externally, or quantitatively, define in adventure contexts. This idea can be seen as another identifying aspect of adventure, as participants might need to figure out for themselves what success means in their given activity. For instance, "summitting Everest" may be about getting up and back down safely, not just reaching the summit. As rules typically do not govern how to win or play in adventure, the structured competition perspective does not provide a very fruitful approach to measure or define skilled or successful performance (Immonen et al., 2017).

In adventure, the functionality of skill (i.e., how effectively task goals are achieved) partially depends on subtle interactions of task and personal constraints such as originality, collective agreement, and interpretation (Immonen et al., 2017). For instance, a climber's attempt to climb a new route using quickdraws as 'holds' for pulling movements might not get recognised as 'successful climbing' among sport climbers. These interactions also concern the physical environment. For example, how a kayaker decides to descent a big rapid is partially about 'reading' the water flows and currents and seeing what the rapid will allow (in terms of affordances, these are examples of socio-cultural tendencies within a form of life which can significantly constrain the behaviours of individuals or reinforce established and preferred ones). Importantly, specific social morals and values (due to historical and social constraints) might emerge to invite participants to function by challenging rules and norms to create their own, distinctive style of movement or unique approaches towards the specific environment. Therefore, development of expertise in adventure requires a deep contextualised understanding of underpinning socio-cultural constraints on functional practices (i.e., based on their usefulness, effectiveness, appropriateness, or adequacy), supported by knowledge of how to diverge from them with innovation and novelty (Immonen et al., 2017).

The fundamental challenge of becoming an expert adventurer is that a typical performance environment is naturally uncertain, unconstrained, dynamic, and often hazardous, meaning that there are not always possibilities to perform and practice safely in that environment. For example, the avalanche hazard in a mountain environment affords no serious mistakes during the learning of skiing locomotion in avalanche-prone territory, due to the obvious reality that any mistake in judgement or decision-making can be fatal. This type of affordance landscape sets a unique requirement that learning environments must allow safe exploration and possibilities to learn through trial and error. Accordingly, boundary conditions of practice and training need to allow these specific skills to be functionally adapted for use in, or transferred to, natural performance environments.

Representative Design in Adventure

Egon Brunswik's (1956) concept, *representative design* refers to conditions and information in psychology experiments. It emphasises that as precisely as participants of an experiment need to be representative of those to which the study wishes to generalise, as rigorously the experimental task constraints must represent the environmental constraints to which they are to be generalised (Brunswik, 1956; Pinder et al., 2011). This idea of representativeness is a particular concern for the study of human behaviour in adventure contexts. From an applied point of view, if experimental tasks do not factor in representativeness of the context, they may not allow the correct analysis of the critical aspects of the skills required. Nor will they allow any further development of intervention or training tasks to achieve these aims (Pinder et al., 2011).

Pinder et al. (2011) further developed Brunswik's original idea and proposed the concept of *representative learning design* (Pinder et al., 2011). It emphasises that for principles of representative design to be applied to the design of functional interventions, practice, and training tasks, it is crucial to acknowledge that different sources of perceptual information present different affordances for different individuals. In other words, there is a high relevance on how adequately the constraints of practice tasks replicate the performance environment so that they allow participants to detect affordances for action and couple actions to key information sources within those specific settings (Pinder et al., 2011).

Recently, Woods and colleagues (Woods et al., 2021) put forth the concept of *representative co-design* to emphasise how experiential knowledge of experienced participants can be utilised in enriching the designs of learning environments. With increasing experience and expertise, performers evolve in their decision-making by becoming increasingly competent at realising the most soliciting or inviting affordances within their ecological niche (Withagen et al., 2012, 2017; Woods et al., 2021). Representative co-design is predicated on Gibson's (1966) distinguishing ideas on *knowledge of* and *knowledge about* the environment. *Knowledge of* the environment refers to understanding of the use of affordances for regulating interactions within a performance environment, analogous to a "first person point of view" (relation of an individual athlete's unique intrinsic dynamics and environment and task constraints). Whereas *knowledge about* the environment facilitates an internalised symbolic manifestation of the environment available (metaphorically, a point of view of a sports commentator analysing performance in climbing competition). It might be especially useful for practitioners to utilise this idea and emphasise this crucial distinction by (co-)designing, with experienced and skilled athletes, representative learning activities that specifically develop each participant's *knowledge of* a performance environment (Woods et al., 2021).

Conclusions and Implications for Research and Practice

An ecological dynamics rationale can help us understand the rich and diverse range of adventure contexts. It provides a holistic, transdisciplinary framework, adaptable to zoom in on multiple perspectives and different time scales and levels of the person-environment system. It can also provide a fruitful point of departure for the application of Adventure Psychology at a level of the human form of life, within a form of life as a specific socio-cultural frame of reference (such as a niche of mountaineers) and, at a more detailed and nuanced, individual level (e.g., when investigating experiences or learning).

Through an ecological framework, it is possible to achieve a nuanced perspective with more detailed definitions of activity categories (such as adventure and extreme sports) and characterisations of specific activities (such as sport climbing and trad climbing). This is especially important when recruiting representative research participants, when comparing data from multiple studies, or when examining behaviours, motivations, cognitions, decision-making or perceptions and actions of humans at an individual level in relation to specific contexts and situations. Adventure can be broadly understood from a multitude of perspectives, capturing different forms of life specific to humans, enabling experiences of freedom from everyday life, opportunities to undergo special transformative experiences, possibilities to explore one's physical and psychological boundaries, and where competition can also play a specific, but not a defining role. It is possible to see that these activities have a potential to be utilised more broadly to enhance psychological and physical health and wellbeing in modern life.

Through the notion of form of life and insights from phenomenological accounts, adventure can also be understood as a "world" in a similar vein to the worlds of science, music, or art, which can offer multiplicity of ways for individuals to experience and perceive the socio-material world in a unique and meaningful way, expanding the perspective to broadly understand each adventure context as a type of form of life specific to being human (Immonen et al., 2018). Therefore, adventure can act as media for humans to engage with the environing world, to experiment with one's physical or psychological capacities and, ultimately, to explore what it inherently and fundamentally means to be a human. This point of view requires a multidisciplinary lens to scrutinise adventure as a form of life specific to humans, clearly distinguishable from traditional and predominantly competitive sports. This point of view also shows why adventure should be fundamental across all human experiences and embedded into systems such as education, health, environment studies, etc.

For researchers it is critically important to get a detailed grasp of historical and socio-cultural constraints of activities under examination. This is a fundamental attribute of the ecological lens, since understanding the situational and contextual horizons of cognitions, perceptions, actions, and experiences of individuals is an essential foundation of the individual–environment scale of analysis. From ontological and epistemological perspectives, there is an evident need for a more balanced composition of methodologies, since positivist baseline assumptions and research paradigms might not, and have not, been able to fully capture the complexity of these issues, and therefore, to appropriately guide the enhancement of sound, evidence-based, practical implications.

When there are potential dangers or hazards to avoid in a performance environment, it is crucial to consider transfer of learning and acquisition of adequate skills (through representative learning designs) required for safe participation. For these designs to be effective, they need to maintain the functional processes of perceptual attunement to information in the environment (affordances) in relation to specific situations and contexts. From the ecological perspective, skilled practitioners are thus required to have a deep and nuanced understanding of the interacting constraints of the specific activity in question.

References

Albrecht, G. (2012). Psychoterratic conditions in a scientific and technological world. In P. H. Kahn, Jr and P. H. Hasbach (Eds.), *Ecopsychology: science, totems, and the technological species* (pp. 241–264) Cambridge, MA: The MIT Press.

Allman, T. L., Mittelstaedt, R. D., Martin, B., & Goldenberg, M. (2009). Exploring the motivations of BASE jumpers: Extreme sport enthusiasts. *Journal of Sport & Tourism*, 14(4), 229–247.

Appelqvist-Schmidlechner, K., Kyröläinen, H., Häkkinen, A., Vasankari, T., Mäntysaari, M., Honkanen, T., & Vaara, J. P. (2021). Childhood sports participation is associated with health-related quality of life in young men: A retrospective cross-sectional study. *Frontiers in Sports and Active Living, 3*, 74.

Araujo, D., Davids, K., & Hristovski, R. (2006). The ecological dynamics of decision making in sport. *Psychology of Sport and Exercise, 7*(6), 653–676.

Breivik, G. (2010). Trends in adventure sports in a post-modern society. *Sport in Society, 13*, 260–273.

Breivik, G. (2011). Dangerous play with the elements: towards a phenomenology of risk sports. *Sport, Ethics and Philosophy, 5*(3), 314–330, https://doi.org/10.1080/17511321.2011.602585

Bronfenbrenner, U. (2005). *Making human beings human: Bioecological perspectives on human development*. Sage.

Brunswik, E. (1956). *Perception and the representative design of psychological experiments*. University of California Press.

Brymer, E., & Gray, T. (2009). Dancing with nature: Rhythm and harmony in extreme sport participation. *Journal of Adventure Education & Outdoor Learning, 9*(2), 135–149.

Brymer, E., & Oades, L. G. (2009). Extreme sports: A positive transformation in courage and humility. *Journal of Humanistic Psychology, 49*(1), 114–126.

Brymer, E., & Schweitzer, R. (2013). Extreme sports are good for your health: A phenomenological understanding of fear and anxiety in extreme sport. *Journal of Health Psychology, 18*(4), 477–487.

Brymer, E., & Schweitzer, R. D. (2017). Evoking the ineffable: The phenomenology of extreme sports. *Psychology of Consciousness: Theory, Research, and Practice, 4*(1), 63.

Button, C., Button, A. J., Jackson, A., Cotter, J. D., & Maraj, B. (2020). Teaching foundational aquatic skills to children in open water environments. *International Journal of Aquatic Research and Education, 13*(1), 1.

Button, C., Seifert, L., Chow, J. Y., Davids, K., & Araujo, D. (2020). *Dynamics of skill acquisition: An ecological dynamics approach*. Human Kinetics Publishers.

Chemero, A. (2018). An outline of a theory of affordances. In K. S. Jones (Ed.), *How shall affordances be refined? Four perspectives* (pp. 181–195). Routledge.

Clough, P., Mackenzie, S. H., Mallabon, L., & Brymer, E. (2016). Adventurous physical activity environments: A mainstream intervention for mental health. *Sports Medicine, 46*(7), 963–968.

Collins, L., & Carson, H. J. (2021). Proposing a new conceptualisation for modern sport based on environmental and regulatory constraints: Implications for research, coach education and professional practice. *Journal of Adventure Education and Outdoor Learning, 22*(3), 228–238. https://doi.org/10.1080/14729679.2021.1902829

Creyer, E., Ross, W., & Evers, D. (2003). Risky recreation: An exploration of factors influencing the likelihood of participation and the effects of experience. *Leisure Studies, 22*(3), 239–253.

Dashper, K., & Brymer, E. (2019). An ecological-phenomenological perspective on multispecies leisure and the horse-human relationship in events. *Leisure Studies, 38*(3), 394–407.

Davids, K., Araújo, D., & Brymer, E. (2016). Designing affordances for health-enhancing physical activity and exercise in sedentary individuals. *Sports Medicine, 46*(7), 933–938.

Frühauf, A., Hardy, W. A., Pfoestl, D., Hoellen, F., & Kopp, M. (2017). A qualitative approach on motives and aspects of risks in freeriding. *Frontiers in Psychology, 8*, 1998.

Frühauf, A., Zenzmaier, J., & Kopp, M. (2020). Does age matter? A qualitative comparison of motives and aspects of risk in adolescent and adult freeriders. *Journal of Sports Science & Medicine, 19*(1), 112.

Gibson. (1979). *The ecological approach to visual perception: Classic edition*. Psychology Press.

Holmbom, M., Brymer, E., & Schweitzer, R. D. (2017). Transformations through proximity flying: A phenomenological investigation. *Frontiers in Psychology, 8*, 1831. doi: 10.3389/fpsyg.2017.01831

Hristovski, R., Davids, K., Araujo, D., & Passos, P. (2011). Constraints-induced emergence of functional novelty in complex neurobiological systems: A basis for creativity in sport. *Nonlinear Dynamics-Psychology and Life Sciences, 15*(2), 175.

Immonen, T., Brymer, E., Davids, K., Liukkonen, J., & Jaakkola, T. (2018). An ecological conceptualization of extreme sports. *Frontiers in Psychology, 9*, 1274.

Immonen, T., Brymer, E., Orth, D., Davids, K., Feletti, F., Liukkonen, J., & Jaakkola, T. (2017). Understanding action and adventure sports participation – an ecological dynamics perspective. *Sports Medicine-Open, 3*(1), 1–7.

Ingold, T. (2002). *The perception of the environment: Essays on livelihood, dwelling and skill*. Routledge.

Kerr, J. H., & Mackenzie, S. H. (2012). Multiple motives for participating in adventure sports. *Psychology of Sport and Exercise, 13*(5), 649–657.

Komar, J., Ong, C. Y. Y., Choo, C. Z. Y., & Chow, J. Y. (2021). Perceptual-motor skill transfer: Multidimensionality and specificity of both general and specific transfers. *Acta Psychologica, 217*, 103321.

Laurendeau, J. (2006). "He didn't go in doing a skydive": Sustaining the illusion of control in an edgework activity. *Sociological Perspectives, 49*(4), 583–605.

Laurendeau, J. (2008). "Gendered risk regimes": A theoretical consideration of edgework and gender. *Sociology of Sport Journal, 25*(3), 293–309.

Mackenzie, S. H., Hodge, K., & Boyes, M. (2011). Expanding the flow model in adventure activities: A reversal theory perspective. *Journal of Leisure Research, 43*(4), 519–544.

Newell, K. (1986). Constraints on the development of coordination. In M. G. Wade, & H. T. A. Whiting (Eds.), *Motor Development in Children: Aspects of Coordination and Control*. Dordrecht: Martinus Nijhoff. http://dx.doi.org/10.1007/978-94-009-4460-2_19

Orth, D., Davids, K., Chow, J., Brymer, E., & Seifert, L. (2018). Behavioral repertoire influences the rate and nature of learning in climbing: Implications for individualized learning design in preparation for extreme sports participation. *Frontiers in Psychology, 9*, 949.

Peacock, S., Brymer, E., Davids, K., & Dillon, M. (2017). An ecological dynamics perspective on adventure tourism. *Tourism Review International, 21*(3), 307–316.

Pinder, R. A., Davids, K., Renshaw, I., & Araújo, D. (2011). Representative learning design and functionality of research and practice in sport. *Journal of Sport and Exercise Psychology, 33*(1), 146–155.

Pyysiäinen, J. (2021). Sociocultural affordances and enactment of agency: A transactional view. *Theory & Psychology, 31*(4), 491–512. https://doi.org/10.1177/0959354321989431

Rietveld, E., & Kiverstein, J. (2014). A rich landscape of affordances. *Ecological Psychology, 26*(4), 325–352.

Ross, E., Gupta, L., & Sanders, L. (2018). When research leads to learning, but not action in high performance sport. *Progress in Brain Research, 240*, 201–217.

Rossi, B., & Cereatti, L. (1993). The sensation seeking in mountain athletes as assessed by Zuckerman's sensation seeking scale. *International Journal of Sport Psychology. 24*(4), 417–431.

Rossing, N. N., Skrubbeltrang, L. S., Bonderup, M. Z., & Karbing, D. S. (2019). Where do elite youth football players come from? *Dansk Sportsmedicin.*

Seifert, L., Dicks, M., Wittmann, F., & Wolf, P. (2021). The perception of nested affordances: An examination of expert climbers. *Psychology of Sport and Exercise, 52*, 101843.

Seifert, L., Orth, D., Boulanger, J., Dovgalecs, V., Hérault, R., & Davids, K. (2014). Climbing skill and complexity of climbing wall design: Assessment of jerk as a novel indicator of performance fluency. *Journal of Applied Biomechanics, 30*(5), 619–625.

Seifert, L., Orth, D., Button, C., Brymer, E., & Davids, K. (2017). An ecological dynamics framework for the acquisition of perceptual–motor skills in climbing. In F. Feletti (Ed.), *Extreme Sports Medicine*. Cham: Springer. https://doi.org/10.1007/978-3-319-28265-7_28

Seifert, L., Wattebled, L., L'Hermette, M., Bideault, G., Herault, R., & Davids, K. (2013). Skill transfer, affordances and dexterity in different climbing environments. *Human Movement Science, 32*(6), 1339–1352.

Self, D. R., De Vries Henry, E., Findley, C. S., & Reilly, E. (2007). Thrill seeking: The type T personality and extreme sports. *International Journal of Sport Management and Marketing, 2*(1–2), 175–190.

Varley, P. J. (2011). Sea kayakers at the margins: The liminoid character of contemporary adventures. *Leisure Studies, 30*(1), 85–98.

Vaughan, J., Mallett, C. J., Davids, K., Potrac, P., & López-Felip, M. A. (2019). Developing creativity to enhance human potential in sport: A wicked transdisciplinary challenge. *Frontiers in Psychology, 10*, 2090. doi: 10.3389/fpsyg.2019.02090

Wagman, J. B., & Stoffregen, T. A. (2020). It doesn't add up: Nested affordances for reaching are perceived as a complex particular. *Attention, Perception, & Psychophysics, 82*(8), 3832–3841.

Wiersma, L. D. (2014). A phenomenological investigation of the psychology of big-wave surfing at Maverick's. *The Sport Psychologist, 28*(2), 151–163.

Willig, C. (2008). A phenomenological investigation of the experience of taking part in Extreme sports. *Journal of Health Psychology, 13*(5), 690–702.

Withagen, R., Araújo, D., & de Poel, H. J. (2017). Inviting affordances and agency. *New Ideas in Psychology, 45*, 11–18.

Withagen, R., De Poel, H. J., Araújo, D., & Pepping, G. (2012). Affordances can invite behavior: Reconsidering the relationship between affordances and agency. *New Ideas in Psychology, 30*(2), 250–258.

Wittgenstein, L. (1953). *Philosophical investigations*. John Wiley & Sons.

Woods, C. T., & Davids, K. (2021). "You look at an ocean; I see the rips, hear the waves, and feel the currents": Dwelling and the growth of enskiled inhabitant knowledge. *Ecological Psychology, 33*(3–4), 279–296, 1–18.

Woods, C. T., Rothwell, M., Rudd, J., Robertson, S., & Davids, K. (2021). Representative co-design: Utilising a source of experiential knowledge for athlete development and performance preparation. *Psychology of Sport and Exercise, 52*, 101804.

7
FEAR IN EXTENDED ADVENTURES
The Case of Expedition Mountaineering

Katrina Kessler and Eric Brymer

From the Point of View of an Adventurer: A Man Walks Alone

A man walks alone on his fifth day traversing the tundra of Alaska. A small airplane has dropped him off several days prior, equipped with just a backpack of bare necessities. He has no gun and no satellite phone, as his quest is to immerse as deeply as possible into the natural world as his ultimate guide in harmony with his innate capacities from many years of experience. He has mastered navigation and deep wilderness survival, and has built up intimate knowledge of the tundra, so he sets off on his spiritual adventure. His mission is to walk the same documented path walked by an aboriginal shamanic healer a century earlier. One day, after an exhausting storm, as the man is checking his navigation and mapped route, he has a feeling that something is not quite right. He repetitively checks his navigation several times over the next few hours, his mind eases somewhat, as he knows cognitively that he is on the right path. Yet he still feels viscerally like something is off-kilter. As the hours pass in the desolate landscape; him as the only human in a radius of perhaps hundreds of hectares, his uneasiness, his sense of the uncanny, the eeriness within him continues to rise despite his frequently checking whether he is still on his planned route. He continues to walk, alone in the vastness of the tundra, knowing if he were to make a mistake in calculations, his bones may very well remain in that tundra indefinitely. He chooses to set up camp for the night; hopefully a good sleep will bring clarity. The next day he rises, shaking from the cold as well as the feeling of fear deep within. His response is to make internal space for the fear, and as he does the fear intensifies, and like a shiver, passes through him, leaving in its wake a clearness of perception that he is actually not on track; he has lost his way, he had incorrectly calculated his navigation the day before. He retraces his steps, taking a full day, and gets back on track, successfully completing his mission. He listened, and fear saved his life.

Fear in Extended Adventures: The Case of Expedition Mountaineering

This chapter discusses the nature of fear in long-haul adventurism, defined as activities requiring several days, weeks, or months to complete, and which typically involve several months or even years of logistics planning, as well as physical and mental preparation. The conceptualisation of the nature of fear discussed in this chapter draws from multiple forms of adventurism, though we focus on expedition mountaineering as an exemplar form of long-haul adventurism to illustrate our hypotheses on the utility of fear in adventure more broadly.

Mountaineering may involve traversing tundra, permafrost, or glaciers; climbing steep mountains covered in snow; or moving through ice caves. Sometimes the term also refers to climbing bare monoliths. The definition of *mountaineering* is evolving, and is increasingly used as an umbrella term for different kinds of activities that use some transferrable skills and equipment within the same kind of geography. For example, climbing up a mountain alpine style (as fast as possible, with as little weight as possible) over the course of several hours, in order to ski down is increasingly referred to as a form of mountaineering (Bortolan et al., 2021). Mountaineers learn to skilfully move through multiple types of terrain, with a focus on safety at all times.

Mountaineering is an inherently dangerous activity, regardless of the skill level of the mountaineer and the general difficulty or ease of any particular venture. Sometimes even relatively easy excursions can suddenly become extremely dangerous when an unanticipated difficulty arises, or when an accident has occurred. Fear is a natural response to mortal danger and the potential for loss of any kind. However, in this chapter we present research which shows that rather than trying to simply endure fear, or push the unpleasant emotion of fear outside of cognitive awareness, expedition mountaineers learn to befriend fear, to listen to fear, and to trust the information given by fear, as doing so not only enhances safety and conserves precious energy, but such a relationship with fear is precisely what allows for the more complex and more extreme forms of expedition mountaineering to be possible at all. This relationship is also apparent in other forms of adventure.

We begin our discussion below with a concise overview of our search for definitions of fear and anxiety in the extant literature; we then condense the common assumptions about the emotion of fear in the context of adventurism. These overviews are followed by a discussion of conclusions drawn from naturalistic research on fear in adventurism, especially mountaineering.

Traditional Definitions of Anxiety and Fear

While it is beyond the scope of this chapter to review the literature in-depth, the following section summarises the traditional positions on anxiety and fear. The fields of animal biology, human neuroscience, and clinical psychology have been studying fear and related concepts, such as anxiety, for at least half a century. Even so, anxiety and fear are still poorly defined, and left entirely undifferentiated in the bulk of the literature in clinical psychology in particular, which some meta-analysts have pointed out is mainly a consequence of psychologists using "fundamentally flawed" measurement tools lacking in construct validity (Sylvers et al., 2011). As one prominent neuroscientist lamented,

> … there is no consensus in the scientific study of fear. Some argue that 'fear' is a psychological construct rather than discoverable through scientific investigation. Others argue that the term 'fear' cannot properly be applied to animals because we cannot know whether they feel afraid. Studies in rodents show that there are highly specific brain circuits for fear, whereas findings from human neuroimaging seem to make the opposite claim.
>
> *(Adolphs, 2013, p. 79)*

However, findings from different fields are not always mutually exclusive, as conclusions seem to intersect on occasion (Sylvers et al., 2011). For example, researchers in multiple fields generally agree that the "main function of fear and anxiety is to act as a signal of danger, threat, or motivational conflict, and to trigger appropriate adaptive responses. For some authors, fear and anxiety are undistinguishable, whereas others believe that they are distinct phenomena" (Steimer, 2002, p. 233).

In the behavioural psychology literature which does differentiate between anxiety and fear, the emotion of fear is purported to be present while the subject is "actively coping with a perceived threat, whereas anxiety results from a threatening situation without an effective means of coping" (Sylvers et al., 2011, p. 124). That is to say, some laboratory-based definitions of anxiety and fear are based entirely on assumptions about the meaning of purely behavioural responses to threats regarding the presence or absence of fight, flight, or freeze responses. Such studies are devoid of phenomenological data that could otherwise be used as a very direct means of testing the veracity of the psychological assumptions based on behavioural observations. In the absence of phenomenological data to verify psychological hypotheses, such studies postulate that the subjects under observation are not experiencing fear, but rather anxiety in the form of hyper-vigilance (Sylvers et al., 2011).

In order to operationalise a differentiation between anxiety and fear, some animal behaviour researchers differentiate according to whether a threat is immediate or anticipated, and whether the same threat is obvious or oblique

(Catherall, 2003). In contrast, some of the neuroscientific literature conceptualises anxiety and fear as distinct emotions involving different neurological pathways and cognitive responses rather than delineation and proximity of threat as the means of differentiation (Sylvers et al., 2011).

More recent research on fear is beginning to include the subjective experience of research participants as part of data collection, though the inclusion of phenomenological data as relevant to theory development is not without criticism from behavioural psychology researchers who are still operating out of an archaic, mechanistic model of human nature (Schaffner, 2020).

In laboratory research in psychology, there is a common practice of treating highly constrained, reductionistic, purely behavioural data as if it were equivalent to psychological data found in real-world, naturalistic conditions which causes problems in general theory formulation (Fink & Keyes, 2017). Some commentators have pointed out that contradictory findings are a frequent occurrence in the behavioural literature partly because there is a general lack of awareness in laboratory researchers that "perception of danger is subjective and can be influenced substantially by individual differences" (Sylvers et al., 2011, p. 125). Although the exact means of differentiating between anxiety and fear varies between the fields of animal biology and behaviour and human neuroscience, there is a general consensus between the fields that there is "an abundance of biological and cognitive research separating fear from anxiety" (Sylvers et al., 2011, p. 124). Disagreements are a matter of interpreting the same data in different ways, which leads to "significant variation in the results of analyses of complex data … even by experts with honest intentions" (Silberzahn et al., 2018, p. 338).

Common Assumptions about Fear in Adventurism

Various common assumptions about the nature of fear in adventurism are propagated by mainstream media, as well as the literature in clinical psychology. For the sake of brevity, the common hypotheses about fear in adventurism can be categorised into three different versions which sometimes overlap: (1) adventurists do not feel fear, (2) adventurists feel fear, but they willfully push it outside of cognitive awareness, as they are focused on seeking thrills that result from wantonly, recklessly taunting death, and/or (3) adventurists have a pathological personality trait that overpowers the emotion of fear, and which may also render the experience of fear as pleasurable (Drane et al., 2017; McEwan, et al., 2019; Roberti, 2004; Tofler et al., 2018; Zarevski et al., 1998; Zuckerman, 1983). The above renditions are based on the assumption that adventure sport participants are driven by a pathological relationship with fear, resulting from a personality disorder, yet these conjectures have never been scientifically substantiated (Brymer & Schweitzer, 2017; Brymer et al., 2020).

Essentially, the popular assumptions have been propagated by personality trait measurement tools, yet such tools have multiple problems regarding construct validity, external validity, and methodological errors or lack of rigour

(Eronen & Bringmann, 2021; Flake et al., 2017; Hopwood & Donnellon, 2010; Hussey & Hughes, 2020; Jackson & Maraun, 1996; Llewellyn & Sanchez, 2008; Toomela, 2021; Uher, 2018). Some methodology analysts maintain that personality tests create fictitious entities, then measure those fictions (Toomela 2010; Uher, 2021). The common assumptions based on personality measurement tools have never been verified through analysis of the extensive empirical data collected in the field by dozens of researchers in various cultures across multiple continents (Brymer & Schweitzer, 2017). For example, researchers who collect field data have never made the claim that adventurists do not feel the emotion of fear. Rather, what has been found is that some adventurists experience fear as an expected emotion to be endured or controlled, while others experience fear as a familiar and trusted guide or messenger who imparts critical information and is extensively relied upon for safety (Brymer & Schweitzer, 2013, 2017; Kessler, 2019). Aside from being a major influence involved in risk assessment for ongoing mitigation of danger, the presence of fear is also valuable for other reasons, such as being requisite for cultivation of courage, as well as being a doorway into a deep level of personal development and spiritual contemplation. In the following section we introduce the concept of fear as a critical factor when making rapid and wise decisions under high pressure and uncertainty, within gravely dangerous situations.

Naturalistic Research on Fear in Adventurism

Until relatively recently, field studies on fear in adventurism have been absent from the literature, and there are still only a small number of studies which have focused on the phenomenon. However, the studies mentioned in our discussion below are based on collection of rich and contextually relevant data collected within naturalistic conditions, combined with long, slow, contemplative data analysis using research methods designed for the purpose of concept development grounded in empirical data. Studies which have utilised field observations, phenomenology, full or partial participatory research, and inferential methodology using field data (e.g., classic grounded theory) are some examples of the means by which adventure psychology is currently moving toward the formulation of a set of hypotheses with a high level of verisimilitude. Current hypotheses tend to contradict those put forth by laboratory researchers who make claims on the psychology of adventurism.

In order to clarify our definition of fear, we begin our discussion below with a differentiation between anxiety and fear as it emerged from a lengthy study on the frontier version of mountaineering – which is regarded as an extreme sport, as venturing into remote terrain where few or no others have ventured before is inherently of high-risk – then we discuss the practical nature of fear as it pertains to mitigation of danger in long-haul adventurism. This discussion is not exhaustive; it is meant to serve as an introductory account of the literature on fear in adventurism, with a focus on extreme sports.

Differentiation between Anxiety and Fear

In order to understand the nature of fear in the difficult, long-haul forms of adventurism, especially extreme sports, it is necessary to first recognise the phenomenological and consequential differences between anxiety and fear; for it is fear, not anxiety, which we maintain is a benevolent presence in outdoor ventures. The following differentiation of anxiety and fear is based on a study of expedition mountaineers consisting of multiple forms of data, including live unstructured interviews, detailed memories of expeditions written by participants, and documentary films on mountaineering (Kessler, 2019).

Fear is an emotion, but anxiety is not an emotion. Anxiety is a state of being. A defining feature of a *state of being*, or simply a *state*, as opposed to an *emotion*, is that a state does not pass by, or pass through oneself in the spontaneous and sometimes fast way that emotions do. States rather linger, sometimes for days, weeks, or even years at a time. States of being have general aesthetic qualities, such as dreariness or jubilance, which are not emotions *per se*, but are the backdrop or atmosphere of different emotions. For example, when people say they are in a "grey state" or an "enlightened state" they are referring to the aesthetic qualities of the fundamental state in which various emotions are continuously passing through. Emotions, in contrast, rather than being a backdrop or atmosphere, tend to be in a more-or-less obvious and direct relationship with personal and environmental features, occurrences, and objects. One of the defining features of *states of being* is that multiple different emotions may pass through states in succession, or simultaneously.

A state of anxiety may *include* the emotion of fear, but anxiety includes other emotions as well. Another defining feature of anxiety is that in contrast to fear, anxiety produces bodily responses that are not necessarily commensurate with the level of danger that can be ascertained through awareness of situational factors. Anxiety is essentially the result of internal fragmentation, often with a disconnect from the present and a shift in focus to the future. In anxiety, the imagination fixates on a series of images depicting possible future misfortunes, sometimes with a concomitant sense of mental and physical paralysis which endures until the wave of anxiety passes, or remains as a constant tension in the background of an anxious state of being. As a byproduct of the ever-increasing industrialisation of modern civilisation, anxiety often accompanies a chronic, low-grade state of mental and physical degradation. In a state of anxiety, the body may be experienced as slightly removed, as being an object rather than the fundament of oneself. In other words, a state of anxiety is a disembodied state; a state that is out of balance between the mental, physical, and emotional realms of the self, and is primarily a cognitively-oriented state with physical responses that signal an organismic fragmentation or disintegration (i.e., the opposite of healing and growth). The primary fact about anxiety which is most relevant in our discussion below is the fact that anxiety is quite different from fear in that anxiety is a state of being, not an emotion.

Etymology and Dictionary Definitions of Fear

In the languages Old English, Middle English, Proto-Germanic, Old Norse, and Dutch, the word fear spelled differently in each language, generally referred to danger, especially sudden danger or attack, and in Proto-Indo-European fear meant "to try, risk" (Harper, n.d.). In those same languages fear also referred not only to being in danger, but also to putting someone else in danger, or plotting against someone, as in lying in wait to ambush (Harper, n.d.). These definitions indicate that fear was thought of as inherent to being in a dangerous place or situation. In the Old Icelandic language fear was thought of also as a presentiment of impending danger not yet present, as in a sense of foreboding (Zoëga, 1910, p. 56). The ancient word sjá referred specifically to seeing danger in the mind's eye ahead of its arrival while also feeling fear before the danger becomes apparent (Zoëga, 1910, p. 363). These definitions seem to indicate that feeling fear is a natural response to being in danger or sensing a future confrontation with danger.

In one modern dictionary fear refers to "apprehension, or alarm caused by impending danger, pain, etc." (Collins, 2012). In an 18th century dictionary fear refers to "dread; horrour; apprehension of danger" and also refers to "a companion" (Johnson, 1770). Another 18th century dictionary defines fear as "apprehension of danger" (Sheridan, 1780). Though the concept of fear has an intriguing history, in our discussion below we have in mind the very simple, straightforward definition, apprehension, or awareness of danger.

Fear as a Messenger and Guide

In contrast to anxiety, fear is an emotion; its nature is to pass through (Chamberlain, 1899). Arduous adventures are filled with many different emotional experiences, both pleasant and unpleasant. There are experiences of physical pain, exhaustion, frustration, and fear. There are also experiences of rapture, deep encounters with oneself, and a profound sense of purification and internal harmony. Like other emotions, fear tends to ebb and flow in long-haul adventures, rather than remaining at the same level of intensity at all times, depending on both internal and external factors relating to fluctuating levels of danger at different points in long-haul expeditions.

Essentially, knowing when a venture would be too dangerous to attempt, or is underway but becoming too dangerous to continue, requires deep self-knowledge about one's strengths and limitations as well as extensive experiential knowledge of the type of terrain being explored. Such knowledge is partly gained through operating on a level that is just slightly frightening, but not for the entire duration of the adventure, for the latter is a signal that one is probably operating too close to the edge or perhaps outside of one's capabilities. Even within ventures that are overall squarely within one's capabilities, sometimes a mountaineer does begin to feel terrified, and this degree or intensity of fear, to the point of feeling terror, which is extreme fear, is usually taken as a signal that it would be best to retreat and abandon the mission. In experienced extreme adventurists, the subjective intensity of fear is a reliable indicator of the objective proportion of sensed danger (Kessler, 2019).

The Importance of Intuition

One power of the intuitive sense is to detect danger, which is felt through the body, where a response and systematic preparation for action originate before the intellect has a chance to ascertain the source of the danger and its various attributes such as immediacy, degree, complexity. For example, sometimes mountaineers intuitively turn their head or shift their eyes toward the origin of sensed danger, before acquiring cognitive knowledge of the exact source of the danger. Intuition, like any other sense, and especially when all the senses are working in harmony, triggers bodily responses to fear before clear factual data is brought into cognitive awareness. The intuitive bodily movements that occur in response to danger are partly what affords an extraordinarily rapid response time in cases when there is perhaps only a fraction of a second available to mitigate or avoid catastrophic danger. Intuition is a sense, like vision and hearing, but which is a felt sense; that is to say, the intuitive sense brings information through embodied feelings rather than through more obvious means such as taste or smell.

Fear as an Integrative Force

Aside from being a source of rapid information relay, fear has the pragmatic function of *integrating* one's internal resources, so that dangers can be addressed immediately and potently, whenever necessary. Fear is a pragmatic force and catalyst which demands a sharpened, narrowed focus of attention and energy toward the source of danger, in preparation for enactment, such as escaping or moving through the danger to restore relative safety once again.

As discussed above, fear is a reliable, interoceptive messenger between the senses and the cognitive faculties, as the information contained within fear pushes its way forward through everything else that may be occupying the mind at the time. Moments of danger require a rapid shift in focus toward the danger, with all other concerns immediately falling by the wayside. The rational realm of the mind plans and calculates responses in coordination with the proprioception of the body and exteroception of the environment. If the environmental information contained in fear were forced to "queue up and wait its turn," so to speak, before it could finally arrive into cognitive awareness, in at least some if not many cases, such a slowing of the time needed to reach cognition would effectively close the window of opportunity in which the danger could have otherwise been sufficiently evaluated and successfully addressed within the timeframe needed for survival. Without integration of the whole self, responses to danger would be too slow to be effective in the context of mountaineering.

Summary

In this chapter we have introduced the hypothesis that fear is a benevolent force or guide which is intermittently felt whenever immediate and potential dangers are sensed in the context of high-risk adventurism, especially extreme sports. The information contained in fear is information used to make wise decisions under extremely dangerous and uncertain conditions. If danger were assessed solely through the cognitive faculties, the process would be insufficient and slow, as the rational realm of the mind cannot possibly detect all the information available in the ever-changing nuances of the natural world all at once, while also fully attending to other practical tasks, while also remaining in a perpetually heightened state of alertness, so that no vital information in the environment is missed. Over-reliance on the rational faculty would quickly exhaust the mind and could make it impossible to carry out a lengthy, intricate adventure if the emotions were not involved as fast carriers of information brought into awareness through the embodied senses.

Without an intimate and harmonious relationship with fear as a familiar and benevolent presence, it is difficult to imagine how expedition mountaineers and other long-haul adventurists could complete their missions, as the intellect would quickly become over-taxed if it were the sole arbiter for ongoing detection and evaluation of the inevitable dangers. Fear is an emotion which brings vital information relating to danger into conscious awareness more quickly than any other means. The nature of fear is to instantly ignite the power of the body and the mind simultaneously, so that there is no delay in executing responses to danger, within a fraction of a second, if necessary. In adventurism, fear is a friend, an essential companion, not something to fear.

References

1770 – A Dictionary of the English Language, Vol. 1, 5th ed, Samuel Johnson, author. London: Strahan.

1780 – A general dictionary of the English language. Thomas Sheridan, author. London: Dodsley.

Adolphs, R. (2013). The biology of fear. *Current Biology, 23*(2), 79–93. https://doi.org/10.1016/j.cub.2012.11.055

Bortolan, L., Savoldelli, A., Pellegrini, B., Modena, R., Sacchi, M., Holmberg, H. C., & Supej, M. (2021). Ski mountaineering: Perspectives on a novel sport to be introduced at the 2026 winter Olympic games. *Frontiers in Physiology, 12*, 737249. https://doi.org/10.3389/fphys.2021.737249

Brymer, E., & Schweitzer, R. (2013). Extreme sports are good for your health: A phenomenological understanding of fear and anxiety in extreme sport. *Journal of Health Psychology, 18*(4), 477–487.

Brymer, E., & Schweitzer, R. (2017). *Phenomenology and the extreme sports experience*. New York: Routledge.

Brymer, E., Araújo, D., Davids, K., & Pepping, G.-J. (2020) Conceptualizing the Human health outcomes of acting in natural environments: An ecological perspective.

Frontiers in Psychology: Movement Science and Sport Psychology, 11, 1362. DOI: 10.3389/fpsyg.2020.013S62

Catherall, D. R. (2003). How fear differs from anxiety. *Traumatology, 9*(2), 76–92.

Chamberlain, A. F. (1899). On the words for "fear" in certain languages: A study in linguistic psychology. *The American Journal of Psychology, 10*(2). 302–305. https://www.jstor.org/stable/1412486

Collins English Dictionary – Complete & Unabridged 2012 Digital Edition © William Collins Sons & Co. Ltd.

Drane, C. F., Modecki, K. L., Barber, B. L. (2017). Disentangling development of sensation seeking, risky peer affiliation, and binge drinking in adolescent sport. *Addictive Behaviors, 66*, 60–65.

Eronen, M. I., & Bringmann, L. F. (2021). The theory crisis in psychology: How to move forward. *Perspectives on Psychological Science, 16*(4), 779–788. https://doi.org/10.1177/1745691620970586

Fink, D. S., & Keyes, K. M. (2017). Wrong answers: When simple interpretations create complex problems. In A. El-Sayed & S. Galea (Eds.), *Systems science and population health* (pp. 25–36). New York: Oxford University Press.

Flake, J. K., Pek, J., & Hehman, E. (2017). Construct validation in social and personality research: Current practice and recommendations. *Social Psychological and Personality Science, 8*(4), 370–378. https://doi.org/10.1177/1948550617693063

Harper, D. (n.d.). Etymology of fear. Online Etymology Dictionary. Retrieved May 5, 2022 from https://www.etymonline.com/word/fear

Hopwood, C. J., & Donnellan, M. B. (2010). How should the internal structure of personality inventories be evaluated? *Personality and Social Psychology Review, 14*(3), 332–346.

Hussey, I., & Hughes, S. (2020). Hidden invalidity among 15 commonly used measures in social and personality psychology. *Advances in Methods and Practices in Psychological Science*, 166–184. https://doi.org/10.1177/2515245919882903

Jackson, J. S. H., & Maraun, M. (1996). The conceptual validity of empirical scale construction: The case of the sensation seeking scale. *Personality and Individual Differences, 21*(1), 103–110.

Kessler, K. V. (2019). Friending fear: A classic grounded theory study of frontier mountaineering (2390612572). Doctoral dissertation, Saybrook University. ProQuest Dissertations Publishing.

Llewellyn, D. J., & Sanchez, X. (2008). Individual differences and risk taking in rock climbing. *Psychology of Sport and Exercise, 9*, 413–426.

McEwan, D., Boudreau, P., Curran, T., Rhodes, R. E. (2019) Personality traits of high-risk sport participants: A meta-analysis. *Journal of Research in Personality, 79*, 83–93.

Roberti, J. W. (2004). A review of behavioral and biological correlates of sensation seeking. *Journal of Research in Personality, 38*, 256–279.

Schaffner, K. F. (2020). A comparison of two neurobiological models of fear and anxiety: A "construct validity" application? *Perspectives on Psychological Science, 15*(5), 1214–1227.

Silberzahn, R., Uhlmann, E. L., Martin, D. P., Anselmi, P., Aust, F., Awtrey, E., … Nosek, B. A. (2018). Many analysts, one data set: Making transparent how variations in analytic choices affect results. *Advances in Methods and Practices in Psychological Science, 1*, 337–356. https://doi.org/10.1177/2515245917747646

Steimer, T. (2002). The biology of fear- and anxiety-related behaviors. *Dialogues in Clinical Neuroscience, 4*(3), 231–249.

Sylvers, P., Lilienfeld, S. O., & LaPrairie, J. L. (2011). Differences between trait fear and trait anxiety: Implications for psychopathology. *Clinical Psychology Review, 31*(1), 122–137.

Tofler, I. R., Hyatt, B. M., & Tofler, D. S. (2018). Psychiatric aspects of extreme sports: Three case studies. *The Permanente Journal, 22*, 17–71. https://doi.org/10.7812/TPP/17-071

Toomela, A. (2010). Quantitative methods in psychology: Inevitable and useless. *Frontiers in Psychology, 29*(1). https://doi.org/10.3389/fpsyg.2010.00029

Toomela, A. (2021). Problems with measurement in psychology – Just a tip of the iceberg. *Theoretical and Philosophical Psychology, 41*(2), 134–138.

Uher, J. (2018). Quantitative data from rating scales: An epistemological and methodological enquiry. *Frontiers in Psychology, 9*. https://doi.org/10.3389/fpsyg.2018.02599

Uher, J. (2021). Psychometrics is not measurement: Unraveling a fundamental misconception in quantitative psychology and the complex network of its underlying fallacies. *Journal of Theoretical and Philosophical Psychology, 41*(1), 58–84. https://doi.org/10.1037/teo0000176

Zarevski, P., Marušić, I., Zolotić, S., Bunjevac, T., & Vukosav, Ž. (1998). Contribution of Arnett's inventory of sensation seeking and Zuckerman's sensation seeking scale to the differentiation of athletes engaged in high and low risk sports. *Personality and Individual Differences, 25*, 763–768.

Zoëga, G. T. (1910). *A concise dictionary of Old Icelandic*. London: Oxford University Press.

Zuckerman, M. (1983). Sensation seeking and sports. *Personality and Individual Differences, 4*(3), 285–293.

8
SUCCESS AND FAILURE IN ADVENTURE

Erik Monasterio

Accident on 'Feeding Time at the Zoo' – An Adventurer's Vignette

My climbing accident on a cliff in New Zealand was serious and potentially fatal. On that day I had not planned to climb, however by midafternoon I determined that if I quickly cleared up a couple of clinical reports I could sneak out for a late afternoon climb. I wanted to climb a route I had failed on the previous week. I rushed out the door of the hospital and threaded my way past the Friday traffic. I racked up the safety equipment to my harness as the evening gave the rock an autumnal honey-orange glow. I needed to warm up quickly. There was no peace of mind as I did this. In the back of my mind the hum of unresolved clinical questions and the pressures of under resourced medical services was unrelenting. I also had a distracting sense that I was rushing but dismissed this as it had become a common feeling from trying to fit in a busy career, family life and staying fit and active in a range of adventure activities.

The warm-up route didn't help to steady my mind as it was very easy and I had climbed it many times. Instead of heading for my intended route I impulsively decided to follow-up with a second warm-up. This 18m route, "Feeding Time at the Zoo" was more serious and committed, and is graded UK E3, 6a, French 6c+ (a moderate technical grade with high overall risk). This route was established 40 years ago, and reflecting the minimalist ethic of that time only had one fixed (security) bolt to clip the rope to, eight meters off the ground to protect from a probable death fall above it. Other removable, traditional protection was sparsely available. Feeding Time at the Zoo requires precise, carefully sequenced climbing to get past the most challenging part of the climb (the 'crux') at six meters. I tied onto the rope and ensured my belayer placed the rope through her belay (security) device.

DOI: 10.4324/9781003173601-11

As this was familiar territory even the first tricky moves did nothing to fix my focus. The steady stream of distracting thoughts hummed even as the route steepened. I ignored the first nut (traditional protection) in a crack to my right and instead jammed my right index and middle fingertips into it. I brought my left foot up high. As I pulled hard on my fingers I was able to bring my right foot up to place the toe-tip on a vertical seam of rock. Pushing off the opposing foot holds I straightened my legs and reached high to jam my left hand into a 'v' shaped crack. By holding body tension, I was able to release my right hand to unclip the nut bundle from my harness. I held this between clenched teeth. I then reached up and held onto a horizontal crack with my right hand. Balanced this way I released the left hand from the 'v' shaped crack, took the nut from my mouth and placed it into the crack. The wedge-shaped nut was too big and instead of securely slotting into the bottom of the crack, sat loosely on top providing substandard security, but I was familiar with the sequence of movements to get past this overhanging section. I clipped the rope to the nut, and without deliberation jammed my left hand back into the 'v' crack. I reached up to the right and with my right hand held onto the base of a wide horizontal crack. I then brought the left hand close to the right and pulling on my arms I cut my feet loose, pushed the tip of my left shoe into a tiny crack and reached up to a very small but sharp diagonal left-hand hold. I swung my right foot up high to push the toe tips into the crack 40cm to the right of my hand. The next move was very awkward and led to the crux. However, I felt physically comfortable. I flagged the free left foot, pulled hard with the left hand and out-stretched, reached up to a tiny right-hand hold. This is the crucial moment of the climb. By stacking (crimping) fingers onto this hold and applying brute force I brought my left foot into the crack where my hands had been. I straightened my left leg to reach for a reasonable left hand hold next to the fixed bolt. This generally completes the 'crux' section, but instead of relief I had the briefest forewarning of doom. It was the only time on the route and that day that my attention was totally focused. I have flashes of flying from the rock. Then a period of darkness.

The next memory is of intense, burning pain in my back, inability to breathe and a sense of crawling out of a cave. As I crawled up the bank where I had fallen past my belayer she emphasised that I should lie still as I had fallen 8 meters. I had been unconscious for a minute, probably from the vertical force up my spine into my brain as I landed on my feet. Emergency services had already been called. I performed a self-neurological screen, and noting full sensation and strength in my legs concluded there was no significant injury to my spinal cord. Due to the intense pain I worried I had ruptured my spleen. Aware that emergency services were at least 1 hour away, I decided to walk and stumble out to meet the ambulance at the road. Lucky to be alive however I sustained a spinal fracture with 40% anterior wedge fractures of Lumbar 1 and 2, and intra-articular fracture of the right wrist.

Erik Monasterio

Success and Failure in Adventure

Introduction

This chapter draws on a combination of personal experiences and reflections, and on extant research literature on personality and psychological factors associated with engagement in the more extreme end of the adventure continuum (mountaineering and BASE jumping) to discuss the psychology of adventure. The two anecdotes are from the author's long trajectory in mountaineering and exploration, and are provided to highlight 'lived experience' in climbing and to set the context to explore how success and failure can be considered in high-performance adventure. While there is a wide range of motivation for adventure participation, with significant leisure and non-competitive participation, this chapter will focus on the more elite dimension of performance, but the concepts can apply to the entire field of adventure activities. The chapter considers what factors can contribute to excessive or naïve ambition, the 'win or succeed at all costs' mentality, and how this can impair decision-making and on occasions lead to catastrophic outcomes. The purpose is to propose alternative considerations of success and failure that can apply to all adventure activities, with the benefits extending well beyond the high-performance environment. This chapter critiques traditional definitions of success and failure, such as the objective achievement of a clearly identified goal, and the pursuit of the fastest and/or most demanding and/or daring activity. Instead, the chapter focuses on opportunities for self-transcendence and personal growth through adventure, and the impact this can have in connecting to and protecting nature. It is hoped that consideration of this can encourage a recalibration of traditional definitions of success and failure in human endeavour.

Integrated Traverse of the Illimani Massif, Bolivia

Sat 68% and HR 120 at rest, and I was only half way ... Shaking the ice from the cocoon of my sleeping bag, I peered into the emerald filaments where the sky met the land and heralded the coming sun. I could not be closer to the stars anywhere else in Bolivia or for that matter in most of the world. On the ridge at 6,250 metres, between the Central and North peaks of Illimani, for what seemed an eternity the night played a physiological cat and mouse game with me, pushing me into different states of awareness. I was not well adapted after only ten days above sea level altitude. As soon as I dropped off to sleep I startled awake gasping for air. The tiny downward shift of my breathing impulse pushed my oxygen levels dangerously low and so I rebounded awake (Cheyne-Stokes breathing). Each time I woke to waves of nausea, panic and confusion; my motivation and judgement sorely tested. Ahead were the three peaks over 6,000 metres that would see us through the integrated traverse of the Illimani Massif. The five-peak traverse from north to south or vice versa has been attempted a number of times but there are only records of four completions.

Parties often get frostbite and altitude problems while spending several days above 6,000 metres.

Who could ask for more? But given a choice, who would want to spend a night in an open-air bivouac, struggling with the physiological profile of a patient in an intensive care unit? At rest on the mountain, my heart rate was 2.5 times faster than my usual base rate and my oxygen saturation was the same as that of a chronic smoker. And I still had three high peaks to go. As is so often the case in high altitude climbing, it was the best and worst that could be hoped for. Leading up to this were 25 years of mountaineering experience, endless ambition and two previous episodes of severe altitude sickness (at similar altitudes). By now however, experience had taught me to better understand the fine balance of reading my physiology at altitude and managing naïve ambition. I was alone in the face of a huge decision. This time, I trusted myself. The traverse is seldom completed, and never without adversity. But I just knew that this time, with my team I would succeed. And we did.

Reflections from Base Camp

From a rational perspective there is little sense to mountaineering and climbing, and overwhelming evidence against it: the higher the altitude and the harder the route, the more compelling the arguments against it. Yet the experience of climbing can be transformational in a way that only deep emotions and hard fought achievements can be. As with adventure more broadly there are primitive instincts at play, and to engage with them is to reconnect to a past that we have largely lost contact with. A past when we were closer to nature. When exploration drove evolution. A past when obeyance to instinct was natural and the natural flow of action liberating. However, in order to achieve and survive in the unforgiving environment of the mountain there has to be uncompromising focus. The distracting, disconnected and erratic inner dialogue, which makes up so much of our internal world has to be far better appreciated and managed. Simple mistakes can have serious consequences and as the focus of attention narrows the senses sharpen. The immediacy of it, the needing to be in the moment, and the connection to nature and a quieter inner world can be transformational, particularly in an increasingly complex world full of distracting experiences, divided attention and alienation from nature.

Personality and Adventure

In previous work the author and associates have examined the role of personality in the more extreme participants of adventure activities which have high morbidity and mortality (Mei-Dan et al., 2012, 2013; Monasterio, 2005). The Temperament and Character Inventory (TCI) has been used in these studies to identify personality factors that contribute to participation, accidents, and stress reactivity in mountaineers and BASE Jumpers. This has helped the author to better understand the attraction to extreme adventure, and factors that contribute to successful performance (Monasterio et al., 2012, 2014, 2016).

Cloninger's Temperament and Character Inventory (TCI)

Personality has been defined as "the dynamic organization within an individual of the psychobiological systems that modulate adaptation to a changing environment" and also as "the way that people learn from experience and adapt their feelings, thoughts, and actions" (Cloninger et al., 1993). The TCI provides a comprehensive account of personality, measuring seven dimensions of personality traits that are moderately heritable and associated with distinct brain networks and psychological characteristics (Cloninger, 1987; Cloninger et al., 1993; Gillespie et al., 2003). The model measures four dimensions of temperament, which involve basic emotional drives or instincts regulated by primitive brain structures (Lennox & Dolan, 2014), and three character dimensions, which involve self-regulation of emotions and attention in order to achieve chosen goals and values, and regulated mainly in the neocortex (Cloninger, 1987; Cloninger et al., 1993; Gillespie et al., 2003). The temperament traits explain how persons respond to novelty, danger or punishment, and reward. *Novelty-Seeking* is a heritable bias in the activation or initiation of behaviours in response to novelty (e.g. impulsive decision-making, exploratory activity); *Harm-Avoidance* is a heritable bias in the inhibition of behaviours (e.g. pessimistic worry, fear of uncertainty); *Reward-Dependence* is a heritable bias in the maintenance of ongoing behaviours (e.g. social attachment, dependence on approval of others); and *Persistence* corresponds to perseverance despite frustration and fatigue. Character involves the conceptual organisation of perceptions which influences behavioural goals and expectancies. The character dimensions are: *Self-Directedness*, which refers to the ability of an individual to control, regulate and adapt behaviour to fit the situation in accordance with individually chosen goals and values, and which encompasses traits such as purposefulness, responsibility; *Cooperativeness*, which refers to the identification with and acceptance of other people and is related to agreeability, empathy, helpfulness to others without selfish domination; and *Self-Transcendence*, which corresponds to a unitive perspective or consciousness where the person is simply aware of being part of a greater whole, and it can be described as acceptance, identification, or spiritual union with nature and its source (Cloninger et al., 1993).

Extensive data on the reliability and validity of the TCI have been reported, and the TCI has been shown to have sound psychometric characteristics (Cloninger et al., 1993).

TCI results in Mountaineers and BASE Jumpers

The authors' findings help to explain the complex interaction between personality, the social environment, the extreme adventure activity and decision-making; all of which are determinant in motivation, and in defining success and failure. While highly influential, many of these factors are not consciously obvious to the participant, and therefore worthy of explicit analysis as part of the skill development process that lead to expertise, satisfaction and maturity (and potentially survival) in the practice of the more extreme adventures. Despite substantial variation in their individual personality profiles (Monasterio et al., 2013, 2014, 2016) there is a consistency of findings across all studies. Mountaineers and BASE Jumpers exhibit an adventurous temperament (high Novelty-Seeking, low Harm-Avoidance and Reward-Dependence) compared to low-risk sports participants and the general population. They are also self-controlled and organised in character (high in Self-Directedness and Cooperation, and low in Self-Transcendence). Different configurations of temperament and character influence the diversity of goals and values derived from these adventures, which are also likely to be shaped by underlying stress reactivity, and resilience to stress and trauma (Monasterio et al., 2016).

Monasterio and Cloninger have highlighted in a previous publication the potential influence of character on the regulation of the dominant risk-taking exploratory impulses of the adventurous temperament present in extreme participants (Monasterio & Cloninger, 2019). While they have been found to have organised character profiles (high Self-Directedness and Cooperativeness, and low Self-Transcendence), which are generally associated with engagement in disciplined, purposeful and socially responsible behaviours irrespective of underlying temperamental biases, extreme participants can also engage in reckless self-serving (walking past acutely sick fellow mountaineers not to forego the chance at reaching a summit and succeeding in an expedition), environmentally destructive (littering and pollution of protected mountain environments), and self-destructive behaviours (high incidence of serious injury and death) in certain critical situations, and in their drive to succeed. It is hypothesised that the character configurations associated with low Self-Transcendence (present in 75–85% of athletes) contributes to this, as the drive of strong ambitiousness is not tempered by altruistic, compassionate and spiritual concerns (conferred by Self-Transcendence). Moreover, at a broader socio-cultural level, the conscious awareness and consideration of Self-Transcendent values is discouraged by the materialistic life that is promoted in social media and in secular societies predominant in the Western world, which promote self-interest, material success, striving for power and celebrity (Cloninger, 2013).

Toward a Broader Definition of Success and Failure in Adventure

The instinctive temperament bias toward engagement in exploratory and adventurous activities, associated with a frequent propensity toward tolerating or under-estimating risk found in adventure sport participants (adventurous temperament), is more pronounced in those participating at the more extreme end of the adventure dimension (Castanier et al., 2010; Fleixanet, 1991; Monasterio et al., 2014, 2016). This instinctive motivator for behaviour therefore is likely to become more influential in decision-making and notions of success and failure, at the more extreme end of adventure (high altitude mountaineering, free-soloing, big wave surfing) and where accidents and mishaps are likely to have much greater consequences (Mei-Dan et al., 2012, 2013; Monasterio, 2005).

The Illimani Traverse anecdote emphasises the intensity of this temperament bias (prevalent in mountaineers) and where the goal of the expedition was to complete the seldom repeated integrated traverse of this massif, despite the author's adverse physiological profile, considerable discomfort and previous episodes of life-threatening altitude sickness. A dominant notion of success based on the achievement of a summit or a predetermined goal strongly contributes to the high rate of injury and death at the more extreme end of mountaineering (Weinbruch & Nordby, 2013). The conscious striving to reach 'the summit at all costs' ethos (emphasised by sponsors, social media and for recognition and celebrity status) adds influence to this, and may contribute to dissatisfaction with any outcome other than the coveted summit.

The psychological factors contributing to the author's accident on Feeding Time at the Zoo are carefully examined in a separate publication (Monasterio & Brymer, 2020). However, for the purpose of the current discussion this anecdote highlights the importance of integrating an appropriate level of focus, concentration and engagement (being present) to climb this style of route safely. The value or kudos given to climbing 'committed routes' (routes with high objective risk), swayed the ill-fated decision by the author to climb this route while struggling with an unfocussed mind-set. The impact of this definition of success, like the Syrens' Song, has led the author to two significant climbing accidents and a number of 'near misses'. This effect is also highlighted in narrative research examining motivation in wingsuit flying, with participants recounting how tragic and unnecessary accidents often occur when pilots are preoccupied with a desire to achieve a spectacular outcome (e.g., fly the most dramatic line before anyone else does and to share the act with the world), and how this impairs engagement with the appropriate wingsuit flying 'processes' that not only mitigates risk but can also lead to personal growth (Arijs et al., 2017).

The traditional value of 'success at all costs' solely determined by the achievement of a coveted objective goal is increasingly challenged from within the adventure community (Arijs et al., 2017; Brymer & Gray, 2009; Brymer et al., 2020). More recently, following the profoundly negative impact of the pressure to succeed in the 2020 Tokyo Olympics and other major events, this has also occurred from within conventional sports which highlight the unacceptable cost to well-being associated with this narrow notion of success (Biles & Osaka, 2021).

As extreme and adventure activities share the common characteristics of skilful physical activity taking place in a natural environment, with research emphasising the importance of the development of a deep relationship with the natural world, these activities provide an opportunity to develop a more positive understanding oneself and place in the natural environment. Recent research highlights that, for a number of high-performance extreme adventure participants from a range of disciplines, success is better defined by the experience of 'tuning into' the present moment, connecting to the natural world as a facilitator to a deeper, more positive understanding of self and the cultivation of meaning and purpose, supported by values that reach beyond the activity and stretch into life (Arijs et al., 2017; Brymer et al., 2020; Monasterio & Brymer, 2020). This research highlights the importance of connecting to the natural environment (such as weather conditions, avalanche propensity and topographical features) leading to improved awareness, acceptance, and regulation of behaviour. For some, nature was described as omnipresent and ubiquitous, and a source of innate power and personal meaning. Findings support the idea that extreme adventure participation can lead to positive relationships with the natural world and pro-environmental behaviours (Brymer et al., 2009; Brymer & Gray, 2010). In this context reframing or better balancing notions of success in adventure provides an opportunity, not only for improving the safety of these activities, but for personal growth and protection of the natural environment. The 'win at all costs' value system can become an impediment to this, where the value of a summit and/or the need to meet the expectation of sponsors or public pressure becomes dominant and distracting. This can not only lead to poor decision-making, engagement in morally questionable behaviours and unnecessary risk-taking (Monasterio & Cloninger, 2019), but also to personal dissatisfaction and exploitation of the natural environment, and a lost opportunity for improvement in well-being and personal growth.

As indicated above, TCI research findings in extreme adventure participant populations have consistently found character configurations associated with low Self-Transcendence (present in 75–85% of athletes). Whereas temperament traits are heritable, moderately stable over time and less amenable to change, character is more dynamic and influenced by life experience, social learning and intentional goals and values (Cloninger, 2013). Character dimensions can regulate emotional impulses and conflicts in such a way that a mature and healthy personality can develop regardless of the temperament. The creative character profile, associated with high scores in Self-Directedness, Cooperativeness and Self-Transcendence, has consistently been found in all human populations to be associated with the most developed capacities for healthy longevity, creativity, transpersonal values, and prosocial behaviours including sacrifice for others to form communities with trust and altruistic support of one another (Cloninger, 2013; Zwir et al., 2021).

Engagement in adventure activities, with their proximity and deep connection to the natural environment can provide avenues for the development of Self-Transcendence, by focusing on this relationship with the natural environment and 'tuning into' the present moment, where awareness extends beyond the individual self to involve a connection to the universe. In the author's opinion, the benefits of this will extend well beyond adventure activity performance and satisfaction, and toward whole personality development and improved well-being, and in all likelihood motivate toward protection of the environment. As modern societies grapple with the negative consequences of excessive materialism, environmental degradation and climate change, and increasing psychological distress, engagement in adventure can potentially provide transformational experiences and a much-needed re-evaluation of our value systems. Therefore, there are many benefits from reframing success to focus on the processes that lead to such experiences rather than the achievement of a coveted outcome at all costs.

Conclusion

The author draws on reflections of 25 years of high-performance mountaineering and research to critique the traditional definitions of success, such as the objective achievement of a clearly identified goal, and the pursuit of the fastest and/or most demanding and/or daring activity in adventure. In doing so, this chapter has considered psychological and social factors that contribute to excessive or naïve ambition, the 'win or succeed at all costs' mentality and how these can impair decision-making, and lead to catastrophic outcomes.

The anecdote of the seldom completed Illimani Traverse is an exemplar of the instinctive drive of the 'adventurous temperament', predominant in adventurers, to choose ambitious and risky expeditions and to pursue these despite considerable personal risks and adversity. The author's reflection on the Feeding Time at the Zoo climb highlights the extent to which the concept of success arising from the kudos given to climbing 'committed routes' can interfere with dynamic aspects of decision-making, satisfaction and lead to serious accidents.

The personality research finds that high-performance adventurers have 'adventurous temperaments' and 'organised character profiles', and with their character profiles mostly associated with low Self-Transcendence. Self-Transcendence is associated with spiritual ideas and experiences, such as searching for something elevated and greater than oneself. Highly self-transcendent people have an outlook of unity and connectedness that motivates them to work in the service of others, instead of being preoccupied with individual accomplishments and self-aggrandisement (Cloninger et al., 1993). Without the moderating effect of Self-Transcendence and its guidance toward altruism, the service of others and a sense of harmony with nature, the adventurous personality characteristics of adventurers may in some (high-stake) situations manifest in callousness, disregard and rationalisation of controversial behaviours (Monasterio & Cloninger, 2019), and adherence to the 'win or succeed at all costs' traditional concept of success. This occurs within a broader socio-cultural context where the conscious awareness and consideration of Self-Transcendent values is discouraged by the materialistic life that is promoted in social media and in secular societies predominant in the Western world, which promote self-interest, material success, striving for power and celebrity (Cloninger, 2013).

Engagement in adventure activities, with their proximity and deep connection to the natural environment can provide avenues for the development of

Self-Transcendence, by focusing on this relationship with the natural environment and 'tuning into' the present moment, where awareness extends beyond the individual self to involve a connection to the universe. Reframing the concept of success to focus on the processes that lead to such experiences rather than the achievement of a coveted outcome at all costs, in the author's opinion is likely to lead to benefits that extend well beyond adventure activity performance and satisfaction, and toward whole personality development and improved well-being, and in all likelihood also motivate toward protection of the environment.

References

Arijs, C., Chroni, S., Brymer, E., & Carless, D. (2017). 'Leave your ego at the door': A narrative investigation into effective wingsuit flying. *Frontiers in Psychology, 8*, 1985.

Biles, S. & Osaka, N. Accessed September 30, 2021 from https://nationalpost.com/news/national/10-3-podcast-how-a-win-at-all-costs-mentality-could-be-harmful-to-athletes

Brymer, E., Feletti, F., Monasterio, E., & Schweitzer, R. (2020). Understanding extreme sports: A psychological perspective. *Frontiers in Psychology, 10*, 3029.

Brymer, E., & Gray, T. (2009). Dancing with nature: Rhythm and harmony in extreme sport participation. *Journal of Adventure Education & Outdoor Learning, 9*(2), 135–149.

Castanier, C., Le Scanff, C., & Woodman, T. (2010). Who takes risks in high-risk sports? A typological personality approach. *Research Quarterly for Exercise and Sport, 81*, 478–484. Retrieved from http://www.aahperd.org/rc/publications/rqes/

Cloninger, C. R. (2013). What makes people healthy, happy, and fulfilled in the face of current world challenges? *Mens Sana Monographs, 11*, 16–24.

Cloninger, C. R. (1987). A systematic method for clinical description and classification of personality variants. A proposal. *Archives of General Psychiatry, 44*(6), 573–588.

Cloninger, C. R., Svrakic, D. M., & Przybeck, T. R. (1993). A psychobiological model of temperament and character. *Archives of General Psychiatry, 50*(12), 975–990.

Frexanet, M. G. (1991). Personality profile of subjects engaged in high physical risk sports. *Personality and Individual Differences, 12*, 1087–1093. DOI: 10.1016/0191-8869(91)90038-D

Gillespie, N. A., Cloninger, C. R., Heath, A. C., & Martin, N. G. (2003). The genetic and environmental relationship between Cloninger's dimensions of temperament and character. *Personality and Individual Differences, 35*, 1931–1946.

Lennox, C., & Dolan, M. (2014). Temperament and character and psychopathy in male conduct disordered offenders. *Psychiatry Research, 215*(3), 706–710.

Mei-Dan, O., Carmont, M. R., & Monasterio, E. (2012). The epidemiology of severe and catastrophic injuries in BASE jumping. *Clinical Journal of Sport Medicine, 22*(3), 262–267.

Mei-Dan, O., Monasterio, E., Carmont, M., & Westman, A. (2013). Fatalities in wingsuit BASE jumping. *Wilderness & Environmental Medicine, 24*(4), 321–327.

Monasterio, E. (2005). Accident and fatality characteristics in a population of mountain climbers in New Zealand. *The New Zealand Medical Journal (Online), 118*(1208).

Monasterio, E., & Brymer, E. (2020). Feeding Time at the Zoo: psychological aspects of a serious rock-climbing accident. *Journal of Adventure Education and Outdoor Learning*, 1–13.

Monasterio, E., &d Cloninger, C. R. (2019). Self-transcendence in mountaineering and BASE Jumping. *Frontiers in Psychology, 9*, 2686.

Monasterio, E., Alamri, Y. A., & Mei-Dan, O. (2014). Personality characteristics in a population of mountain climbers. *Wilderness & Environmental Medicine, 25*(2), 214–219.

Monasterio, E., Mei-Dan, O., Hackney, A. C., Lane, A. R., Zwir, I., Rozsa, S., & Cloninger, C. R. (2016). Stress reactivity and personality in extreme sport athletes: The psychobiology of BASE jumpers. *Physiology & Behavior, 167*, 289–297.

Monasterio, E., Mulder, R., Frampton, C., & Mei-Dan, O. (2012). Personality characteristics of BASE jumpers. *Journal of Applied Sport Psychology, 24*(4), 391–400. DOI: 10.1080/10413200.2012.666710

Weinbruch, S., & Nordby, K. C. (2013). Fatalities in high altitude mountaineering: A review of quantitative risk estimates. *High Altitude Medicine & Biology, 14*(4), 346–359.

Zwir, I., Del-Val, C., Hintsanen, M., Cloninger, K. M., Romero-Zaliz, R., Mesa, A., et al. (2021). The evolution of genetic networks for human creativity. *Molecular Psychiatry*. https://doi.org/10.1038/s41480-021-0197-y

9

SISU

Answering the Call of Adventure with Strength and Grace

Emilia Elisabet Lahti

An Adventurer's Point of View: Crazy Baptism

My first experience with Sisu was in 2007 when I signed myself up to run The Canadian Death Race (CDR), a 72-mile ultramarathon race in the mountains of Grande Cache, Alberta. The CDR was my first experience of an ultramarathon and the first moment where I realised I was capable of more if I just dared to try.

Most recently, I had qualified for the Boston Marathon, leaving me with newfound confidence to attempt something so crazy after only a few months of running at a serious level. While the Boston Marathon is a badge of honour in the running community, the Canadian Death Race was on a different level in my mind. Although I had little experience running marathons, it was not impossible to think that I could accomplish this goal myself and maybe even go further. At this time, ultrarunning was still an obscure, niche and unknown sport that had an almost mystical allure in the runner's world, so I struggled to think that this was something that I could be a part of.

Regardless of my feelings, or maybe because of them, I decided to take on this challenge and attempt an adventure with high uncertainty of the outcome. I believe it's fair to say that the adventure didn't find me, I went looking for it. Most people believe that it was the act of running that helped me get through this turbulent time in my life, however, running was the medium that expressed my desire to lose myself in the great outdoors. It was the opportunity I saw to face my battles with bravery and resilience, seeking out an adventurous life. I underestimated how hard I would struggle on this new path I was on, but at the same time, I underestimated my ability to fight through the doubt and pain.

So it was in this crazy ultramarathon race that I received my baptism, the rebirth of this new side of me that would from then on choose to not run away from obstacles and chaos, but instead run towards them with the tenacity to conquer what's ahead.

On my first attempt at this notoriously difficult race, I didn't finish. But this was a result of slipping at a creek at 0200 still with 12 miles to go in freezing temperatures. With the threat of hyperthermia I rationally decided to DNF, but nothing would be the same after that unparalleled moment of calling myself to action. Instead of feeling defeated like I once might have, I came home thrilled and excited, having discovered an untapped source of potential that was hidden inside of me all along.

The next year, without hesitation, I came back to the race with this new mindset. This time I placed ninth female overall, resulting in me winning my age group and consequently winning the female category of the Alberta Ultra Running series. Adventure has taught me endless lessons in my life. Most importantly, to never doubt my abilities in hardship, that I can overcome anything if I just dare.

Norma Bastidas

Sisu: Answering the Call of Adventure with Strength and Grace

Just as one of the main premises of all scientific inquiry is to increase collective understanding of life and its phenomena, one purpose of adventure is to voyage toward the unknown edges of our experience and unlock knowledge about ourselves and the world. In the Finnish language, a little-known word called *sisu* is used to refer to the kind of relentless doggedness in the face of extraordinary adversity that is often needed in adventurous pursuits. The significance and meaning of sisu has undergone transformations, and while there have been fluctuations in how it has been regarded in its native country (reflecting Finland's socio-economic times, history, and sports success), it has been more and less part of the ongoing popular discourse of the country. Etymologically, sisu derives from *sisus* which refers to the internal organs of a human or animal body (literally, the guts), or it can mean the interior of an object. Dating back to the 16th century, when the first written remarks about sisu occurred, the word referred to a quality or inherent tendency. It is a deeply personal thing however, and there can be many ways of experiencing it. It is embodied by those who endure severe stress in their daily lives, who do not give up in the face of challenges, or who choose to stand up against injustice despite the threat. What unites expressions of sisu is the notion that sisu "will enable you to cut through even a stone wall" (Tokoi, 1957): as goes the old Finnish phrase about not giving up.

While having been a central part of the Finnish folklore and national identity for about half a millennium (Häkkinen, 2004), sisu has remained elusive in popular discourse and under-researched as a psychological construct. It has been described as a tough-to-translate, near spiritual quality (Aho, 1994; Lucas

& Buzzanella, 2004) that helps the individual push through what is seemingly unbearable. In a reader survey from 1942 by *Uusi-Suomi* newspaper, that for over half a century remained the most comprehensive attempt to understand the meaning of sisu, one reader defined sisu as a "hidden possibility within our being," while another respondent wrote that sisu "in a crucial moment enables the individual to flex beyond their usual capacity for action and resistance" (Mitä on sisu?, 1942). Recently, sisu has become the subject of systematic empirical research and is defined as a universal quality of extraordinary perseverance, action mindset, and latent power in the face of extreme adversity (Lahti, 2019). It can become harmful or beneficial to the individual and their environment depending on how it is harnessed (Lahti, 2013, 2019, 2022). In this chapter, four angles to sisu are offered as levers "to go knowingly into the unknown," as the framework for the novel field of Adventure Psychology posits and do so from an internal orientation that is conducive to not only strong and powerful action, but action that is long-sighted, harmonious, and elevating even for those who coexist with us. The elements associated with sisu that are presented here are extraordinary perseverance, latent strength, gentle power, and systems intelligence (Lahti, 2019, 2022).

Extraordinary Perseverance—Accessing Strength When There Seems to Be None Left

> A death blow is a blow of life to some
> Who, till they died, did not alive become,
> Who, had they lived, had died, but when they died,
> vitality begun.
>
> *Emily Dickinson*

Sisu in its most simple form, stated once by my father, is about exceeding our preconceived capacities. As we pass the checkpoints of our known ability, we peer into the various unknowns of our mental, physical, and social landscapes. As part of my doctoral dissertation to examine the lived experience of sisu, I implemented a field study using phenomenological and auto-ethnographic research frameworks in which I ran and cycled 1500 miles across the length of New Zealand in 50 days (Lahti, 2022). Extraordinary perseverance for me in New Zealand meant discovering repeatedly what William James (1914) over a century ago referred to as the "second wind." He wrote in *The Energies of Men*:

> I have mused on the phenomenon of second wind, trying to find a physiological theory. It is evident that our organism has stored-up reserves of energy that are ordinarily not called upon, but that may be called upon: deeper and deeper strata of combustible or explosible material,

discontinuously arranged, but ready for use by anyone who probes so deep, and repairing themselves by rest as well as do the superficial strata. Most of us continue living unnecessarily near our surface.

(p. 8)

As I accessed my second, third, and fourth winds through ultrarunning and wandered into the various unknown edges of my mental, physical, and social landscapes, it appeared to me that the start point of sisu is subjective and often changes as we change through our experiences. Over time and through training for example, a six-mile run that would leave me completely wiped out was replaced with a reality of running sometimes even two six- to ten-mile training runs the same day with ease and quick recovery. In more philosophical terms, extraordinary perseverance could be described as an experience of "becoming-into-being" (Broad, 1923, p. 68) in that what becomes-to-be is a more expanded experience of our capacities in a point where the two opposite realities of "giving up" and "going onwards" both linger a mere breath away. James (1907) further wrote about the second wind that "[m]ental activity shows the phenomenon as well as physical" and continued:

> …in exceptional cases we may find, beyond the very extremity of fatigue-distress, amounts of ease and power that we never dreamed ourselves to own, sources of strength habitually not taxed at all, because habitually we never push through the obstruction, never pass those early critical points.
>
> *(p. 4)*

Research supports the idea that the threshold of one's assumed maximum effort seems not to be fixed. In a 2008 study, Pollo et al. found that subjects who were given a placebo but told it was caffeine were able to lift more weight. Clark et al. (2000) discovered a similar effect in a simulated 40-km bicycle time trial. The placebo effect has also been illustrated for pain and movement disorders (Amanzio & Benedetti, 1999; Pollo et al., 2011), and there is evidence to suggest that the effect is related to individuals' expectations and beliefs. Amanzio and Benedetti (1999) showed that placebo analgesia (pain relief) could be induced with verbal suggestions, and Dweck and colleagues' decades of research on mindset suggests that the beliefs individuals hold about their abilities impact their future behaviour and even willpower (Job et al., 2010; Yeager & Dweck, 2012). Research participants who *believed* that their willpower is limited and fixed were more likely to give up than those who believed that willpower is self-renewing. They named this optimistic way of looking at ourselves and others the "growth mindset." Six decades ago, American runner Roger Bannister became the first person to run a mile in under four minutes. A deed that was long deemed impossible and even dangerous has since been lowered by almost 17 seconds and is now the standard of all male professional middle-distance runners.

In a 2019 article, I labelled one aspect of sisu as action mindset (Lahti, 2019) because it denotes an active, courageous approach toward challenges that seem substantially greater than our current reserves, opportunities, or capacities. Whereas action mindset can enable action against very slim odds and summit the literal and proverbial mountains that test our capacities, extraordinary perseverance enables an adventurer to keep moving onwards during potential breaking points. Sisu as action mindset is about the beliefs and emotions we bring into endeavours that are especially thorny and uncertain or outright overwhelming because of their scale. Modulating our responses to these emotions that unfold (see Gross, 1998, 2001 for emotion regulation) can mean the difference between success and failure. Sisu is about venturing beyond what we thought we are capable of and transcending what until then indicated the boundaries of our action repertoire as our new frontiers. Mälkki (2011) has labelled the threat and discomfort one might feel when approaching these boundaries as "edge-emotions." Mälkki and Green (2016) describe edge-emotions "as a signal that our assumptions are being challenged and our meaning perspectives threatened" and that "thus, we may feel a number of unpleasant emotions including anxiety, fear, anger" (p. 175). This phenomenon is demonstrated easily by a toddler for whom the world is different from their caregiver and who yet sets afoot (or a crawl) toward their personal unknown despite the emotional signals of instant danger due to leaving the adult companion. Edge-emotions are a key element within the "interaction amongst the emotional, cognitive and social dimensions of experience" (Mälkki & Green, 2016, p. 174). To go toward our edge-emotions and past the comfort-boundaries is to go to the place where growth and learning happen (Mälkki, 2011). This far edge of personal unknown—be it the toddler or their new parent, or a mountain climber—is where the adventure begins and there the occasional visit to the zone of sisu.

Sisu overlaps with certain endurance aspects of qualities such as perseverance and grit but differs in its emphasis on short-term intensity rather than long-term stamina. Most of the examples of sisu in my data involved determination and doggedness typical to grit but without the passion or pursuit of a dominant superordinate life goal (Duckworth & Gross, 2014). Furthermore, though "being gritty" and persevering means to keep on going despite adversities along the way, it does not necessarily require a singular adverse incident to initiate it (Collins et al., 2016). One of the essential features of sisu, however, is the experience of adversity. In the survey data, sisu was rarely described in relation to the pursuit of goals. One response defined sisu as "[p]ressing onward when you feel you cannot keep going, reaching beyond your limit, having resoluteness when facing an insurmountable obstacle, and sticking to your word," and another, more descriptive response went as: "blood and guts to go through the shit that life heaves on your shoulders, whether it's wars, disabling accidents or diseases, financial ruination, death of loved ones, divorce, or having to turn a swamp into productive farmland" (Lahti, 2019, p. 66). Sisu in the Finnish cultural sense is less about "achievement for achievement's sake" and more about responding to a challenge with our best and most honest effort—be this situation a self-selected extreme challenge like the 72-mile ultramarathon across mountains in the example shared by Norma Bastidas, or an unexpected hardship hurled at us by life.

Latent Strength—Unearthing Hidden Reserves

> Remember that what pulls the strings is the force hidden within; there lies the power to persuade, there the life—there, if one must speak out, the real man.
>
> *Marcus Aurelius*

While extraordinary perseverance incorporates nuances from concepts such as perseverance and grit with their connection to beliefs and mindset, a more unique theme based on the survey data is sisu as a kind of latent strength, or "intestinal fortitude," as described by a respondent (Lahti, 2019, p. 74). It brought sisu closer to what James (1914) worded as a "different type of vital endurance" (p. 21) and invited me to form an inquiry into fortitude as something closer to somatic or "embodied toughness" rather than mental or psychological toughness.

Latent power denotes a visceral quality (meaning it is more about the responses of the body as opposed to intellect, cognition, and sheer will) of the stored-up inner strength that then manifests as extraordinary perseverance in the face of adversity. This reserve lies dormant, is normally not accessed, and becomes available through the gateway of an extraordinary challenge. It denotes the side of sisu that is sometimes shorthanded as a "magical" or "mind-boggling power" that has made sisu so elusive and hard to describe (Lahti, 2019, p. 68). In the words of one survey respondent, "[sisu] is what defines us and is almost like magic in the sense that with it, you can do what others think is not possible" (p. 71) and another, "sisu is the fire that does not fade, no matter what. A driving force, deep inside ones [sic] soul, big strong feisty energy that makes one go pursuing the set goal" (p. 68). Latent power echoes the etymological origin of sisu as the "innermost part" or the "guts." In 1745, Daniel Juslenius defined *sisucunda* in his dictionary as the specific location in the human body where strong affects originate (Länsimäki, 2003).

Furthermore, while the ancient Greeks two millennia ago entertained the idea of stomach as the seat of humanly inner strength and Greco-Roman poet and satirist Persius (34–62 AD) mused that "Magister artis ingenique largitor venter" [That master of the arts, that dispenser of genius, the belly.] (Ramsay, 1920, line 10, p. 310), most research on the determinants of human behaviour has traditionally been overshadowed by the notion of actions emanating from the mind. In the last few decades, an idea has been promoted in cognitive science to view the body as having a central role in shaping our mind, actions, and emotions. Wilson and Galonka (2013) describe embodied cognition as the radical hypothesis that "the brain is not the sole cognitive resource available to us to solve problems" (para. 3). This view is in alignment with and builds upon the pioneering work of husband-and-wife J. J. Gibson and E. J. Gibson of cognition as an embodied experience that offered an innovative way to overcome the dichotomy of the mind and body dilemma present in traditional psychology (see J. J. Gibson, 1929, 1950; E. J. Gibson, 2002; also see Maturana & Varela, 1988, for the embodied approach to the mind). "Our bodies and their perceptually guided motions through the world do much of the work required to achieve our goals" (para. 3), Wilson and Galonka further continue. Understanding the gut–brain connection took a leap forward with the discovery of the enteric nervous system (ENS) in the middle of the 19th century (Furness, 2006). Because of its complexity, size, and similarity to the central nervous system (CNS), the ENS has become described not only as the brain in the gut but our first evolved or original brain. Preclinical evidence suggests that gut microbes are part of the unconscious system regulating our behavioural responses related to stress, pain perception, emotions, and social interactions (Dinan et al., 2015; Foster et al., 2017; Moloney et al., 2014). While coming from the direction of neuroscience, study by Paulus et al. (2009) on extreme environments that require optimal cognitive and behavioural performance suggests that "individual variability with respect to optimal performance in extreme environments depends on a well 'contextualised' internal body state that is associated with an appropriate potential to act" (p. 1080).

While embodied cognition is still finding its way as a research methodology and unified theoretical framework (Zwaan, 2021)—a challenge not unique to embodied cognition—and while it is not yet clear how the microbiome alters the brain or how the ENS influences our behaviour through emotions, preliminary research within these developing disciplines offers interesting future directions regarding the role of the body in the cognitive and non-cognitive processes and the nature of the mind–body integration. It may allow a look into potential connections between the gut and for example courage, sisu, grit, and the like with perhaps inquiries into something as organic as individual dietary interventions to enhance life energy through supporting the gut's microbial composition (see Frame et al., 2020). In a culture that has long praised the power of the mind at the expense of the somatic side of the human experience, sisu—like embodied practices such as breathwork, dance, and cold-water therapy—can support an exploration toward more holistic research-backed dialogue regarding the nature of inner strength.

Gentle Power—The Necessity of Graceful Strength

> This is the moment when what we need most is enough people with the skill, heart, and wisdom to help us pull ourselves back from the edge of breakdown and onto a different path.
>
> *Otto Scharmer*

Endurance athletes, expeditioners, and adventurers are often applauded for their willpower, dogged mental endurance, and resilience that allow them to navigate and excel amidst the most unimaginable circumstances. Sisu however goes beyond mere stamina and resolve and invites us to discern not just *what* we do but *how* we do what we do. In today's super-connected world, the impact of our behaviour and the ripples of our example travel far. Therefore, any socially conscious discussion around fortitude must include an inquiry into how our mighty actions influence not only our own life but the lives of those around us, as well as the social systems at large.

While sisu can be a positive driving force that is central to both survival and high performance, perhaps even giving rise to a kind of "brave entrepreneurialism" (Lahti, 2013, p. 54), too much sisu can lead to stubbornness, foolhardiness, inflexible thinking, and even mercilessness toward others (Lahti, 2019). Three main themes around harmful sisu were generated as a result of a survey: (1) sisu that leads to extreme mental stress and overextending the body in ways that lead to physical injury, accidents, and burnout; (2) sisu that causes harm to others as a result of an obsession over a task at the expense of others, ignoring people's perspectives, failing to sympathise with their struggles, as well as being cold and ruthless toward colleagues, family, and friends; and finally (3) sisu that impairs the individual's ability to think, reason, and discern a healthy course of action. The last mentioned can lead to poor judgment, inability to see the big picture of things, evaluate one's capacities, ask for help, and know when to quit or pivot (Lahti, 2019).

Most respondents of the survey were keen to acquire more sisu but were also concerned how one can know when to continue in the face of hardship and when to release the effort. "[Too much sisu leads to] denying the realities of life, as well as the limits of human strength, therefore denying the very core of our humanity in ourselves and others," one respondent wrote (Lahti, 2019, p. 68). Even though the majority (58%) of the respondents (n = 1,036) indicated that they wished they had more sisu, the case was not so clear when the respondents were asked to choose between being more intelligent (43%) or having more sisu (36%). One response stated that "If you have intelligence but lack sisu, you are going nowhere" (Lahti, 2013, p. 39). The third response option, "something else," yielded interesting comments as some examples of the qualities the respondents indicated they wished to gain were emotional intelligence, wisdom, empathy, compassion, and in fact, the ability to have both sisu and intelligence in a healthy balance along with an understanding of when and how to use these qualities. This speaks to the idea that sisu itself is neither "good" nor "bad" but is a tool that one needs to learn to master.

Gentle power, I propose, is the *higher octave* expression of sisu that is not blind and obsessive but adaptive, conscious, and harmonious and while not necessarily *of* reason, it is *informed* by reason (Lahti, 2022). It can also mean the strength to find acceptance and contentment in a moment when we are facing insurmountable headwind and even cease from further action if this leads to more beneficial long-term outcomes. This notion aligns with research by Vallerand et al. (2003) who wrote that, "[w]hether a passion will foster positive affect and healthy persistence depends on whether it is harmonious or obsessive" (p. 757). Descartes (2015), in his treatise on the *Passions of the Soul* distinguishes even between 'virtuous' and 'vicious' humility. Sisu, too, can become an expression of either polarity. This way, healthy sisu is ultimately a call for self-examination. While sisu is indeed about exceeding our assumed limits, it is also about learning to notice when our power turns into force and even having the courage to let go of our pursuit when needed.

Comte-Sponville (2002) writes that gentleness is "courage without violence, [its] strength without harshness, [its] love without anger" and that, "gentleness is, to begin with, a kind of peace, either real or desired" (p. x). To Aristotle (1934), gentleness was a virtue of temperance and the observance of mean between anger and "lack of spirit" and it was to not be led by emotion and "irascibility" (book 2, chapter 7). Gentleness therefore is not to be interpreted as weakness or fragility but rather as the courage to yield and the power to regulate one's emotional response to adapt when needed. While grand feats of adventure and even trauma can act as a pathway to growth and resilience (see Tedeschi & Calhoun, 2004, for posttraumatic growth and Chapter 11), seeking to thread our adventures from a place of self-awareness, balance, and harmony is the lantern to guide our steps. "A person possessing sisu must also possess grace and kindness. It is a fine line to walk," another respondent wrote (Lahti, 2019, p. 68). Since sisu can become either harmful or beneficial depending on how it is wielded, I propose developing it as a reserve of strength for adventure through the "humanly tuned" practice of *systems intelligence* (Hämäläinen & Saarinen, 2007, p. 4). This way rendering sisu as a balanced reserve of strength that is not only powerful to the individual, but gentle and elevating to those around the peculiar forces of nature that extreme athletes and adventurers often are.

Systems Intelligence—To Consciously Create Excellence in How We Think and Overcome

Systems intelligence, developed by professors Raimo Hämäläinen and Esa Saarinen at the Aalto University in Finland, describe systems thinking as "a key form of human behavioural intelligence" and success through the concrete efforts of self-inquiry (Saarinen & Hämäläinen, 2004, p. 9; see also Hämäläinen & Saarinen, 2007). Systems intelligence can be increased when the person consciously pauses to examine their belief structures and the systems of the environment that might need to be changed. "Thinking about thinking is a meta-level capability fundamental to man as a self-corrective system" (Saarinen & Hämäläinen, 2004, p. 18). As demonstrated by researchers such as Carol Dweck and her colleagues, beliefs held by an individual form the blueprint that to a great extent defines their future action (see Job et al., 2010; Yeager & Dweck, 2012). While sisu points to something embodied rather than just cognitive, as interconnected and holistic systems, our thinking is an inseparable part of our functioning. The beliefs held by an adventurer in a challenging, strenuous moment that triggers survival mode and therefore limits access to cognitive reserves when the adventurer needs it the most are of crucial importance.

Systems intelligence is an invitation to "challenge ourselves and improve on a daily basis" (Hämäläinen et al., 2014, p. 22), and this reflective inquiry is done within the eight domains of systems intelligence that are labelled as systemic perception, attunement, reflection, positive engagement, spirited discovery, effective responsiveness, wise action, and positive attitude (see Hämäläinen et al., 2014; Törmänen et al., 2016, 2021).[1] This same idea—to overcome limiting conditionings through conscious practice—is at the heart of my approach to sisu. The four assumptions from which I draw upon in this context are:

1. People are naturally systems intelligent (Hämäläinen et al., 2014, p. 50).
2. People are naturally equipped with sisu (Lahti, 2019) and "strength habitually not taxed at all" (James, 1907, p. 8).
3. Human systems and their respective structures are created by the underlying forces of mental models (Monat, 2018, pp. 4–5; Saarinen & Hämäläinen, 2004, pp. 17–18).
4. The key to creating change (including fostering systems intelligence and sisu) lies in our self-reflective ability to *think about our thinking* and reflect on these mental models (Hämäläinen et al., 2014; Saarinen & Hämäläinen, 2004, pp. 17–18).

Hämäläinen et al. (2014) present that success and survival involve something beyond the intelligence of the individual. This something is the system, i.e., the "big picture" consisting of the environment, context, situation, and our internal dialogue with which we are in a constant conversation. For someone sailing across the Atlantic Ocean or summiting Kilimanjaro, it is the changing weather conditions (or the terrain in mountaineering), the dynamics among the team, and how consciously we can navigate all this dynamism. Just like sisu, systems intelligence is assumed as an innate quality and therefore people will naturally sometimes 'hit home,' i.e., make systems intelligent choices and respond to significant hardships with fortitude. The point, according to Hämäläinen, Jones, and Saarinen, however, is not to rely on manifesting our innate systems intelligence randomly here and there, if we're lucky, but to make systems intelligence systemic by engineering it into our daily lives. They write in *Being Better Better* (2014):

> Few of us, however, push ourselves to test the limits of our capacities within systems. Yet, there is little doubt that with just minimal effort we could make much more intelligent choices with respect to the contexts we find ourselves in. We can make ourselves better at being better.
>
> *(p. 17)*

In systems thinking, our potentiality is accessed through improving the quality of our thinking, which then bridges to the quality of our actions. According to Saarinen & Hämäläinen (2004, pp. 18–19), thinking about our thinking involves the following:

- Acknowledging that one's action and behaviour are the result of one's thinking (mental models, beliefs, assumptions, and interpretations).
- Acknowledging that one's thinking is likely to be highly one-sided and a far cry from an accurate grasp of the bigger picture; the holistic system around self is likely to be reflected in one's thinking only partially and possibly in a distorted form ("How well do I know what I don't know?").
- To act more intelligently in systemic environments, one must engage in meta-level thinking regarding their thinking ("How do I use my thinking?").
- One's framing of the environment and its interconnected systems likely reflects their subjective assumptions. Reflection on how I frame and look at things is an intelligent path to life in systems ("How do my beliefs guide my thinking?").

Systems intelligence provides a conceptual platform to investigate and talk about how one's thinking can be used better to create better results in unusually demanding, strenuous, or even risky undertakings in which adventurers might find themselves in but it is of course abundant everywhere from regular daily activities to the uncommon situations of extreme sports. Because systems often share many similar characteristics, it is possible "to transfer successful strategies and approaches from one system to another" (Hämäläinen et al., 2014, p. 107) such as the exchange between strategies of resilience in athletics and music performers (Clark & Williamon, 2011) or for example the best practices in rock climbing and ethical leadership or business (Bischak & Woiceshyn, 2015). Lessons learned for example through patience required in parenthood or sisu needed to manoeuvre big setbacks of daily life (being laid off from work, experiencing loss, illness, or an existential crisis) can translate into strategies for adventure and vice versa: overcoming hardships in adventure and extreme sports can contribute to practices for dealing better with daily life. The promise of systems intelligence lies in its ability to invite and prime adventurers to tune into the "ordinary magic" of everyday experiences as training ground for the deep-seated fortitude of sisu and to develop a blueprint of inner strength that serves them throughout their daily lives—both *on and off* the beaten track.

Conclusion

Sisu is about the hidden strength that lies beyond the edges of our assumed capacities and it carries a message to all explorers to not shy away from the call of the adventure: there is more strength to us than meets the eye. While sisu shares overlapping features with qualities like perseverance, resilience, and grit, its most pronounced aspect is about tapping into a reserve of previously unexpressed strength that seems more embodied than mental. While neither sisu nor the better thinking advocated by systems intelligence alone is enough to produce our highest expression in extreme situations, these two combined could be used to develop fortitude that not only helps adventurers excel and achieve their goals but ascend on a personal level too. It is no secret that the world as we know it is breathing heavily under the current transformations in the many arenas of human life from political, social, and health to environmental and technological. Within this, we are confronted with both the urgency and opportunity to explore the boundaries of our presently known world. Be they expeditions of athleticism, activism, adventure, or inner awareness, the relentlessness with which humans are able to seek "the examined life," as Socrates articulated millennia ago, that is engaged with "truth" and "goodness" of things, is the ultimate adventure of a lifetime, and what to me holds the hope of our future. In this chapter, I discussed the Finnish construct of sisu through some of its expressions—extraordinary perseverance, latent strength, and gentle power—and highlighted systems intelligence as a tool to support the balanced cultivation of this quality, so that we may not only survive and be triumphant in our adventures but become better through these feats.

Note

1 The systems intelligence inventory is available at http://salserver.org.aalto.fi/sitest/en/

References

Aho, W. R. (1994). Is sisu alive and well among Finnish Americans? In M. G. Karni & J. Asala (Eds.), *The best of Finnish Americana* (pp. 196–205). Penfield Press.
Amanzio, M., & Benedetti, F. (1999). Neuropharmacological dissection of placebo analgesia: Expectation-activated opioid systems versus conditioning-activated specific sub-systems. *Journal of Neuroscience, 19*(1), 484–494. https://doi.org/10.1523/JNEUROSCI.19-01-00484.1999
Aristotle (1934). *Aristotle in 23 Volumes, Vol. 19*. Translated by H. Rackham. Harvard University Press.
Bischak, D. P., & Woiceshyn, J. (2016). Leadership virtues exposed: Ethical leadership lessons from leading in rock climbing. *Journal of Leadership & Organizational Studies, 23*(3), 248–259. https://doi.org/10.1177/1548051815617629
Broad, C. (1923). *Scientific thought*. Harcourt, Brace, and Company, Inc.
Clark, V. R., Hopkins, W. G., Hawley, J. A., & Burke, L. M. (2000). Placebo effect of carbohydrate feedings during a 40-km cycling time trial. *Medicine & Science in Sports & Exercise, 32*(9), 1642–1647. https://doi.org/10.1097/00005768-200009000-00019
Clark, T. A., & Williamon, A. (2011). Evaluating a mental skills training program for musicians. *Journal of Applied Sport Psychology, 23*(3), 342–359. https://doi.org/10.1080/10413200.2011.574676
Collins, D., MacNamara, A., & McCarthy, N. (2016). Super champions, champions, and almosts: Important differences and commonalities on the rocky road. *Frontiers in Psychology, 6*, 1–11. https://doi.org/10.3389/fpsyg.2015.02009

Comte-Sponville, A. (2002). *A small treatise on the great virtues*. Metropolitan Books.

Descartes, R. (2015). *The passions of the soul and other late philosophical writings*. Edited by M. Moriarty. Oxford: Oxford University Press.

Dinan, T. G., Stilling, R. M., Stanton, C., & Cryan, J. F. (2015). Collective unconscious: How gut microbes shape human behavior. *Journal of Psychiatric Research, 63*, 1–9. http://doi.org/10.1016/j.jpsychires.2015.02.021

Duckworth, A. L., & Gross, J. J. (2014). Self-control and grit: Related but separable determinants of success. *Current Directions in Psychological Science, 23*(5), 319–325. https://doi.org/10.1177/0963721414541462

Foster, J. A., Rinaman, L., & Cryan, J. F. (2017). Stress and the gut-brain axis: Regulation by the microbiome. *Neurobiology of Stress, 19*(7), 124–136. https://doi.org/10.1016/j.ynstr.2017.03.001

Frame, L. A, Costa, E., & Jackson, S. A. (2020). Current explorations of nutrition and the gut microbiome: A comprehensive evaluation of the review literature, *Nutrition Reviews, 78*(10), 798–812. https://doi.org/10.1093/nutrit/nuz106\

Furness, J. B. (2006). *The enteric nervous system*. Blackwell Publishing.

Gibson, E. J. (2002). *Perceiving the affordances: A portrait of two psychologists*. Lawrence Erlbaum Associates.

Gibson, J. J. (1929). The reproduction of visually perceived forms. *Journal of Experimental Psychology, 12*, 1–39. https://doi.org/10.1037/h0072470

Gibson, J. J. (1950). *The perception of the visual world*. Houghton Mifflin.

Gross, J. (1998). The emerging field of emotion regulation: An integrative review. *Review of General Psychology, 2*(3), 271–299.

Gross, J. (2001). Emotion regulation in adulthood: Timing is everything. *Current Directions in Psychological Science, 10*(6), 214–219.

Häkkinen, K. (2004). Nykysuomen etymologinen sanakirja [the etymological dictionary of modern Finnish]. Juva: WSOY.

Hämäläinen, R., Jones, R., & Saarinen, E. (2014). *Being better better: Living with systems intelligence*. CreateSpace Independent Publishing Platform.

Hämäläinen, R. P., & Saarinen, E. (Eds.) (2007). *Systems intelligence in leadership and everyday life*. Systems Analysis Laboratory. Helsinki University of Technology. https://sal.aalto.fi/publications/pdf-files/systemsintelligence2007.pdf

James, W. (1907). The energies of men. *Science, New Series, 25*(635), 321–332. www.jstor.org

James, W. (1914). *The energies of men*. Moffat, Yard and Company.

Job, V., Dweck, C. S., & Walton, G. M. (2010). Ego depletion – Is it all in your head? Implicit theories about willpower affect self-regulation. *Psychological Science, 21*(11), 1686–1693. https://doi.org/10.1177/0956797610384745

Lahti, E. (2013). *Above and beyond perseverance: An exploration of sisu*. Unpublished master's thesis. University of Pennsylvania, Philadelphia, United States.

Lahti, E. (2019). Embodied fortitude: An introduction to the Finnish construct of sisu. *International Journal of Wellbeing, 9*(1), 61–82. https://doi.org/10.5502/ijw.v9i1.672

Lahti, E. (2022). Sisu as guts, grace and gentleness: A way of life, growth, and being in times of adversity. Doctoral thesis. Aalto University, Finland.

Länsimäki, M. (2003, March 11). *Suomalaista sisua* [Finnish sisu]. Helsingin Sanomat.

Lucas, K., & Buzzanell, P. M. (2004). Blue-collar work, career, and success: Occupational narratives of sisu. *Journal of Applied Communication Research, 32*(4), 273–292. https://doi.org/10.1080/0090988042000240167

Mälkki, K. (2011). Theorizing the nature of reflection. Unpublished doctoral thesis. University of Helsinki, Helsinki, Finland.

Mälkki, K., & Green, L. (2016). Ground, warmth, and light: Facilitating conditions for reflection and transformative dialogue. *Journal of Educational Issues, 2*(2), 169–183. http://doi:10.5296/jei.v2i2.9947

Maturana, H. R., & Varela, F. J. (1988). *The tree of knowledge: The biological roots of human understanding.* Shambhala Publications, Inc.

Mitä on sisu? [What is sisu?] (1942, November 22). Uusi-Suomi. Copy in possession of the author.

Moloney, R. D., Desbonnet, L., Clarke, G. Dinan, T. G., & Cryan, J. F. (2014). The microbiome: Stress, health and disease. *Mammalian Genome, 25,* 49–74. https://doi.org/10.1007/s00335-013-9488-5

Monat, J. P. (2018). Explaining natural patterns using systems thinking. American Journal of Systems Science, *6(1), 1–15.* http://doi:10.5923/j.ajss.20180601.01

Paulus, M. P., Potterat, E. G., Taylor, M. K., Van Orden, K. F., Bauman, J., Momen, N., Padilla, G. A., & Swain, J. L. (2009). A neuroscience approach to optimizing brain resources for human performance in extreme environments. *Neuroscience & Biobehavioral Reviews, 33*(7), 1080–1088. https://doi.org/10.1016/j.neubiorev.2009.05.003

Pollo, A., Carlino, E., & Benedetti, F. (2008). The top-down influence of ergogenic placebos on muscle work and fatigue. *European Journal of Neuroscience, 28*(2), 379–388. https://doi.org/10.1111/j.1460-9568.2008.06344.x

Pollo, A., Carlino, E., & Benedetti, F. (2011). Placebo mechanisms across different conditions: from the clinical setting to physical performance. *Philosophical Transactions of the Royal Society, 366*(1572), 1790–1798. https://doi.org/10.1098/rstb.2010.0381

Ramsay, G. G. (1920). *Juvenial and Persius.* G. P. Putnam's Sons.

Saarinen, E., & Hämäläinen, R. P. (2004). Systems intelligence: Connecting engineering thinking with human sensitivity. In R. P. Hämäläinen & E. Saarinen (Eds.), *Systems intelligence: Discovering a hidden competence in human action and organizational life* (pp. 9–37). Helsinki University of Technology, Systems Analysis Laboratory, Research Reports A88. https://sal.aalto.fi/publications/pdf-files/systemsintelligence2004.pdf

Tedeschi, R. G., & Calhoun, L. G. (2004). Posttraumatic growth: Conceptual foundations and empirical evidence. *Psychological Inquiry, 15*(1), 1–18. https://doi.org/doi:10.1207/s15327965pli1501_01

Tokoi, O. (1957). Sisu, even through a stone wall: The autobiography of Oskari Tokoi. Robert Speller & Sons.

Törmänen, J., Hämäläinen, R. P., & Saarinen, E. (2016), Systems intelligence inventory. *The Learning Organization, 23*(4), 218–231. https://doi.org/10.1108/TLO-01-2016-0006

Törmänen, J., Hämäläinen, R. P., & Saarinen, E. (2021). Perceived systems intelligence and performance in organizations. *Human Resource Development Quarterly,* 1–24. https://doi.org/10.1108/TLO-04-2021-0045

Vallerand, R. J., Blanchard, C., Mageau, G. A., Koestner, R., Ratelle, C., ... Marsolais, J. (2003). Les passions de l'âme: On obsessive and harmonious passion. *Journal of Personality and Social Psychology, 85*(4), 756–767. https://doi.org/10.1037/0022-3514.85.4.756

Wilson, A. D., & Galonka, S. (2013). Embodied cognition is not what you think it is. *Frontiers in Psychology, 4*(58), 1–13. https://doi.org/10.3389/fpsyg.2013.00058

Yeager, D. S., & Dweck, C. S. (2012). Mindsets that promote resilience: When students believe that personal characteristics can be developed. *Educational Psychologist, 47*(4), 302–314. http://doi.org/10.1080/00461520.2012.722805

Zwaan, R. A. (2021). Two Challenges to "embodied cognition": Research and how to overcome them. *Journal of Cognition, 4*(1), 14. https://doi.org/10.5334/joc.151

SECTION II
Transformational Impact of Adventure

10

HOW CAN ADVENTURE CHANGE OUR CONSCIOUSNESS? AN EXPLORATION OF FLOW, MINDFULNESS, AND ADVENTURE

Susan Houge Mackenzie

An Adventurer's Point of View – Tranquility by Fabio Brunazzi

In the Summer of 2020 I crossed the North Atlantic Ocean from West to East solo on a 29-foot sailboat.

This voyage came unexpectedly, even if I had dreamed of it many times before.

Today I want to present an experience I went through on this trip, which has a special meaning for me. I am talking about the so called "oceanic feeling", a concept which made its way into academic discussion in the late 1920s through the correspondence between Sigmund Freud and French novelist Romain Rolland.

I will always remember tonight. I am quite in the middle of my trip as I already passed Bermuda. Earlier I turned off all lights on Tranquility, even navigation lights, to let my eyes adapt to the night. The risk of collision is minimal and I am on deck anyway, fully awake and attuned to my surroundings.

The breeze is pushing the boat along nicely at 4 knots on a completely flat sea. The pressure of the wind on the sails is keeping the boat on a gentle and stable beam reach.

Tranquility's heading is perfectly en route with the imaginary line that connects where we are with the Azores. The autopilot steadily steers the boat in the right direction.

I recall the feeling of fresh air on my bare skin. I stay completely naked on deck, there are no bugs to torment me, no noise, no worries, just myself on the boat and the stars above and bioluminescence sparkling in green dots all around Tranquility's wake. It is like stardust of the ocean, green sparkles of aquatic life.

In the safety of the cockpit I raise my head to the sky and start to observe the stars.

There is no moon in sight and the entirety of the sky unfolds in any direction. Only the foresail hides part of it.

I walk to the bow. There, behind the canvas wing, the Milky Way opens in front of me, immense and clear against the dark.

Here, one hundred miles or so north of Bermuda, on a flat North Atlantic Ocean, I realise that a moment with my head up looking at the stars is the experience of a lifetime.

I don't have to do anything special to experience this moment. I don't need to power a device, to open the pages of a book or to be doing something. Thinking becomes also unnecessary. I realise I am simply part of it. The inner and outer parts of what I consider myself blend seamlessly.

The choices made and actions taken created this very night, the ripples propagate from this now to the infinity, going even beyond the local and finite existence of my ego. Words and images are not enough to grasp this feeling, yet I recall the various degrees of euphoria, satisfaction and belonging that flow through my attention.

In this joyful state I can perceive the connections in my life, all the people that helped or antagonised me, and potentially every condition that brought me where I am, inscribed within a larger world or network.

On the background of a North Atlantic starry night, I perceive the fabric that connects everything, of which I am but a small knot, a whole containing all at once where I come from, where I am and where I am going.

Nothing but this memory, perhaps these words, will remain as the wake of my ship wanes in the calm ocean.

Fabio Brunazzi

How Can Adventure Change Our Consciousness? An Exploration of Flow, Mindfulness, and Adventure

Introduction

Athletes across a range of sport and adventure activities and experience levels often report being *in the zone*, a psychological state in which they are highly focused and frequently able to accomplish their greatest performances (Jackson & Csikszentmihalyi, 1999). In the psychological literature, this state is referred to as *flow*. Flow is an intrinsically rewarding optimal psychological state wherein individuals experience total absorption in an activity and a high sense of control, often in challenging situations (Csikszentmihalyi, 2002; Jackson et al., 2010). Flow has been extensively investigated in the domains of sport (Stamatelopoulou et al., 2018) and exercise (Jackman et al., 2019), and has been associated with optimal sporting performance and experience (Jackson et al., 2001; Swann et al., 2012), increased exercise motivation, and long-term exercise adherence (Jackman et al., 2019).

In addition to traditional sport contexts, flow has been identified as a key motivation for, and characteristic of, participants' experiences across diverse adventure activities (Csikszentmihalyi & Csikszentmihalyi, 1990; Houge Mackenzie et al., 2011, 2013). Flow experiences have been reported as motivational for both novice and expert adventure participants. There may be unique stages, facilitators and characteristics of flow in adventure contexts such as immersion in nature and exercising skills to control and reduce risks (Boudreau et al., 2022b). Flow also appears to be linked to a range of positive adventure outcomes, including enhanced well-being, intrinsic motivation, optimal performance, spiritual development and progression, as well as some potentially negative consequences, such as increased risk-taking and addiction (Boudreau et al., 2020, 2022a).

Given that flow appears to be so integral to the adventure experience, this chapter will first explore what flow is, from the perspective of consciousness and attention, and present the traditional model of flow. Emergent models of flow will then be presented and discussed in adventure contexts. Next, the relationship between flow and mindfulness will be considered and tensions in the literature related to these two experiences discussed. Finally, potential links between adventure activities, mindfulness, and flow will be explored alongside directions for future research and implications for enhancing human and environmental well-being.

The Nature of Flow and Consciousness

Rather than pre-emptively defining the positive experience state known as 'flow', the origins of this positive experience state, which is rooted in cognitive processes collectively termed 'consciousness' (Csikszentmihalyi, 1988), will first be explored. This understanding will be important to inform the discussion of mindfulness and flow further on in the chapter.

The concept of flow stemmed from intrinsic motivation research, particularly work by Lepper and Greene (1978), Deci (1975) and deCharms (1968). Seminal flow investigations (Csikszentmihalyi, 1975) went beyond asking why people participated in activities with no extrinsic rewards, to asking how intrinsic rewards *felt*. What began as an attempt to understand the experiences and motivations of artists generated an extensively studied construct for understanding consciousness and enjoyment that has been foundational to our understanding of sport and adventure activities (Jackson & Csikszentmihalyi, 1999; Jones et al., 2000, 2003; Massimini & Carli, 1988).

In its essence, flow theory was an attempt to link the structure of consciousness to positive experiential states. Csikszentmihalyi (1988), the originator of flow theory, posited that consciousness evolved as a way to convert physiological instincts to subjective understanding and viewed it as the accumulation of all our experiences. Consciousness is composed of three basic systems: attention, awareness and memory. Attention denotes immediate information and is temporally limited. Awareness refers to any processes occurring after information is attended to, such as emotions and evaluation. Finally, memory stores relevant information that has passed through consciousness. Through this process, "awareness of the self" emerges (Csikszentmihalyi, 1988, p. 20).

As reflected in Maslow's (1968) theory of self-actualisation and in more well-developed psychological theories (e.g., self-determination theory; Deci & Ryan, 2012), the self has a variety of needs beyond basic survival. One key role of the self is to determine which goals or needs to fulfil, based on genetic, cultural and idiosyncratic information (Csikszentmihalyi & Csikszentmihalyi, 1988). Foremost, the self will attempt to duplicate states of consciousness that are congruent with the goals of the self, and therefore pleasant, and avoid states that conflict with the goals of the self and thereby threaten it. Flow theory underscores the key role of consciousness in determining self-actualising goals; "What [people] want to do does not depend directly on outside forces, but... on the priorities established by the needs of the self" (Csikszentmihalyi, 1988, p. 16). According to Csikszentmihalyi, psychic entropy is caused by activities which conflict with individual goals and thereby produce disorder in consciousness (e.g., boredom or anxiety). Conversely, psychic negentropy, the ordering of consciousness, or flow, is created by activities congruent with the goals of the self. "[Flow is obtained] when all the contents of consciousness are in harmony with each other, and with the goals that define the person's self" (Csikszentmihalyi, 1988, p. 24). Csikszentmihalyi's (1975, 1988) initial research supported these principles. He found that pleasant emotional experiences occurred when consciousness was ordered and congruent with the goals of the self.

Flow theory has robustly demonstrated that people enjoy, and are intrinsically motivated by, activities that present an optimal balance between perceived challenges and the perceived skills necessary to meet that challenge (Csikszentmihalyi & Csikszentmihalyi, 1988). Further, this balance must spiral infinitely upward in order to continually exceed personal averages and thereby facilitate flow experiences. Jackson and Csikszentmihalyi (1999) referred to this continual (re)balancing that facilitates flow as the challenge/skill balance. However, flow occurs only when a balance of challenge and skills is perceived; not necessarily when it is 'objectively' achieved. This means that flow is determined by the subjective experience of an activity, which means that objective measures of skill versus challenge may be extraneous to this experience. While Csikszentmihalyi (1975) originally identified six flow dimensions that facilitated this ordered state of consciousness, sport-based studies (Jackson, 1992, 1996; Jackson et al., 1998, 2001; Marsh & Jackson, 1999) expanded the original six flow dimensions to the following nine (Jackson & Csikszentmihalyi, 1999; Jackson et al., 2010):

1. *A challenges/skill balance.* Flow occurs when perceived challenges are balanced with perceived skills. This balance, however, must exist at a level higher than the individual's normal level of functioning. Readers should also note at this point that the term 'balance' does not always indicate an exact matching of

challenges and skills, but rather that perceived challenge and skills tends to fluctuate or hover around this balance point.
2. *Merging of action and awareness.* In flow, actions merge with awareness and a feeling of oneness with the action is experienced.
3. *Clear goals.* Flow is characterised by coherent demands for action, or goals.
4. *Unambiguous feedback.* In flow, an individual's actions are met with clear and unambiguous feedback.
5. *Total concentration on the task at hand.* Individuals demonstrate intense concentration centred on the activity at hand during flow.
6. *Sense of control.* A strong sense of being in control of actions and the environment is reported during flow.
7. *Loss of self-consciousness.* In flow, the 'self' disappears from awareness. Although the self is fully functioning, it is not aware of itself doing so, and therefore attends only to the present task.
8. *Transcendence of time.* During a flow experience, an individual's sense of time is altered. Generally, hours seem to pass by in minutes and, less commonly, seconds stretch to what seems like eternity.
9. *Autotelic experience.* The end product of the above elements is an autotelic experience. Flow is so intrinsically rewarding and enjoyable that individuals will participate simply for the sake of doing it.

Flow in Adventure Contexts

Flow researchers have often lamented the difficulty of isolating and predicting 'flow activities' in everyday settings, (Ellis et al., 1994; Massimini & Carli, 1988). However, research has shown that flow dimensions may be more pronounced when participants engage in adventurous, challenging, intrinsically rewarding activities, such as adventure pursuits (Csikszentmihalyi, 1975, 1988; Csikszentmihalyi & Csikszentmihalyi, 1990; Delle Fave et al., 2003; Jones et al., 2000, 2003). Flow has been studied in adventure contexts such as rock climbing (Csikszentmihalyi, 1975) since its inception, and has since been identified as an important source of enjoyment and motivation across a range of land and water-based adventure activities (Houge Mackenzie et al., 2011, 2013; Morgan & Coutts, 2016; Motl, 1996; Nerothin, 2017; Partington et al., 2009).

A recent meta-analysis of flow states in adventure recreation contexts identified four key facets of this flow literature: antecedents and inhibitors, flow characteristics, consequences, and conceptual differences (Boudreau et al., 2020). The antecedents of flow in adventure include challenge perceptions; context (i.e., risk reduction, immersion in nature, appropriate experience level); goals (both exploratory goals and fixed, objective goals); exploration; and confidence. Conversely, flow is inhibited in adventure contexts by factors such as anxiety, lack of confidence, and self-consciousness. The characteristics of flow in adventure (i.e. during the experiential state of flow) include some of the traditional flow dimensions such as time transformation (e.g., faster or slower), increased sense of control and focus on the activity, and effortlessness. Concentration on, and absorption in, the task at hand, and focus on specific stimuli were prevalent across studies of flow in adventure, which appeared linked to a loss of self-consciousness (Boudreau et al., 2020, 2022b). This finding is particularly relevant to our discussion of how mindfulness might be linked to flow and adventure further on.

Consequences of flow in adventure include a range of positive as well as negative outcomes. In terms of positive consequences, flow experiences have been linked to enhanced performance, skill development, well-being, motivation, and spirituality (Boudreau et al., 2020; Houge Mackenzie & Hodge, 2020). Although current evidence precludes establishing causal links between flow and improved performance in adventure contexts, studies suggest that these experiences may be related. For example, adventure participants have reported perceiving that their performance exceeded expectations and/or feeling highly accomplished as a result of flow (Partington et al., 2009; Swann et al., 2017). Future research could further explore if flow in adventure settings is associated with enhanced performance based on objective performance indicators. In addition, as a handful of studies have identified potential negative consequences of flow, in relation to both underestimating risk (Schüler & Nakamura, 2013) and addictive behaviours (Partington et al., 2009), further research on the potentially negative consequences of flow in adventure contexts is also needed.

Finally, Boudreau et al. (2020)'s meta-analysis reflected a key tension which has emerged in the flow literature over the last decade in both adventure and sport contexts. Specifically, adventure and sport literature has challenged traditional conceptualisations of flow as a singular state. For instance, studies in the adventure context have identified evidence of distinct optimal states based on participant goals. These include a state of 'paratelic flow', wherein participants reported lowered arousal levels and lacked a clearly defined outcome goal, and 'telic flow', characterised by clear, important outcome goals and heightened arousal levels (Houge Mackenzie et al., 2011, 2013). In the adventure context, the natural environment may also play a role in these distinct states (e.g., expanded awareness of the natural environment was linked to paratelic flow, whereas narrowed awareness limited to the immediate adventure task/challenge was linked to telic flow). Houge Mackenzie et al. (2011, 2013) argued that their findings were congruent with Csikszentmihalyi's original conceptualisation of flow as an ordering of consciousness created by activities congruent with the goals of the self. In these studies, the authors identified that multiple goal states could produce distinct flow states in the adventure contexts, and that these distinct states were often experienced in several phases, as part of the holistic adventure experience. In the sport domain, Swann et al. (2017) have similarly posited two distinct optimal states characterised by distinct goal states. These are the flow state, which has commonalities with the concept of paratelic flow in that it is associated with exploratory or open goals, and the clutch state, which has commonalities with telic flow in that it is associated with important outcome goals.

Emerging evidence from both the adventure and sport contexts suggests that there are either distinct types of flow states or distinct optimal experiences (e.g., flow and clutch) that have previously been presented as a single state within the literature. For instance, clutch scholars, such as Swann et al. (2017), posit that flow entails being completely absorbed in what one is doing and performing a task effortlessly (i.e. 'letting it happen'), whereas clutch states are experienced as 'making it happen', in the sense that individuals purposefully increase the level of effort and concentration exerted to achieve important performance outcomes. Swann et al. (2017) proposed the following as characteristics as being unique to flow: effortless attention, positive feedback about progress, absence of critical thoughts, optimal arousal, and automatic experience. Boudreau et al. (2020) suggested that, in adventure recreation, definitions of flow should also include time transformation, sense of control, focus on the activity, and effortlessness.

Clearly further research is needed to identify, define and measure flow states, and/or related optimal experiences and outcomes, in adventure contexts. However, these investigations should be guided by the often overlooked conceptual and empirical underpinnings of flow theory, which from the outset detailed evidence of potentially distinct flow states. For example, pursuits which required limited skills and presented "very low challenge levels" were termed "microflow activities" (Csikszentmihalyi, 1975, p. 141). Microflow activities mirrored "deep flow" activities in that they involved some goals and procedures, which enabled concentration on a limited stimulus field and provided feedback. It was the degree of task challenge and complexity that distinguished 'microflow' from 'deep flow' in initial models. Csikszentmihalyi (1975) originally argued that, "the flow model suggests that flow exists on a continuum from extremely low to extremely high complexity" (p. 141), and reported differences in flow experiences and outcomes related to distinct activities, such as housework versus rock climbing. While participants reported flow in a range of goal-oriented activities, such as housework, they did not report that these flow experiences contributed to personal growth, or were as rewarding, intense, or personally meaningful as more intense forms of flow. These findings are reflected in early flow models, which posited that the greatest potential for personal growth arose when challenges were above average (Csikszentmihalyi, 1990, 1993). Conceptually, some of these distinct flow experiences identified in early flow research are congruent with more recent propositions regarding distinct states of paratelic flow, telic flow, and/or clutch. These terms reflect more fine-grained attempts to capture important differences in similar types of highly absorbing and engaging optimal experiences, based on attributes such as the nature of attentional focus, preferred arousal levels, goal states and, potentially, activity types.

Mindfulness, Meditation, Flow and Adventure

The previous section identified how flow experiences are rooted in the way we experience consciousness, which is comprised of our attention, awareness and memory. When we conceptualise flow in these terms, we begin to see that the ways in which we direct our attention and awareness are fundamental to flow experiences, and the consequences of those experiences. Not only does this help us to understand how multiple flow states might be possible in adventure contexts (e.g., in relation to what we are focused on), but it also suggests that there may be important parallels between flow and the concepts of mindfulness and meditation. Therefore, we will next examine mindfulness and meditation and how they may relate to the concept of flow, as well as considering how these states may play a role in adventure experiences.

Mindfulness is "non-elaborative, non-judgmental, present-centred awareness in which each thought, feeling, or sensation that arises in the attentional field is acknowledged and accepted as is" (Bishop et al., 2004, p. 31). As such, it involves fully focusing on your present experience as it unfolds. While there are numerous perspectives on how mindfulness and meditation differ, they both seek to alter one's consciousness through attentional focus. There are also myriad meditation practices detailed in the literature, generally categorised into two basic types: concentrative meditation and mindfulness (or insight) meditation (Marlatt & Kristeller, 1999). Concentrative practices narrow and direct attention to a specific focus, such as breath or physical sensations, to the exclusion of everything else. In contrast, mindfulness practices are focused on expanding attention and creating an accepting, non-judgemental awareness of imagery, feelings, and all the physical and mental sensations. The regulation of attention is central to all forms of meditation (Cahn & Polich, 2006).

These definitions suggest that there are overlaps between flow, mindfulness and meditation. They all entail altered attentional focus (e.g., narrowed, expanded), involve full engagement in the present moment or current activity, and are all associated with optimal experiences and well-being (Landhäußer & Keller, 2012; Marlatt & Kristeller, 1999; Weinstein et al., 2009). Conceptually, there also appears to be the potential for connections between the distinct types of flow that have been proposed in adventure contexts (e.g., narrow, outcome focus of telic flow; expanded, process focus of paratelic flow) and some of the distinct attentional foci associated with mindfulness and different meditation practices.

Some research provides initial support for these propositions. For example, in sport contexts, mindfulness interventions have been positively associated with enhanced performance and flow (Kaufman et al., 2009). Mindfulness training has also been shown to enhance flow in sport, particularly when focused on developing clear goals and a sense of control (Aherne et al., 2011). While there is relatively sparse research on intentional or formalised mindfulness and meditation practices in adventure contexts, evidence from adventure education contexts suggests that adventure experiences are conducive to mindfulness (Kirwin et al., 2019; Mutz & Müller, 2016). However, it remains unclear whether the adventure activities themselves, the natural environments they unfold in, or some combination therein, facilitates mindfulness. Research suggests that simply being in nature fosters mindfulness and this is reflected in practices that combine mindfulness and nature (forest bathing, forest therapy; Ambrose-Oji, 2013; Shin et al., 2010). In addition, positive relationships have been identified between experiencing a sense of connection to nature and increased mindfulness (Howell et al., 2011).

Of most relevance to our consideration of relationships between flow, mindfulness and adventure is evidence that nature can cultivate directed attention due to the unique sensory environment (Hartig et al., 2014; Mayer et al., 2008). Attention restoration theory (Kaplan, 1995) helps to explain why natural environments may cultivate mindfulness: they have unique characteristics that hold our attention and interest, which helps to restore, rather than deplete, our attention (Kaplan & Berman, 2010). Specifically, the fact that adventure unfolds in natural environments means that there are at least three key ways these activities can change our attentional focus, based on Kaplan's model of attention and the natural environment. These are: (1) novel, engaging environments that are different to our everyday surroundings (e.g., forests, green/blue spaces); (2) fascinating objects that are effortless to observe and capture our attention (e.g., plants, clouds); and (3) an inherent human affinity for the natural environment and the opportunities it affords us. A growing body of literature supports this account of how time in nature is linked to enhanced directed attention, which is a key characteristic of flow, mindfulness and meditation (Berto, 2005; Mayer et al., 2008).

Despite conceptual similarities between states of mindfulness and flow, and the seemingly enhanced capacity of adventure contexts to facilitate these states, some scholars suggest that these relationships are not as straightforward as they may seem. Sheldon, Prentice, and Halusic (2015), for instance, argue that flow and mindfulness are fundamentally incompatible states. Key to their argument is the fact that, traditionally, flow has been characterised by a loss of self-awareness while engaged in an activity, while "mindfulness is characterised by maintaining self-awareness throughout or even despite an activity" (p. 276). Sheldon et al. hypothesised that mindfulness would be negatively associated with flow because mindfulness involves striving for sustained self-awareness, which could prevent us from losing ourselves in an activity and thereby experiencing flow. They use a metaphor from William James to illustrate this potential paradox:

> …mindfulness seems to entail standing on the bank of the stream without falling in; in contrast, flow entails jumping into the stream and tackling a challenging task or problem. In this sense, the two states might even be viewed as antagonistic, with mindfulness tending to bring one back to the bank of the stream, precluding flow.
>
> *(Sheldon et al., 2015, p. 276)*

Sheldon et al.'s (2015) argument is bolstered by examining the neurological correlates of these states. Research has suggested that transient hypofrontality may be the neurological correlate of flow (i.e., frontal and medial temporal lobes are temporarily suppressed, which decreases deliberative thought) (Dietrich, 2004; Peifer, 2012). In contrast, mindfulness training has been shown to increase frontal lobe function (e.g., increasing left versus right frontal asymmetry; Moynihan et al., 2013; Travis & Arenander, 2004). These neurological studies suggest that flow and mindfulness are expressed in opposing ways in the frontal lobe.

While Sheldon et al. (2015) found empirical evidence supporting their hypothesis in relation to attentional absorption (i.e. increasing someone's mindfulness abilities during an activity could undermine absorption), they also found that dimensions of flow related to a sense of control were non-associated or positively associated with mindfulness. What does this mean? These two dimensions of flow appear incompatible with mindfulness. These challenging findings could also be considered as support for emerging models of flow detailed earlier, based on distinct attentional foci and characteristics, which could be used to inform future adventure-based research. Scholars might find it useful, for example, to compare how flow is related to concentrative meditation and mindfulness (or insight) meditation, respectively, to determine if these distinct approaches to changing consciousness provide evidence of distinct flow-like experiences in adventure contexts. These unresolved tensions highlight the need for further research on potential links between flow, mindfulness and meditation, particularly in adventure contexts.

Conclusion

While this chapter only provides an initial exploration of some key tensions in the relationships between flow, mindfulness, meditation and adventure, even this brief enquiry highlights the deep psychological complexity that can accompany adventure activities. Adventure activities have a profound potential to support our psychological health by facilitating unique experiences and states of consciousness (Houge Mackenzie & Hodge, 2020). Experiencing these optimal states in adventure activities, which inherently unfold in absorbing natural environments, has also been linked to the development of eco-centric perspectives and pro-environmental behaviours (Brymer et al., 2014; Brymer & Gray, 2010). By cultivating enhanced states of consciousness and connections to the natural world, adventure activities offer a wide range of untapped research avenues and health-promotion opportunities in service of both human and planetary health (Clough et al., 2016; Maller et al., 2006). While we are still seeking to understand how adventure can change our consciousness, it is clear that this context provides a fertile combination of challenging physical activities and engaging natural environments, which can combine to facilitate unique and highly desirable states of consciousness. Integrating research on flow, mindfulness, and mediation may help to further elucidate and inform our understanding of how adventure changes our consciousness in unique and fulfilling ways.

References

Aherne, C., Moran, A. P., & Lonsdale, C. (2011). The effect of mindfulness training on athletes' flow: An initial investigation. *Sport Psychologist, 25*, 177–189.

Ambrose-Oji, B. (2013). *Mindfulness practice in woods and forests: An evidence review.* Research Report for The Mersey Forest, Forest Research. Alice Holt Lodge Farnham, Surrey, UK.

Berto, R. (2005). Exposure to restorative environments helps restore attentional capacity. *Journal of Environmental Psychology, 25*(3), 249–259.

Bishop, S. R., Lau, M., Shapiro, S., Carlson, L., Anderson, N. D., Carmody, J., ... Devins, G. (2004). Mindfulness: A proposed operational definition. *Clinical Psychology: Science and Practice, 11,* 230–241.

Boudreau, P., Houge Mackenzie, S., & Hodge, K. (2022a). Adventure mindset and COVID-19: Using adventure-based skills to maintain psychological well-being during the coronavirus pandemic. *Psychology of Sport and Exercise, 62,* 102245.

Boudreau, P., Houge Mackenzie, S., & Hodge, K. (2022b). Optimal states of flow and clutch in advanced climbers. *Psychology of Sport and Exercise, 60.* https://doi.org/10.1016/j.psychsport.2022.102155

Boudreau, P., Houge Mackenzie, S. & Hodge, K. (2020). Flow states in adventure recreation: A systematic review and thematic synthesis. *Psychology of Sport and Exercise, 46.* https://doi.org/10.1016/j.psychsport.2019.101611

Brymer, E., Davids, K., & Mallabon, E. (2014). Understanding the psychological health and well-being benefits of physical activity in nature: An ecological dynamics analysis. *Journal of Ecopsychology, 6*(3), 189–197.

Brymer, E., & Gray, T. (2010). Developing an intimate "relationship" with nature through extreme sports participation. *Leisure/Loisir, 34*(4), 361–374.

Cahn, B. R., & Polich, J. (2006). Meditation states and traits: EEG, ERP, and neuroimaging studies. *Psychological Bulletin, 132*(2), 180–211.

Clough, P., Mackenzie, S. H., Mallabon, L., & Brymer, E. (2016). Adventurous physical activity environments: A mainstream intervention for mental health. *Sports Medicine, 46*(7), 963–968.

Csikszentmihalyi, M. (1975). *Beyond boredom and anxiety: Experiencing flow in work and play.* Jossey-Bass.

Csikszentmihalyi, M. (1988). The flow experience and its significance for human psychology. In M. Csikszentmihalyi & I. S. Csikszentmihalyi (Eds.), *Optimal experience: Psychological studies of flow in consciousness* (pp. 15–35). Cambridge University Press.

Csikszentmihalyi, M. (1990). *Flow: The psychology of optimal performance.* Cambridge University Press.

Csikszentmihalyi, M. (1993). *The evolving self.* New York: Harper & Rowe.

Csikszentmihalyi, M. (2002). *Flow: The classic work on how to achieve happiness.* Random House.

Csikszentmihalyi, M., & Csikszentmihalyi, I. S. (Eds.) (1988). *Optimal experience: Psychological studies of flow in consciousness.* Cambridge University Press.

Csikszentmihalyi, M., & Csikszentmihalyi, I. S. (1990). Adventure and the flow experience. In J. C. Miles & S. Priest (Eds.), *Adventure education* (pp. 149–155). Venture.

deCharms, R. (1968). *Personal causation: The internal affective determinants of behavior.* Academic Press.

Deci, E. (1975). *Intrinsic motivation.* Plenum.

Deci, E. L., & Ryan, R. M. (2012). Self-determination theory. In P. A. M. Van Lange, A. W. Kruglanski, & E. T. Higgins (Eds.), *Handbook of theories of social psychology* (pp. 416–436). Sage Publications Ltd.

Delle Fave, A. A., Bassi, M. A., & Massimini, F. A. (2003). Quality of experience and risk perception in high-altitude rock climbing. *Journal of Applied Sport Psychology, 15*(1), 82–98.

Dietrich, A. (2004). Neurocognitive mechanisms underlying the experience of flow. *Consciousness and Cognition: An International Journal, 13,* 746–761.

Ellis, G., Voelkl, J., & Morris, C. (1994). Measurement and analysis issues with explanation of variance in daily experience using the flow model. *Journal of Leisure Research*, 26(4), 337–356.

Hartig, T., Mitchell, R., De Vries, S., & Frumkin, H. (2014). Nature and health. *Annual Review of Public Health*, 35, 207–228.

Houge Mackenzie, S., & Hodge, K. (2020). Adventure recreation and subjective well-being: A conceptual framework. *Leisure Studies*, 39(1), 26–40.

Houge Mackenzie, S., Hodge, K., & Boyes, M. (2011). Expanding the flow model in adventure activities: A reversal theory perspective. *Journal of Leisure Research*, 43(4), 519–544.

Houge Mackenzie, S., Hodge, K., & Boyes, M. (2013). The multi-phasic and dynamic nature of flow in adventure experiences. *Journal of Leisure Research*, 45(2), 214–232.

Howell, A. J., Dopko, R. L., Passmore, H., & Buro, K. (2011). Nature connectedness: Associations with well-being and mindfulness. *Personality and Individual Differences*, 51(2), 166–171.

Jackman, P. C., Hawkins, R. M., Crust, L., & Swann, C. (2019). Flow states in exercise: A systematic review. *Psychology of Sport and Exercise*, 45, 101546.

Jackson, S. A. (1992). Athletes in flow: A qualitative investigation of flow states in elite figure skaters. *Journal of Applied Sport Psychology*, 4(2), 161–180.

Jackson, S. A. (1996). Toward a conceptual understanding of the flow experience in elite athletes. *Research Quarterly for Exercise and Sport*, 67(1), 76–90.

Jackson, S. A., & Csikszentmihalyi, M. (1999). *Flow in sports*. Human Kinetics.

Jackson, S. A., Eklund, R. C., & Martin A. J. (2010). *The FLOW manual*. Mind Garden Inc.

Jackson, S. A., Kimiecik, J. C., Ford, S., & Marsh, H. W. (1998). Psychological correlates of flow in sport. *Journal of Sport and Exercise Psychology*, 20(3), 358–378.

Jackson, S. A., Thomas, P. R., Marsh, H. W., & Smethurst, C. J. (2001). Relationships between flow, self-concept, psychological skills, and performance. *Journal of Applied Sport Psychology*, 13(2), 129–153.

Jones, C., Hollenhorst, S., & Perna, F. (2003). An empirical comparison of the four channel flow model and adventure experience paradigm. *Leisure Sciences*, 25(1), 17–31.

Jones, C., Hollenhorst, S., Perna, F., & Selin, S. (2000). Validation of the flow theory in an on-site whitewater kayaking setting. *Journal of Leisure Research*, 32(2), 247–261.

Kaplan, S. (1995). The restorative benefits of nature: Toward an integrative framework. *Journal of Environmental Psychology*, 15(3), 169–182.

Kaplan, S., & Berman, M. G. (2010). Directed attention as a common resource for executive functioning and self-regulation. *Perspectives on Psychological Science*, 5(1), 43–57.

Kaufman, K. A., Glass, C. R., & Arnkoff, D. B. (2009). Evaluation of Mindful Sport Performance Enhancement (MSPE): A new approach to promote flow in athletes. *Journal of Clinical Sport Psychology*, 3, 334–356.

Kirwin, M., Harper, N. J., Young, T., & Itzvan, I. (2019). Mindful adventures: A pilot study of the outward bound mindfulness program *Journal of Outdoor and Environmental Education*, 22(1), 75–90.

Landhäußer, A., & Keller, J. (2012). Flow and its affective, cognitive, and performance-related consequences. In S. Engeser (Ed.), *Advances in flow research* (pp. 65–85). Springer.

Lepper, M. R., & Greene, D. (Eds.) (1978). *The hidden costs of reward: New perspectives on the psychology of human motivation*. Lawrence Earlbaum.

Maller, C., Townsend, M., Pryor, A., Brown, P., & St Leger, L. (2006). Healthy nature healthy people: 'Contact with nature' as an upstream health promotion intervention for populations. *Health Promotion International*, 21(1), 45–54.

Marlatt, G. A., & Kristeller, J. L. (1999). Mindfulness and meditation. In W. R. Miller (Ed.) *Integrating spirituality into treatment: Resources for practitioners* (pp. 67–84). American Psychological Association.

Marsh, H. W., & Jackson, S. A. (1999). Flow experience in sport: Construct validation of multidimensional, hierarchical state and trait responses. *Structural Equation Modeling: A Multidisciplinary Journal, 6*(4), 343–371.

Maslow, A. (1968). *Toward a psychology of being*. Van Nostrand.

Massimini, F., & Carli, M. (1988). The systematic assessment of flow in daily experience. In M. Csikszentmihalyi & I. S. Csikszentmihalyi (Eds.), *Optimal experience: Psychological studies of flow in consciousness* (pp. 266–287). Cambridge University Press.

Mayer, F. S., Frantz, C. M., Bruehlman-Senecal, E., & Dolliver, K. (2008). Why is nature beneficial? *Environment and Behavior, 41*(5), 607–643.

Morgan, J. D., & Coutts, R. A. (2016). Measuring peak experience in recreational surfing. *Journal of Sport Behavior, 39*(2), 202–217.

Motl, R. W. (1996). *Enjoyment of High- and low-risk activities: Personality and environmental influences*. University of Wyoming.

Moynihan, J. A., Chapman, B. P., Klorman, R., Krasner, M. S., Duberstein, P. R., Brown, K. W., & Talbot, N. L. (2013). Mindfulness-based stress reduction for older adults: Effects on executive function, frontal alpha asymmetry and immune function. *Neuropsychobiology, 68*, 34–43.

Mutz, M., & Müller, J. (2016). Mental health benefits of outdoor adventures: Results from two pilot studies. *Journal of adolescence, 49*, 105–114.

Nerothin, P. H. (2017). *A phenomenological investigation of lifestyle surfers from San Diego*. Prescott College.

Partington, S., Partington, E., & Olivier, S. (2009). The dark side of flow: A qualitative study of dependence in big wave surfing. *The Sport Psychologist, 23*, 170–185.

Peifer, C. (2012). Psychophysiological correlates of flow-experience. In S. Engeser (Ed.), *Advances in flow research* (pp. 139–164). Springer.

Sheldon, K. M., Prentice, M., & Halusic, M. (2015). The experiential incompatibility of mindfulness and flow absorption. *Social Psychological and Personality Science, 6*(3), 276–283.

Shin, W. S., Yeoun, P. S., Yoo, R. W., & Shin, C. S. (2010). Forest experience and psychological health benefits: The state of the art and future prospect in Korea. *Environmental Health and Preventive Medicine, 15*(1), 38.

Stamatelopoulou, F., Pezirkianidis, C., Karakasidou, E., Lakioti, A., & Stalikas, A. (2018). Being in the zone: A systematic review on the relationship of psychological correlates and the occurrence of flow experiences in sports' performance. *Psychology, 9*(8), 2011–2030.

Swann, C., Crust, L., Jackman, P., Vella, S. A., Allen, M. S., & Keegan, R. (2017). Psychological states underlying excellent performance in sport: toward an integrated model of flow and clutch states. *Journal of Applied Sport Psychology, 29*(4), 375–401.

Swann, C., Keegan, R. J., Piggott, D., & Crust, L. (2012). A systematic review of the experience, occurrence, and controllability of flow states in elite sport. *Psychology of Sport and Exercise, 13*(6), 807–819.

Travis, F., & Arenander, A. (2004). EEG asymmetry and mindfulness meditation. *Psychosomatic Medicine, 66*, 147–148.

Weinstein, N., Brown, K. W., & Ryan, R. M. (2009). A multi-method examination of the effects of mindfulness on stress attribution, coping, and emotional well-being. *Journal of Research in Personality, 43*, 374–385.

11
ADVENTURE, POSTTRAUMATIC GROWTH, AND WISDOM

Hanna Kampman and Petra Walker

An Adventurer's Point of View: A New Me

Ocean Sailing was a way to uncover parts of myself that I never knew existed. I joined the race as a last resort to bring myself out of the dark pit I had found myself in after the death of my sister, the loss of my job and a toxic relationship I'd just managed to get out of. Nothing else had worked. I'd tried therapy, travelling, going out with friends. Nothing seemed to shake me out of the darkness. I joined the race with a sense of "What's there to lose? Worst case scenario, I'll lose my life, no big deal". I was in despair. Yet, throughout the training, I found that I was gradually gaining increments of self confidence, little by little. I was good at this new sport! I was useful to others on board as well, a feeling that had been somehow wiped out of me in the previous rough years. When the race begun, I found myself enjoying the tranquility of the sea and the never-ending blue horizon. It was a chance for me to pause and step out of the spinning whirl that my life had become. I found the moments to truly listen to myself and my needs. I also found support. Plenty of support! From mentors, like the captain, and the other crew. We were a team; we were a family. And the best interest of the team was something that took away the focus from my own problems and nudged me to focus on something greater than myself: the wellbeing of others and our boat. I found that being surrounded by people who believed in me and believed I could do this ocean racing more than I believed in myself at that time; one of the most valuable aspects of the adventure. I entered this race a broken person, defeated by life. But being tested and tried in new things that I seemed to get hold of and being encouraged by a supportive team worked wonders on my fragile self-esteem. As the adventure progressed and the oceans became colder, wilder and more dangerous, my skills gradually grew and by the end of my journey, I could not recognise the person I'd become.

I'd taken on a huge challenge and came out the other end as a winner. After the race I had a newfound appreciation for life, and concentrated on the things I had, rather than the things that were missing. I transferred the attitude of "nothing is impossible" to my everyday life and kept pushing myself to more challenging situations, expanding what I thought was possible for me. I achieved a lot more in the years after the race, than all the previous years of my life. The best though was the life stance I was left with: happier about myself and my life, grateful for who and what I had, more sure of myself. People who saw me months after the race commented on how I now radiated a healthy confidence. My life has truly been transformed because of this Ocean Adventure.

Memnia Theodorou

Adventure, Posttraumatic Growth, and Wisdom

I am currently pondering about the northern lights. You cannot know if they exist or if you just see them. Everything is very uncertain, and exactly that makes me calm.

Tuutikki

The notion of growth through adventuring is not new. People have gone on adventures throughout history, exploring and processing deep meaningful questions in their lives. As early as 1908, a seminal anthropological work by Arnold van Gennep, "The Rites of Passage" highlighted the idea of spending time in the wilderness (often alone) in a *vision quest* to grow and gain wisdom (van Gennep et al., 2019). Echoing this, Naor and Mayseless (2020) recently noted that immersing oneself into the wilderness has been used as a ritual across many cultures to aid contemplation around life's purpose and meaning.

Facing the dark side of life, such as adversity and trauma, requires an individual to contemplate questions that perhaps previously could be avoided (e.g., mortality). Research has suggested that adventure often involves substantial risks and (un)expected challenges (e.g., Ewert, 1989; Fletcher, 2010) which can also create adverse experiences. Equally, adventures aid individuals to tap into previously unknown resources, realise their potential, and experience awe and wonder at the natural world as they "go knowingly into the unknown" (Reid & Kampman, 2020, p. 3). Therefore, it appears that one of the various motives behind why people adventure is to both contemplate on existing challenges in their lives, and to grow from inherent challenges and opportunities that the adventuring poses.

This chapter explores posttraumatic growth (PTG) and adventure from these two often interconnected perspectives, namely: the potentially positive role of adventure when journeying forwards after trauma; and the growth and wisdom gained through adventuring. It is important to note that there is of course also a lot of evidence for growth through adventure without the disruption of trauma, for example due to the disruption via "peak experience(s)." This can be seen in the many descriptions and quotes in other chapters of this book (such as Chapter 12 on transformation or transcendence). However, this chapter is particularly exploring how individuals potentially grow from adversities.

Defining Adventure, Trauma and Posttraumatic Growth

There are various ways to define "adventure" (e.g., see overview in Reid & Kampman, 2020). However, in this chapter, we conceptualise adventure as: "to go knowingly into the unknown on expeditions, travels and experiences that are unusual or daring, and that involve opportunities for taking risks, whilst demanding commitment and responsibility" (Reid & Kampman, 2020, p. 9). Both the "unknown" and "risks" create the potential for highly challenging life situations, which can test the individuals beyond their previous level of physiological and psychological functioning as illustrated in this quote: "*I think it was an adventure because it pushed my emotional limits, physical limits, it pushed every single limit I had.*" (Emma in Reid & Kampman, 2020, p. 4; (see also reference to Sisu and going beyond one's perceived limits in Chapter 9).

However, as suggested, sometimes individuals embark on these adventures *because* they have faced adversity, even trauma (e.g., Burke & Sabiston, 2012; Theodorou & Kampman, 2021.), and choose to go knowingly into the unknown after this trauma. For us to be able to discuss why this might be, we must first define and discuss adversity and trauma.

In this chapter, we define trauma and adversity within the framework of PTG as a "highly challenging life event" which is out of the ordinary for most people, producing "psychological difficulties not in a vulnerable few, but in large numbers of people exposed to them" (Janoff-Bulman, 1992, p. 50). However, we also recognise the subjective nature of trauma. This means that similar experiences might be traumatising for some whilst not for others. Correspondingly, what is "unusual or daring" and "involves a risk" is also subjective, therefore adventure and the challenges it poses to individuals could mean different things to different people.

Going through trauma or severe adversity is always an embodied experience, impacting the individual's nervous system, biopsychology and relationship with one's body (Hefferon & Kampman, 2021; Kampman, 2021; Levine, 2008, 2010; van der Kolk, 1996). To give an example, the body reacts to a psychological and emotional threat as much as it does to a physical threat (e.g., flight, fight) with accompanying chemicals (e.g., cortisol) and with potentially altered neural pathways. As humans we also interpret the world through our bodies (Hefferon & Kampman, 2021; Merleau-Ponty, 2013), thus, the body becomes an essential aspect of exploring growth following trauma and adventure. How we adventure, and what an adventure is for us, depends on our bodies and we often choose our adventures according to the body (e.g., adaptive sailing, rock climbing) and experience the adventuring and growth through our bodies (Ellingson, 2017; Hefferon et al., 2009; Hefferon & Kampman, 2021; Kampman et al., 2015; Kampman & Hefferon, 2020). Therefore, the body will also be given a "meaningful presence" throughout this chapter (Ellingson, 2017, p. 1; Hefferon & Kampman, 2021).

Posttraumatic Growth

The struggle with the above mentioned, unforeseen "seismic events" which "seriously challenges or shatters an individual's assumptive world" (p. 4) can, in some situations, and *with time*, also turn into "positive psychological changes" (Tedeschi, et al., 2018, p. 3). This positive "cognitive, emotional, behavioural, and, more recently, biological" transformation is most commonly referred to as posttraumatic growth (PTG; Tedeschi et al., 2018, p. 25). This chapter subscribes to the position that PTG can be seen both as a process and an outcome, which unfolds with personal pace and with time (e.g., see discussions around alternative perspectives Jayawickreme & Blackie, 2014; Joseph & Linley, 2008; Wadey et al., 2021). Journeying forwards after trauma is first and foremost a personal endeavour, and we want to emphasise that it is completely normal not to experience PTG, nor should this be expected from oneself or others. All too often, when people struggle with the aftermath of adversity, this is viewed as an "abnormal response" to a stressful event rather than "adaptive responses to abnormal events" (Janoff-Bulman, 1992, p. 95). Therefore, we want to highlight that growth is only one potential trajectory after adversity, it is not the only one.

Equally, it would be harmful to solely tell stories of enduring distress as many individuals recognise transformative changes in themselves after navigating these highly challenging times. Individuals identifying with posttraumatic growth after adversity often notice positive changes in their *personal strength* (e.g., they are stronger in some ways than before) or in the way they *relate to others* (e.g., they develop more close, authentic relationships). People also report *recognising and experiencing new possibilities* (e.g., finding new hobbies and careers), *appreciating life more* (e.g., appreciating the uniqueness of one's life) and changes in their *spiritual and existential* perspectives (e.g., feeling they are part of wider humanity) (Hefferon et al., 2010; Kampman et al., 2015; Tedeschi et al., 2017, 2018). More embodied outcomes are also reported, such as "a new awareness of the body" (Hefferon, 2012; Hefferon et al., 2010; Hefferon & Kampman, 2021), as well as embodied versions of the previously cognitively perceived outcomes, such as personal strength, physical strength, or recognising and appreciating the diversity of bodies and abilities (Kampman, 2021) and superior performance among athletes (Howells et al., 2017). Indeed, we should include the "body into all explorations and models of growth" (Kampman, 2021, p. 261).

These transformative changes can be eventually witnessed in an individual's actions, as their behaviour shifts according to these changes in their thinking (Hobfoll et al., 2007; Kampman & Hefferon, 2020). One of these transformative changes could lead to actions such as going on an *adventure,* for example, as part of *recognising and experiencing new possibilities* as illustrated in a beautiful qualitative study of breast cancer survivors who climbed Mount Kilimanjaro by Burke and Sabiston:

> I was terrified of dying. It wasn't until I began to talk about death and dying and came to terms with the fact that I would die, whether it was a year from now or ten years from now, that I made a shift and my perspective of life changed. I began thinking of what I wanted to do with my life and I started setting goals for myself. I really enjoy taking on new challenges and striving toward a goal. And climbing Mt. Kilimanjaro is one of those goals.
>
> *(Bonnie in Burke & Sabiston, 2012, p. 8)*

Equally these changes might evolve during the adventure, for example people could feel *stronger* as they navigate their adventures: "*Sometimes I liken myself to becoming Lara Croft when I'm adventuring because I just become her. I'm tougher and wiser and more capable without the cotton-wool stuff that I get at home*" (Lara in Reid & Kampman, 2020, p. 6). Growth may also occur after the journey as people explore and contemplate the changes which the adventure has initiated, such as *changed spiritual and existential* perspectives as illustrated in Reid and Kampman: "*the journey just became bigger than me*" the adventure "*gifted me a pathway to help people*" (Ted in Reid & Kampman, p. 6).

It is key to recognise that different traumas and trauma profiles (Kira, 2021) can also lead to different outcomes and the context in which the growth evolves matters (e.g., Chopko et al., 2013; Kampman, 2021; Karanci et al., 2012; Kira et al., 2013; Kılıç et al., 2016; Shakespeare-Finch & Armstrong, 2010; Shuwiekh et al., 2018).

These changes can also take time, and therefore, PTG is not seen as reactive, but rather the process and outcomes evolve as the individual develops new ways of "thinking, feeling and behaving" (Tedeschi et al., 2018, p. 5). Even if the outcomes might be "akin to an epiphany about life" (Tedeschi et al., 2018, p. 6) and seem quite sudden, the meaning and implications of this epiphany will still be processed with unfolding time, potentially long after the adventuring itself. It is not the event itself that produces the growth, it is the individual working hard to make sense of the aftermath of it, and its implications to their life. Therefore, for some individuals, this process might be initiated and/or facilitated by adventuring, as this participant in a wilderness canoe expedition discovered:

> You are out there in the wilderness … you don't worry about watches … is your tie straight and that stuff. It helped me finalize priorities. It helped me focus on what my priorities are and what's important and what's not.
>
> *(Participant, Anderson & Schleien, 1997, p. 225)*

Process of Posttraumatic Growth

According to the theory of PTG the initial adverse event(s) are evaluated by the individual and if the individual's worldview provides context to what has happened, the emotional distress can be mitigated by the beliefs and coping mechanisms employed to potentially facilitate and experience resilience. Resilience is defined here as a dynamic process *before*, *during* and *after* adversity leading to a positive adaptation (Chmitorz et al., 2018; IJntema et al., 2019; Tedeschi et al., 2018). Often adventuring provides opportunities to utilise and develop resilience as individuals push themselves beyond their imagined limits, challenging their mental and physical skills, to redefine what is possible: *"I've learned to toughen up. Strategies and tactics with coping and dealing with stuff and don't sweat the small stuff"* (Lara in Reid & Kampman, 2020, p. 6).

However, there are times when reality comes even closer, either in life in general or during the adventure, when something fundamental is shattered, causing distress and challenging core beliefs that the individual holds. This initiates an automatic and intrusive rumination, requiring the individual to work through the challenge, engage in self-analysis and reflection, manage emotional distress, and employ coping strategies (Tedeschi et al., 2018). The fundamental challenge and mortality awareness is captured by one adventurer in the following quote: *"The possibility of dying changed my whole attitude on things"* (Jessica in Burke & Sabiston, 2012, p. 10).

Here is where adventuring could serve people in several ways. People might choose to go on a solo adventure, to detach themselves from their everyday life and other people to be able to engage in self-analysis and reflection. Participants in a qualitative study by Kalisch et al. (2011) described this desire, stating both, *"I couldn't wait to be alone and reflect on my life"* (p. 7) and *"I knew it was my time to relax and think about things"* (p. 7). Alternatively, people might choose to travel with others and gain opportunities for self-disclosure and shared stories away from normal life, as illustrated by Stuart, who participated in inclusive adventure training:

> … maybe one of the benefits is giving guys a chance to meet other guys who've been through something like they have. That's why I'm talking about this to you today I suppose, so someone else might hear something in my story that fits their life, that makes them feel like they're not going through stuff alone.
>
> *(Stuart in Carless et al., 2013, p. 127)*

Adventure can also offer ample opportunities to rewrite personal narratives, co-create a new embodied story and deliberately change schemas around oneself and the body after trauma, as beautifully expressed by Bonnie in Burke and Sabiston (2012):

> This experience is part of my self-realisation or my self-discovery. It is helping me realise how strong I really am. I am not a mountain climber. I

don't see myself as a climber. But I really surprised myself at how much I could do. I look at other things in my life and say to myself "if I can climb that mountain, then I can deal with this too." I have much more faith in myself. I am more aware that I can face just about any challenge and that is very satisfying.

(Bonnie in Burke & Sabiston, 2012, p. 11)

Nature, wilderness, and adventure can potentially provide an environment and an experience where individuals can reframe their initial traumatic experiences including vulnerability, danger, or helplessness and rewrite their stories to include alternative narratives of safety, strength, and perseverance (e.g., see Harper et al., 2014). A personal narrative around "a hurt, disabled body" can become "a skilled adventuring body" with new abilities and skills.

These examples help us to understand how the process of growth can be facilitated by adventuring: equipping people with tools to accept the changes in their world and enable them to grow. Growth often dances together with the challenges; therefore, some enduring distress might still be present even when people recognise growth in some areas. Adventure can, at its best, give tools for the individual to navigate the challenging thoughts and feelings when these re-emerge, for example, Chris, a veteran with PTSD, uses images from his diving adventures to calm himself elsewhere: *"If I have to go back to a place of stillness or quietness, then I can go back to those images."* (Chris in Walker & Kampman, 2021, p. 6). People can therefore emerge from their adventures as more resilient (e.g., Reid & Kampman, 2020), with expanded coping strategies and knowledge (e.g., Craig et al., 2020; Naor & Mayseless, 2020; Reid & Kampman, 2020), increased wisdom (e.g., Naor & Mayseless, 2020; Reid & Kampman, 2020), and compassion for others and for nature (e.g., Burke & Sabiston, 2012; Walker & Kampman, 2021).

The body should be acknowledged as an essential travel companion, as the body is at the centre of these adventures, pushed to the limits, challenged, whilst getting stronger and discovering new abilities. *"I would say that the physical challenges of it as well also made a difference in my life because it's not always going to be easy and things might not always go the way you planned"* (Wassif, 2014, p. 107).

Finally, it is essential to acknowledge that both the process and growth are continuously evolving (Kampman, 2021). Each adventure comes with different contexts (e.g., wilderness vs motorbikes) and different intra- and interpersonal challenges (e.g., solo vs group) potentially facilitating different aspects of growth (e.g., process and outcomes). Personal growth from adventuring is a journey that starts when the individual *prepares for the adventure* (e.g., planning, practising skills, "going knowingly"), continues *during the adventure* (e.g., facing new challenges, skill acquisition and utilisation, pushing limits, challenging old narratives) and *after the adventure* (e.g., reflection, further narrative revisions, and behavioural changes).

The potential benefits of adventuring to an individuals' wellbeing are well recognised within several therapeutic practices and are used in different variations to help individuals to navigate challenging times. Some examples of these include the Integrated Outdoor Adventure Programme (Anderson et al., 1997), Wilderness Therapy (Bettmann et al., 2016), Adventure-based counselling (Fletcher & Hinkle, 2002), Adventure-based group therapy (Norton & Tucker, 2010), Adventure-based group work and interventions (Norton & Tucker, 2010), and Adventure- and recreation-based group interventions (Voruganti et al., 2006). Some researchers suggest these should be grouped together under Adventure Therapy (Norton & Hseih, 2011; Tucker & Norton, 2013) or grouped more broadly alongside non-therapeutic adventuring under Adventure Psychology as proposed by Reid & Kampman in 2020 (p. 9) although it is important to acknowledge that each has distinct elements in them. Meanwhile, the research around embodiment, and adventuring in the context of PTG is still sparse, therefore what follows is mainly theoretical and will hopefully offer a point of departure to new adventures within research.

Common Facilitators of Posttraumatic Growth

Before we examine Adventure and the various ways it could facilitate PTG, it is important to introduce some known facilitators from earlier studies. A meta-analysis by Prati and Pietratoni (2009) suggested that optimism, social support, and active coping strategies (religious, acceptance and reappraisal) all had significant positive effects on PTG, as did spirituality, which they equated with religion but which has also been defined as "a personal journey to understanding the world, the environment and a person's place in it" (Tedeschi et al., 2018, p. 116). Physical activity, sport and leisure have also been identified as facilitators for growth (Kampman et al., 2015; Wadey et al., 2021). Of course, these factors often combine. For example, a search for meaning combined with physical activity, and reappraisal coping, can result in the creation of a new identity, possibly as an athlete (Kampman & Hefferon, 2020), or an adventurer. It is also possible that these facilitators of PTG could enable post-adventure growth in those who have not previously experienced trauma.

Potential Facilitators of Growth in Adventuring

As briefly mentioned before, adventuring has the potential to facilitate both the processes and outcomes of growth *before* (preparing), *during* (adventuring) and *after* (assimilating and accommodating) the adventure. Adventure can enable growth and wisdom through: reducing negative symptoms associated with trauma; stabilising, calming, and grounding; and producing positive embodied, action-oriented psychological phenomena. The following section will explore the developing research around adventure, growth, and PTG. The section is not intended as an exhaustive list of the potential facilitators of growth in adventuring. However, the aim is to start a conversation among adventure, growth and PTG researchers. Therefore, it also ends with suggestions for future research.

Reducing

> You feel so free out there, you don't worry about anything, you don't think about the bills you've got to pay or your life problems, you're just kind of free of thought. That's kind of what makes it all worthwhile, just for that whatever, 5 min of freedom.
>
> *(Participant 1, Brymer & Schweitzer, 2013, p. 868)*

Being away from everyday life appears to decrease everyday anxieties as well as severe symptoms of trauma. For example, the level of clinical symptoms of posttraumatic stress disorder (PTSD; a trauma and stressor-related disorder) and trait anxiety have been shown to reduce during a sailing intervention (Gelkopf et al., 2013); when engaging in physical activity and sport (Caddick & Smith, 2014), and whilst Scuba diving. Peter who suffers from PTSD contrasts the peace of the underwater world with his normal life saying: *"There is no noise, there is no bangs, there's no cracks, there's nothings that trigger people like me"* (Peter in Walker & Kampman, 2021, p. 6). Therefore, adventuring provides the opportunity to be away from everyday hassles and potential trauma reminders, being fully present whilst often engaging in physical activity which is a known facilitator of PTG (e.g., Day, 2013; Kampman & Hefferon, 2020; Kampman, 2021; Wadey et al., 2021; Wadey & Day, 2018).

Adventuring can reduce some of the negative symptoms, carving space for calm and further awareness of what is possible (Kampman, 2021). *"You are thinking in the present moment instead of thinking about previous invasive thoughts that you get on top of the water"* (Chris in Walker & Kampman, 2021, p. 6). Through this reduction of negative symptoms, an adventure experience can help stabilise the body and the mind; giving the individuals' attention a new purpose.

Stabilising, Calming, and Grounding

Silence: In their empirical and theoretical literature review on solo wilderness experiences, Naor and Mayseless (2020) suggested that silence had a significant role in allowing the mind to rest from cognitive processing. For the process of PTG this could mean an opportunity to move from intrusive rumination into a more purposeful place of reflection and contemplation. The solitude and wilderness appeared to offer a unique opportunity for "tranquillity, peace" and "cognitive freedom" to engage in self-analysis and reflection – essential for the process of growth to evolve. Time spent in solitude offers a break from "daily demands" and "human interference" (p.9) and adventuring in nature, can become "a sanctuary for the healing process, partially because it is non-judgmental" (Dustin et al., 2011, p. 331). This could offer insights into why individuals quite organically sometimes choose to adventure after trauma. As Jack describes this: *"You've just cut out all the background noise"* (Jack in Reid & Kampman, 2020, p. 5).

Even when adventuring together with others, the natural environments can offer "soft fascination" for the adventurers – it can hold their attention without demanding it (Duvall & Sullivan, 2016; Kampman, 2022; Kaplan & Kaplan, 1989). This can offer individuals and their attention a break and facilitate mindfulness and flow experiences. This focus on the present, instead of the daily basic life struggles, has already been found useful in veteran populations (Walker & Kampman, 2021; Wassif, 2014). An example of this is given by Ben a diver who suffers from PTSD: "*When you enter the water, it's not like you are in threat, but you are in a situation where you have to focus and so your mind calms down … it's almost like mindfulness, you become in the moment*" (Ben in Walker & Kampman, 2021, p. 4).

Adventuring can therefore become an embodied mindfulness experience where the individual is engaging with the experience through the body and employing different senses. Again, a quote from Ben, a diver, illustrates this: "*The world seems to slow down because you are completely fixated on physical senses*" (Ben in Walker & Kampman, 2021, p. 6).

Producing

Wellbeing: through (adaptive) physical activity and sport. Adventuring can increase subjective positive affective states and quality of life (Caddick & Smith, 2014; Reese et al., 2019), facilitate psychological wellbeing through increasing inner strength and motivation and provide opportunities for achievements, social wellbeing and ecotherapy (Caddick & Smith, 2014).

Silence and wilderness can aid contemplation around purpose and meaning in life (Naor & Mayseless, 2020). For example, climbing Mt. Kilimanjaro was found to provide an opportunity for women who had survived cancer, to (a) nurture priorities, (b) foster self-belief, and (c) cultivate connections (Burke & Sabiston, 2012). The women were able to embrace physical and mental challenges, physical discomfort, and push themselves beyond initial limits. These findings were echoed in Reid and Kampman (2020) where new physiological and psychological skills were found and developed through "pushing boundaries" during the adventure. This then created a wider toolkit of skills, thereby, "expanding their capacities and capabilities for stronger functioning in future" (Reid & Kampman, 2020, p. 6). The transference of skills and ideas into life outside of adventure is described beautifully in the following quote: "*I consider myself a perfectionist in certain things, and after the first trip, I realised that perfection cannot be a part of the wilderness experience. I wanted the chance for that in my everyday life*" (male, 43 years old, cerebral palsy in Anderson & Scheien, 1997, p. 225).

"Meaningful activities" (Burke & Sabiston, 2012, p. 13) and "meaningful leisure engagement" (Kampman et al., 2015, p. 290; Kampman, 2021) such as adventure, sport, art, high altitude mountain trekking, can facilitate personal growth and transformation through to discovering of "new abilities, hidden talents, and rediscover existing skills in a new way" (Kampman et al., 2015, p. 290). Meaningful leisure, such as adventure, can aid independence after trauma and provide new meaningful relationships, camaraderie, and offer opportunities to ask for help (Kampman, 2021; Walker & Kampman, 2021).

New relationships: preparing for an adventure or going for an adventure with other people can produce new meaningful relationships with camaraderie and shared wisdom. As it is not uncommon for people to adventure after adversities, individuals might organically find role models from the adventure community and offer each other opportunities for self-disclosure and schema change. Rewriting cognitive, emotional, behavioural, and embodied pathways through adventuring evolves with time and the adventure community can potentially offer ample examples of individuals who have travelled similar paths.

Concluding Thoughts

What we have hopefully provided here is a point of departure for research adventures around PTG. We want to emphasise that we are not considering adventuring as a panacea for trauma and adversity. Researchers should carefully consider some of the challenges that adventuring can pose for individuals journeying forward after trauma (e.g., further injuries and trauma, avoidance behaviours, etc.). However, there is age old wisdom and cumulating psychological research around the benefits of adventuring for growth experiences, and we can learn a lot from this thriving community to enable us to consider alternative ways of journeying onwards after challenging times.

Key Considerations for Future

Inclusivity: adventure and adventuring belong to everyone; we must consider who we are including/excluding with our definitions of adventure. There are elements in adventure that are subjective and we should be mindful that the definition does not become another aid for discrimination.

Diversity: it would be essential to explore adventure and growth within different racial, ethnic, and cultural groups. Contemporary adventure is still often attached to the affluent white hetero man, despite its strong indigenous and global history. Therefore, it would be valuable to listen to the unheard voices within adventuring and growth, whose stories are we not listening to?

Embodied perspectives: the body must become a meaningful presence in our endeavours to explore adventuring, growth, and posttraumatic growth. Various bodies with different abilities adventure, we need to give these bodies a presence in our research endeavours. When exploring this area, we could embrace more embodied ways to research (e.g., adventuring together).

Acknowledgement: The authors of this chapter want to acknowledge the pioneering researchers in the area of posttraumatic growth and adventuring for enabling many of the insights discussed in this chapter. Thank you.

References

Anderson, L., Schleien, S. J., McAvoy, L., Lais, G. & Seligmann, D. (1997). Creating positive change through an integrated outdoor adventure program. *Therapeutic Recreation Journal, 31*(4), 214–229.

Bettmann, J. E., Gillis, H. L., Speelman, E. A., Parry, K. J., & Case, J. M. (2016). A meta-analysis of wilderness therapy outcomes for private pay clients. *Journal of Child and Family Studies, 25*(9), 2659–2673. https://doi.org/10.1007/s10826-016-0439-0

Brymer, E., & Schweitzer, R. D. (2013). The search for freedom in extreme sports: A phenomenological exploration. *Psychology of Sport and Exercise, 14*(6), 865–873.

Burke, S., & Sabiston, C. (2012). Fostering growth in the survivorship experience: Investigating breast cancer survivors' lived experiences scaling Mt. Kilimanjaro from a posttraumatic growth perspective. *The Qualitative Report*. https://doi.org/10.46743/2160-3715/2012.1783

Caddick, N., & Smith, B. (2014). The impact of sport and physical activity on the well-being of combat veterans: A systematic review. *Psychology of Sport and Exercise, 15*(1), 9–18. https://doi.org/10.1016/j.psychsport.2013.09.011

Carless, D., Peacock, S., McKenna, J., & Cooke, C. (2013). Psychosocial outcomes of an inclusive adapted sport and adventurous training course for military personnel. *Disability and Rehabilitation, 35*(24), 2081–2088. https://doi.org/10.3109/09638288.2013.802376

Chmitorz, A., Kunzler, A., Helmreich, I., Tüscher, O., Kalisch, R., Kubiak, T., Wessa, M., & Lieb, K. (2018). Intervention studies to foster resilience – A systematic review and proposal for a resilience framework in future intervention studies. *Clinical Psychology Review, 59*, 78–100. http://dx.doi.org/10.1016/j.cpr.2017.11.002

Chopko, B. A., Palmieri, P. A., & Adams, R. E. (2013). Associations between police stress and alcohol use: Implications for practice. *Journal of Loss and Trauma, 18*(5), 482–497.

Craig, P., Alger, D., Bennett, J., & Martin, T. (2020). The transformative nature of fly-fishing for veterans and military personnel with posttraumatic stress disorder. *Therapeutic Recreation Journal, 54*(2). https://doi.org/10.18666/TRJ-2020-V54-I2-9965

Day, M. C. (2013). The role of initial physical activity experiences in promoting posttraumatic growth in Paralympic athletes with an acquired disability. *Disability and Rehabilitation, 35*(24), 2064–2072. https://doi.org/10.3109/09638288.2013.805822

Dustin, D., Bricker, N., Arave, J., Wall, W., & Wendt, G. (2011). The promise of river running as a therapeutic medium for veterans coping with post-traumatic stress disorder. *Therapeutic Recreation Journal, 45*(4), 326–340.

Duvall, J., & Sullivan, W. C. (2016). How to get more out of the green exercise experience: Insights from attention restoration therapy. In J. Barton, R. Bragg, C. Wood, & J. Pretty (Eds.), *Green exercise* (1st ed., pp. 37–45). Routledge.

Ellingson, L. L. (2017). *Embodiment in qualitative research*. Taylor & Francis.

Ewert, A. W. (1989). *Outdoor adventure pursuits: Foundations, models, and theories*. Publishing Horizons.

Fletcher, R. (2010). The emperor's new adventure: Public secrecy and the paradox of adventure tourism. *Journal of Contemporary Ethnography, 39*(1), 6–33.

Fletcher, T. B., & Hinkle, J. S. (2002). Adventure based counseling: An innovation in counseling. *Journal of Counseling & Development, 80*(3), 277–285.

Gelkopf, M., Hasson-Ohayon, I., Bikman, M., & Kravetz, S. (2013). Nature adventure rehabilitation for combat-related posttraumatic chronic stress disorder: A randomized control trial. *Psychiatry Research, 209*(3), 485–493.

Harper, N. J., Norris, J., & D'astous, M. (2014). Veterans and the outward bound experience: An evaluation of impact and meaning. *Ecopsychology, 6*(3), 165–173. https://doi.org/10.1089/eco.2013.0101

Hefferon, K. (2012). Bringing back the body into positive psychology: The theory of corporeal posttraumatic growth in breast cancer survivorship. *Psychology, 3*(12), 1238–1242. https://doi.org/10.4236/psych.2012.312A183

Hefferon, K., Grealy, M., & Mutrie, N. (2009). *Post-traumatic growth and life threatening physical illness: A systematic review of the qualitative literature*, 343–378. https://doi.org/10.1348/135910708X332936

Hefferon, K., Grealy, M., & Mutrie, N. (2010). Transforming from cocoon to butterfly: The potential role of the body in the process of posttraumatic growth. *Journal of Humanistic Psychology, 50*(2), 224–247. https://doi.org/10.1177/0022167809341996

Hefferon, K., & Kampman, H. (2021). Taking an Embodied approach to posttraumatic growth research and sport. In R. Wadey, D. Melissa, & K. Howells (Eds.), *Growth following adversity in sport a mechanism to positive change* (pp. 131–144), 1st ed. Routledge.

Hobfoll, S. E., Hall, B. J., Canetti-Nisim, D., Galea, S., Johnson, R. J., & Palmieri, P. A. (2007). Refining our understanding of traumatic growth in the face of terrorism: Moving from meaning cognitions to doing what is meaningful. *Applied Psychology, 56*(3), 345–366. https://doi.org/10.1111/j.1464-0597.2007.00292.x

Howells, K., Sarkar, M., & Fletcher, D. (2017). Can athletes benefit from difficulty? A systematic review of growth following adversity in competitive sport. In *Progress in brain research* (Vol. 234, pp. 117–159). Elsevier. https://doi.org/10.1016/bs.pbr.2017.06.002

IJntema, R. C., Burger, Y. D., & Schaufeli, W. B. (2019). Reviewing the labyrinth of psychological resilience: Establishing criteria for resilience-building programs. *Consulting Psychology Journal: Practice and Research, 71*(4), 288–304. https://doi.org/10.1037/cpb0000147

Janoff-Bulman, R. (1992). *Shattered assumptions: Towards a new psychology of trauma*. Free Press.

Jayawickreme, E., & Blackie, L. E. R. (2014). *Post-traumatic growth as positive personality change: Evidence, Controversies and future directions, 28*(4), 20. https://doi.org/10.1002/per.1963

Joseph, S., & Linley, P. A. (2008). *Trauma, recovery, and growth: Positive psychological perspectives on posttraumatic stress* (pp. xi, 372). John Wiley & Sons Inc.

Kalisch, K. R., Bobilya, A. J., & Daniel, B. (2011). The outward bound solo: A study of participants' perceptions. *Journal of Experiential Education, 34*(1), 1–18. https://doi.org/10.5193/JEE34.1.1

Kampman, H. (2021). Exploring the complex relationship between posttraumatic growth, sport, and athletes with acquired disabilities. Ph.D. Thesis University of East London School of Psychology. https://doi.org/10.15123/uel.89w7z

Kampman, H. (2022). How to prepare for adversity. In C. Van Nieuwerburgh & P. William (Eds.), *From surviving to thriving: A student's guide to feeling and doing well at university*. SAGE.

Kampman, H., & Hefferon, K. (2020). 'Find a sport and carry on': Posttraumatic growth and achievement in British Paralympic athletes. *International Journal of Wellbeing, 10*(1), Article 1. https://doi.org/10.5502/ijw.v10i1.765

Kampman, H., Hefferon, K., Wilson, M., & Beale, J. (2015). "I can do things now that people thought were impossible, actually, things that I thought were impossible":

A meta-synthesis of the qualitative findings on posttraumatic growth and severe physical injury. *Canadian Psychology/Psychologie Canadienne, 56*(3), 283–294. https://doi.org/10.1037/cap0000031

Kaplan, R. & Kaplan, S. (1989). *The experience of nature: A psychological perspective*. Cambridge University Press.

Karanci, A. N., Işıklı, S., Aker, A. T., Gül, E. İ., Erkan, B. B., Özkol, H., & Güzel, H. Y. (2012). Personality, posttraumatic stress and trauma type: Factors contributing to posttraumatic growth and its domains in a Turkish community sample. *European Journal of Psychotraumatology, 3*(1), 17303.

Kira, I. A. (2021). Taxonomy of stressors and traumas: An update of the development-based trauma framework (DBTF): A life-course perspective on stress and trauma. *Traumatology*. https://doi.org/10.1037/trm0000305

Kira, I. A., Aboumediene, S., Ashby, J. S., Odenat, L., Mohanesh, J., & Alamia, H. (2013). The dynamics of posttraumatic growth across different trauma types in a Palestinian sample. *Journal of Loss and Trauma, 18*(2), 120–139. https://doi.org/10.1080/15325024.2012.679129

Kılıç, C., Magruder, K. M., & Koryürek, M. M. (2016). Does trauma type relate to posttraumatic growth after war? A pilot study of young Iraqi war survivors living in Turkey. *Transcultural psychiatry, 53*(1), 110–123.

Levine, P. A. (2008). *Healing trauma*. ReadHowYouWant.com

Levine, P. A. (2010). *In an unspoken voice: How the body releases trauma and restores goodness*. North Atlantic Books.

Merleau-Ponty, M. (2013). *Phenomenology of perception*. 1st ed. Routledge.

Naor, L., & Mayseless, O. (2020). The wilderness solo experience: A unique practice of silence and solitude for personal growth. *Frontiers in Psychology, 11*, 547067. https://doi.org/10.3389/fpsyg.2020.547067

Norton, C. L., & Hsieh, C.M. (2011). Cultural bridging through shared adventure: Cross-cultural perspectives on adventure therapy. *Journal of Adventure Education and Outdoor Learning, 11*(2), 173–188, DOI: 10.1080/14729679.2011.633390

Norton, C. L., & Tucker, A. R. (2010). New Heights. *Groupwork, 20*(2), 24–44.

Prati, G., & Pietratoni, L. (2009). Optimism, social support and coping strategies as factors contributing to posttraumatic growth: A meta-analysis. *Journal of Loss and Trauma, 14*, 364–388. https://doi.org/10.1080/15325020902724271

Reese, R. F., Hadeed, S., Craig, H., Beyer, A., & Gosling, M. (2019). EcoWellness: Integrating the natural world into wilderness therapy settings with intentionality. *Journal of Adventure Education and Outdoor Learning, 19*(3), 202–215. https://doi.org/10.1080/14729679.2018.1508357

Reid, P., & Kampman, H. (2020). Exploring the psychology of extended-period expeditionary adventurers: Going knowingly into the unknown. *Psychology of Sport and Exercise, 46*, 101608. https://doi.org/10.1016/j.psychsport.2019.101608

Shakespeare-Finch, J., & Armstrong, D. (2010). Trauma type and posttrauma outcomes: Differences between survivors of motor vehicle accidents, sexual assault, and bereavement. *Journal of Loss and Trauma, 15*(2), 69–82.

Shuwiekh, H., Kira, I. A., & Ashby, J. S. (2018). What are the personality and trauma dynamics that contribute to posttraumatic growth? *International Journal of Stress Management, 25*(2), 181–194. https://doi.org/10.1037/str0000054

Tedeschi, R. G., Cann, A., Taku, K., Senol-Durak, E., & Calhoun, L. G. (2017). The posttraumatic growth inventory: A revision integrating existential and spiritual change: posttraumatic growth inventory and spiritual change. *Journal of Traumatic Stress, 30*(1), 11–18. https://doi.org/10.1002/jts.22155

Tedeschi, R. G., Shakespeare-Finch, J., Taku, K., & Calhoun, L. G. (2018). *Posttraumatic growth theory, research, and applications.* Routledge.

Theodorou, M., & Kampman, H. (2022). "Taking the helm of life": Exploring the role of "blue" adventure in the experience of post traumatic growth in women who participated in ocean racing sailing after the loss of a loved one. [Manuscript in preparation] Department of Psychology, University of East London.

Tucker, A. R., & Norton, C. L. (2013). The use of adventure therapy techniques by clinical social workers: Implications for practice and training. *Clinical Social Work Journal,* 41(4), 333–343. https://doi.org/10.1007/s10615-012-0411-4

van der Kolk, B. A. (1996). The body keeps score: Approaches to the psychobiology of posttraumatic stress disorder. In *Traumatic stress: The effects of overwhelming experience on mind, body, and society* (pp. 214–241). Guilford Press.

van Gennep, A., Kertzer, D. I., Vizedom, M. B., & Caffee, G. L. (2019). *The rites of passage* (2nd ed.). University of Chicago Press.

Voruganti, L. N., Whatham, J., Bard, E., Parker, G., Babbey, C., Ryan, J., … & MacCrimmon, D. J. (2006). Going beyond: An adventure-and recreation-based group intervention promotes well-being and weight loss in schizophrenia. *The Canadian Journal of Psychiatry,* 51(9), 575–580.

Wadey, R., & Day, M. (2018). A longitudinal examination of leisure time physical activity following amputation in England. *Psychology of Sport and Exercise, 37,* 251–261. https://doi.org/10.1016/j.psychsport.2017.11.005

Wadey, R., Day, M., & Howells, K. (2021). *Growth following adversity in sport: A mechanism to positive change* (Vol. 1). Routledge.

Walker, P. A. & Kampman, H. (2021). "It didn't bring back the old me but helped me on the path to the new me": Exploring posttraumatic growth in British veterans with PTSD. *Disability and Rehabilitation,* 1–9. https://doi.org/10.1080/09638288.2021.1995056

Wassif, J. A. (2014). *The utilization of adventure based programming to foster posttraumatic growth within a veteran population: A mixed methods study.* https://doi.org/10.33915/etd.6920

12
ADVENTURE AND THE SUBLIME
A Quest for Transformation or Transcendence?

Chris Loynes and Amy Smallwood

An Adventurer's Point of View: The Cave

The Pembrokeshire coast is dramatic – big cliffs, deep caves, stormy seas, spectacular skies, rainbows, winds, sunrises and sunsets.

A group of adults made their way along the foot of the cliffs; coastal traversing for three days, bivouacking as they went, facing various and progressive challenges of climbing, jumping, swimming, caving, in search of seal pups.

On the second day, one scrambler shared his fear of moving water with the guide and explained that, given how close the group were to an increasingly disturbed sea, he thought this might be the chance to face his fear. He asked that, if he spotted an opportunity, would the guide support him and the guide agreed. The next day the sea was rough and waves were breaking up to, and over, the party. The scrambler spotted a sea stack set out amongst the waves with a slab connecting it to the cliff base. They asked to sit with the guide on the stack until nerves settled.

It was a sublime moment with the awe, wonder and terror of a dynamic sea very close sometimes breaking over the couple as they sat. After a while they returned to the group and continued on their way to the seal cave. Later, when the trip was over, the guide asked the group for any moments of transformation. Among the stories told was that of overcoming fear of the moving water. It was explained as a deep fear, a symbolic fear of something else in life, that had been faced and could now be lived with in a different way.

★ ★ ★

Another participant spoke of their time in the seal cave.

The cave was entered by swimming into a very narrow gap at low tide. Beyond the entrance the cave opened into an expanding long tunnel with an eerie green light cast by the low sun shining through the entrance filtered by the waves as they pulsed along the passage. A ledge gave a safe harbour to watch and feel the rhythmic pulse of the waves pushing through the entrance with a whoosh of trapped air, followed by a rushing green wave sinking just below the shelf to break on the shingle beach.

They spoke of not wanting to leave the cave; mesmerised by the water, the light, the sounds and the new born life of the seal pups in such a fragile setting, and yet so resilient and calm.

This had the effect of shifting their whole point of view from one centred on themselves to one aware of the wider world on which they were such a small thing. An egocentric person had found transcendence in that sublime moment that altered perspective on identity, family, role and a relationship with the world as a dynamic and vibrant place. A value of care, for human and non-human life, and a relational rather than transactional sense of a place in the world was born in that instant.

Adventure and the Sublime: A Quest for Transformation or Transcendence?

Introduction

Outdoor adventures have emerged as recreational and educational experiences alongside the development of modern western cultures. Adventures both reflect and challenge societies norms. Can they lead to opportunities for new attachments to nature that tends towards greater appreciation, concern and care in these times of environmental crisis? In this chapter we suggest that the narratives of adventure experiences fall into two main sets, those that are understood to be transformational and those that are understood as transcendental. Both versions are, we claim, rooted in the western Romantic idea of the sublime that arose as a counter narrative to the industrial revolution and the consequent objectification of nature. However, we think transformational adventures instrumentalise nature and largely focus on the benefits to humans. We explore in what way transcendental adventures are different and whether this offers any possibilities for better human–nature relations.

Human–nature relations have also evolved during modernity. The industrial revolution in both North America and Europe changed where people lived, what work they did, their standard of living and their relationships with nature. We propose that human–nature relations in the modern western world can be understood as three broad phases linked to these societal changes. The first phase was adversarial, whether it was the conquest of the west in North America or of the lands of the new colonies by Europeans. The second phase was one of exploitation, both of nature and of the people of these newly acquired lands for the resources and the labour needed to fuel the industrial revolution. Finally, the Romantic counter movement challenged the objectification of nature, and primed a trend towards conservation that led to the setting up of National Parks in North America and Europe.

Adventure had a foot in all three of these phases and, to this day, is influenced by approaches that draw on the very different attitudes they illicit. These approaches also align with the cultural trends of the day. Two adventurous trails emerged, both drawing on the sublime idea of dramatic land and seascapes: adventure as transformation, exemplified by its appearance in the educational systems of the west; and adventure as transcendence, found for example in extreme outdoor sports, allowing people to develop a relationship with nature, albeit, we will argue, taking a new form congruent with the modern way of life. Finally, we discuss whether these insights could lead to nature based adventure experiences that can address the issue of the exclusiveness enjoyed by those who can access the outdoors, and the issue of nature as 'other', that leads to the separation of humans and nature, a split that many claim lies at the heart of the current environmental crises. In the next section we take a broad view of the changes in human–nature relations in the West during modernity.

New Relations

In Europe, in the nineteenth century, the industrial revolution rapidly displaced the majority of people from rural settings and a working relationship with the land. As farms revolutionised food production in the countryside so the growing number of jobs in manufacturing attracted working people to urban centres. This disruption eventually made substantially qualitative differences to people's lives and changed the relationship of the majority of people to nature as well as to society. Better health, longer lifespans, disposable income, education and recreational time became the privilege of more and more of the population. For example, in the UK, newly wealthy people followed in the footsteps of Queen Victoria who adopted the habit of summers at Balmoral, a Scottish estate where the royal family could hunt and fish. The new rich bought land and built summer homes in the most attractive places. Increasingly, and spurred on by cheap forms of travel made possible by the railways, middle- and working-class people returned to the rural landscapes of their past to enjoy the fresh air, the open spaces, the views and the recreational activities. These destinations were quickly commercialised.

The history of North American settlement by European immigrants provides a different perspective on the human relationship with the natural world, how it was perceived by the western world, and how this perception changed over time. Roderick Nash (2001) who, in his seminal work *Wilderness and the American Mind*, provides a narrative history of the North American understanding of the idea of wilderness as a cultural phenomenon. Nash catalogues the various perceptual changes that have taken place, starting with early attempts to conquer and tame a threatening landscape. When the first Europeans arrived on the shores of North America, the natural environment they encountered was not exactly hospitable. In the onslaught of a harsh New England winter, they struggled desperately to survive. These early settlers sought to tame this wild new land (including the 'savages' they found already living here) with rifles and towering wooden walls. Thus, the human relationship to nature was perceived as adversarial (Nash, 2001).

As the new world was expanded and explored, these early Americans began to discover valuable resources – timber, furs, coal, and minerals. Extraction and export of these resources provided stability and greater independence, and the natural world became a commodity. In fact, the abundance of resources pushed the expansion into the west, and the US economy began to grow by measure. The human relationship to place became economical, and the management of land and resources became pragmatic (Nash, 2001).

During the peak of resource extraction, a few voices began to challenge the rate by which beautiful landscapes were depleting. Transcendental thinkers like Thoreau, Emerson, and John Muir wrote eloquently about the sublime wilderness – that which evokes awe and wonder – and the need to protect its pristine state. Humankind was now the enemy, a parasite that needed containment.

In both the European and American cases, the industrial revolution transformed the relationships with the land of most people from one of a parochial working place to an expansive recreational space, and nature from a productive home for many to a recreational escape for the privileged. In the meantime, those now owning and still working the land turned it into an extractive farmed landscape leaving only the most remote and marginal land, sometimes protected, for other purposes. Inevitably, a counter movement emerged. The Romantics offered a new way of seeing and experiencing the wilder natural landscapes as places of sublime encounters to be cherished.

The Sublime and Protected Landscapes

As in North America, a counter movement sprang up in Europe pushing back against some of the implications of modernity and the relationship with nature it promulgated. Often described as the Romantic movement, artists and thinkers across Europe and in North America countered the view of nature as an objectified natural resource with a new vision of sublime and picturesque landscapes to be found both at home and further afield. This movement emerged as traditional religions were in retreat from scientific explanations of the world. The Darwinian turn extended the explanatory power of science to nature, its origins, diversity and evolution. At the same time early geologists became more confident in explaining the story of the earth and life upon it in the context of geological rather than biblical time. As science contributed to the objectification of nature so the romantics countered by acknowledging human emotional responses restoring subjective, inspirational awe and wonder towards the natural world. Nature, for some, became a secular religion worthy of intrinsic and aesthetic value, providing transcendental experiences and in need of protection from the rational, industrial world. To these artists and thinkers an 'awful' land or seascape, mountains, canyons and oceans, was not as a modern person might understand the term, but a landscape full of awe providing joy and terror in equal emotional measures.

This led to the development of National and State parks and wilderness areas, the first, Yellowstone National Park in the USA in 1872 whilst the UK was late to this trend setting up the Lake District in 1951. The places perceived as the most beautiful were catalogued, set aside, and preserved so that future generations could enjoy sublime landscapes without fearing the effects of the human parasite. While these early preservationists helped in recognising the natural world for its intrinsic value, nature was still understood for the ways in which it benefited humans for recreation, leisure, and personal renewal (Nash, 2001).

In both continents the landscapes of the sublime became tourist destinations, initially for the wealthy and time rich, who travelled seeking out the mountains, glaciers, waterfalls and canyons for the promised moments of the sublime. Within North America, as in Europe, travel companies promoted and exploited these destinations for business purposes. In the USA, rail companies, capitalising on the newly found desire to protect wilderness, promoted destinations, such as Yellowstone in order to create income streams to finance their push to the west and the Pacific coast. In the UK Wordsworth, the globally famous romantic poet, spoke out against the coming of the railway to Windermere, something he saw as an abomination bringing the working classes to the Lake District, a landscape he had made popular through his poetry. He thought they would not have the eyes to appreciate it.

These romantic thinkers challenge us to consider the nature of a sublime experience and the kind of human–nature relationship that results. Clewis (2019), while acknowledging that the meaning of sublime is elusive, defines it as 'a complex feeling of intense satisfaction, uplift, or elevation, felt before an object or event that is considered awe-inspiring, (p. 1). This definition focuses solely on the positive aspects of sublime, but for Kant, who wrote prolifically about the sublime, there also exists what he called negative pleasure. The pleasure comes from the expansion of our imagination and an awareness of our moral capacities (e.g. freedom, reason). The negative comes from frustration over our ability to understand or take in what we are exposed to (e.g. formlessness, mathematical impossibilities) and the recognition of our physical helplessness (Brady, 2013, p. 84). The sublime forces us to consider our own frailty, brevity, and insignificance in the vastness of wild and untamed nature. Elements not dissimilar to our understanding of the concept of awe.

Nash (2001), in his reflections on wilderness, understands place as a cultural rather than just a material phenomenon, and claims that humans perceive place based on their political and physical environments. Viewed this way, the three phases of human–nature relations mentioned above, adversarial, exploitative and protective, appear largely anthropocentric in nature, although the last suggests a slight movement towards eco-centrism. The current cultural climate in Europe and the United States continues to engage in all three of these forms of human–nature relationships. From reality TV (Survivor, Man vs. Wild) that perpetuates nature as adversary, to timber, mining, and oil industries. Even in the romantic and conservation movements that sprung from transcendental thinkers, there remains (arguably) a distinct separation between humans and nature. Nature becomes conflated with the landscapes of remote and sublime land and seascapes preserved as reserves or parks at a, sometimes, considerable distance from people. The parks, and by default nature, become far off destinations for human enjoyment. This analysis does not offer a construction of the human relationship with nature as equitable and mutualistic. It is not one that automatically understands or cares for nature. Adventure, as one modern expression of the human relationship with nature, is caught up in and is central to this narrative.

Adventure

Adventure is often equated with risk, initially the financial risk of a merchant venture to bring spices back from the Far East. However, it is also understood as a much broader concept involving new experiences, uncertainty of outcome and heightened degrees of personal agency – the freedom of the hills linking directly to Clewis's (2019) positive elements of the sublime idea. In this formulation of adventure, risk is a secondary consequence to be managed rather than the outcome being sought. Travelling to new places on ventures with uncertain outcome was increasingly common for business, scientific and religious reasons. Over time, the hierarchy of adventurers, as they were considered by their cultures, was increasingly judged by the risks they took, how hard, how far, how dangerous, how wild. It is worth noting that many must have disappeared without their stories ever being heard. It is also worth noting that many women were also involved in exploration, though it was considered inappropriate for their stories to be told. It was not long before people, mainly men, set off on adventures for their own sake.

The cultural appropriation of adventure. Emerging democracies, in need of symbols of a good citizen willing to transform the expectations of a previous generation and contribute in new and innovative ways to a rapidly changing economy and society, jumped on the masculine and heroic symbols of early explorers. Their exploits, often justified on commercial and scientific grounds, became, on return, best-selling adventure stories. Fictional adventure stories, such as Robinson Crusoe by Daniel Defoe published in 1719, followed close behind. The polar expeditions of both European and American explorers are good examples of this trend lasting well into the early twentieth century. The race to the north and south poles involved lots of money and human capital, with little reward other than some scientific achievements and adventure for adventure's sake.

This trend readily entwined with the quest for sublime landscapes, no longer viewed as settings where the observer is passive and nature dynamic, but engaged with by actors such as mountaineers or sailors, etc, in which both the landscape and the human are active in an embodied, emotional and relational experience. The culturally dominant narratives about these adventure experiences became that of challenges overcome, of discoveries and 'conquests' in which nature was subjugated to man's[1] will. The respect for nature implied by the awe-inspiring sublime was replaced by an anthropocentric concept of the adventurer, a man worthy of character and as a symbol of the ideal citizen for the new world triumphant over nature – and other cultures.

Adventure therefore broke the emerging eco-centric shifts encouraged by the Romantics by adopting the earlier adversarial approach building on the negative pleasure of Kant's concept of the sublime. A proving ground for the men of the new society was established, a space onto which these men could conduct their own hero's journeys, writing their own narratives of conquest and achievement that transformed the state of awareness of their moral capacities.

Adventure as Education

Adventure maintained its transformational relationship with emerging democratic cultures throughout the 20th century. The historical roots of combining education with the out-of-doors varies by context and culture. In North America, origins are traditionally traced back to several sources, including The Great Age of Exploration (Ewert & Sibthorp, 2014), European Romanticism, and the influence of aesthetics and adventure tourism (Martin et al., 2017). Perhaps the first programmes to intentionally utilise outdoor adventure educationally were the Scout Movement (1907) and Outward Bound (1941) both founded in Great Britain. Pedagogically, a connection can be seen between Kant's idea of 'negative pleasure' and the character development aims of traditional Adventure Education programmes. The negative emotion exposes a power struggle, human survival versus nature, and sets the stage for exercising courage and tenacity in the face of something much more powerful and incomprehensible. Additionally, when programmed as a group experience, there often results the sense of unity, comradery, and interdependence William James calls for in his moral equivalent to war which was a primary aim of Kurt Hahn in his founding of Outward Bound. The result is that Adventure Education has traditionally located programming in sublime locations. As Roberts notes, 'the educational journey often involves a trip to another place … and that place is often the location of a more powerful, sublime, and thus transcendent experience' (2012, p. 45). To our minds, this experience is more appropriately described as transformative, a youth to adult rite of passage (Loynes, 2008). Throughout the 20th century western societies co-opted adventure as an experience and sublime landscapes as spaces in which to build character epitomised by Mortlock (1987) in his book the Adventure Alternative in which he makes the case for the relationship between adventure and moral development.

In considering human relations with the more-than-human world, we question, as does Mortlock (2001) in his later writing, the quality of relationship that is being formed from these kinds of experiences. The seemingly singular focus on character development suggests a relationship that is adversarial - nature provides a worthy opponent for *homo sapiens*, who has risen to the top of the food chain to create a tame and ordered world. Looking beyond character, locating Adventure Education in sublime places also serves to emphasise the otherness of more-than-human nature. The sheer alterity of the wilderness, it's wildness, inscrutable depth and breadth, its space, set an ideal stage for the development of tenacity, courage, and determination. However, alongside the widely applauded transformational adventure experiences, transcendental adventures remained discreet and were increasingly understood to offer something else, which we explore next.

Transformative Experiences

Many of the early adventure education programmes shared common aims for combining education and the out-of-doors (Macleod, 1983). Lord Robert Baden-Powell founded The Boy Scouts to address a perceived decline in the physical and moral character of modern civilisation (MacDonald, 1993). Similarly, Kurt Hahn helped create Outward Bound partly as an attempt to realise William James's challenge for a moral equivalent to war. Hahn's programmes were developed around his definition of the five declines of modern civilisation, which were understood as moral failures of society contributing to an overall lack of character (Hahn, 1960).

Both Outward Bound and the Boy Scouts were also heavily influenced by the realities of war. Baden-Powell, a British hero of the Boer War, was inspired by the war-zone maturity of army scouts and recycled a manual he wrote for these British soldiers as an outdoor skills manual for young boys. Hahn, stymied by the high casualty rate of younger (presumably stronger and healthier) British castaways during World War II, concluded that these younger sailors relied too heavily on technology and lacked the experience and the craft of seamanship (Martin et al., 2017). Both saw the crucible of war as a key influence in the development of character.

Additionally, these programmes were founded on the heels of the industrial revolution and during a dramatic increase in urbanisation and changes in wealth distribution and power. The assumption was that modernisation and the progressive movement produced men who were physically, mentally, and morally weak as compared to their ancestors (Cronon, 1996; Phelps, 1980). Fuelled by a desire to reverse these damages and address the issue of moral decline, the outdoors became the new crucible – a place to test one's limits and strengthen moral values. Adventure was valued for its transformative power, both for the individual and then, through that individual, society.

Transcendental Experiences

It would be wrong to give the impression that the sole purpose of Adventure Education (AE) was transformative in approach constructing nature as an adversary to be overcome. Too many people provide accounts of transcendental experiences in classically sublime land and seascapes enabled by programmes of AE provided by organisations such as Outward Bound. In *Beyond Learning by Doing*, Roberts (2012) notes romantic transcendentalism as one of five theoretical currents that have shaped Outdoor AE pedagogy, specifically highlighting the influential voices of Emerson, Thoreau, and Muir. Experience of the sublime in nature is a common theme that runs throughout the transcendental literature of these particular authors. Wildness is often used interchangeably with sublime, juxtaposed with the ordered beauty of a well-kept English garden. The romantics argue for the intrinsic value of wild, unordered nature which evokes feelings of the sublime and is different from (and often described in opposition to) the aesthetic experience of a cultivated landscape. Adventure as transcendence remained alive and well if hidden from wider anthropocentric social constructions of human–nature relations.

One way to understand the difference between adventures that are transformative and those that are transcendental lies in the writings of Martin Buber best known for what he called 'a philosophy of dialogue'. Buber's work points to two different kinds of relational receptivity: I/It and I/Thou. He describes I/It as a sort of monologue:

> ... when we behold what confronts us in the world, we deal with it by treating it as an object which can be compared and assigned a place in an order of objects, described and analysed objectively, filed away in our memory to be recalled when needed.

By contrast, an I/Thou interaction is a dialogue; one that recognises the reciprocity and mutuality of relationship. Buber calls this an encounter and ties it to the Hebrew word for 'to know'. We cannot relate to the other without an intimate knowledge of our reciprocal influence and a mutual understanding of what it means to be 'other.' This encounter, particularly with the natural world, means that we embrace the 'other' lovingly, not to exploit, use up, exhaust, or ravish. The link is between knowing and loving, rather than knowing and doing.

Brymer et al. (2009) captures the motivation of 'extreme' adventurers in ways that resonate with Buber's ideas rather than the cultural constructions of heroes dominating and conquering, overcoming risks in order to persevere. For the adventurers he interviews controlling risk, as discussed earlier, is an essential but secondary element of the desired experience. The primary motive is to encounter their chosen element, to find a flow state in which there is a loss of self in a deep embodied and dynamic relationship with the elements involved, a sublime and sustained moment of an active relationship with nature. Brymer found the same outcomes amongst mountain bikers, free divers, wing suit base jumpers and white water kayakers. The experience was frequently described as a sense of the universal, of the power of nature and of being intimately a part of nature. A respect for nature was universally implied and often expressed in spiritual terms. These new extreme adventurers have broken away from the cultural narratives of adventure as character building, as anthropocentric. Instead, they offer a highly personal account of their transcendence of themselves restoring the romantic movement's idea of the sublime but in a way that encounters nature as equally as active as the humans involved. If there is a meaningful power relationship in an experience that is often described as a sense of oneness and a loss of self, then it is an equitable one.

Adventure and Wellbeing

Human wellbeing and experience in nature are increasingly linked. Less commonly, the wellbeing of nature is also considered. Adventure, in both its transformative and transcendental forms, tangles with these different ideas of human wellbeing. A *hedonic* model defines human wellbeing as that which gives us pleasure and satisfies desire. This approach recognises an affective component (the presence of positive emotions) and a cognitive component (articulating something as satisfying). A contrasting approach to human wellbeing is the *eudaemonic* model, which defines wellbeing as that which connects to our values and helps us realise our full potential. The *eudaemonic* model is often described as an approach based on human flourishing. Some psychologists have categorised this into six areas of self-actualisation: mastery, life purpose, autonomy, self-acceptance, positive relatedness, and personal growth (Capaldi et al., 2014).

From these two perspectives, aspects of the natural world have instrumental value by contributing to human pleasure (hedonistic model) or to human flourishing (*eudaemonic* model). However, James (2019) argues that this fails to acknowledge the intimacy of certain human–nature relationships such as those described by Brymer (2009). James provides an example of Katherine Smith, a 1970s Navajo activist who refused to leave her land even if she were relocated to one that provided her with more amenities and an easier life. For her, there was no substitute for the land of her dwelling. This snapshot of a surviving pre-industrial human–nature relationship might offer a bridge from the pre-modern to the current transcendental forms of adventure and the human–nature relationship this strives to achieve. For James, one possible approach is to understand human–nature relations in terms of meanings rather than instrumentation. In short, stemming from an assumption that nature has meaning that varies based on context, we can conclude that nature contributes to our wellbeing because of the meaning that it offers. James calls this conception a *semiotic-constitutive* model (James, 2019).

James Raffan has also been interested in human attachments to place that extend beyond an instrumental model. In his research regarding 'Land as Teacher' (1993), Raffan explores the types of connections that people establish with certain places over a long period of time. Specifically, he decides to locate his research in the Thelon Game Sanctuary of the Northwest Territories of Canada. Raffan discusses land conflicts in this particular area, asserting that the conflicts are necessarily fights about land use, but are ultimately disagreements about what land means. He distinguishes between our perceptions of land as commodity, recreation, peaceful haven, energy potential, and part of a God-given (i.e. transcendent) universe. Through his ethnographic research, he identified four different types of a sense of place: toponymic, narrative, experiential, and numinous. Toponymic connections have to do with things like place names, indicating both knowledge and attachment to a certain place. Narrative connections were evident through the stories embedded in the culture regarding how the land came to be, history of the land, and even gossip about events that occurred over the years. An experiential connection is different than toponymic or narrative in that it is a first-hand encounter with a particular place. Within the experiential connection, Raffan notes a distinct difference between the experiences of those who were dependent upon the land for survival (hunters, trappers, and the like) and those who experienced the land for more leisurely reasons (a canoe trip). Those who were dependent upon the land were able to recall the land in much more detail (wind direction, flow of water, etc). The last connection identified by Raffan's research is that of the numinous.

> Numinous connections to place are all that is awe-inspiring, all that transcends the rational, all that touches the heart more than the mind, all that goes beyond names, stories, and experience and yet still plays a significant role in the bond that links people and place'.
>
> *(p. 44)*

Raffan concludes his article by contending that these types of a 'sense of place' are intimately associated with identity. 'Because it appears that sense of place, in varying degrees, constitutes an existential definition of self. For many consultants to this study, you take away the land or break the connection to land, you prevent them from being who they are' (p. 45).

Brymer's (2009) adventurers could be described as having both an experiential (in Raffan's leisure sense) and a numinous relationship but with a more universal idea of the elements rather than a located idea of a place. Perhaps some extreme sportspeople do become attached to a place as well as an element. However, the evidence suggests that most travel to experience their chosen element in various places, sometimes following repeated seasonal patterns, a neo-nomadic life not rooted or settled in place. Transcendental adventure offers a deeply meaningful experience understood as a mutual relationship between adventurers and their elements. However, it is not a return to a pre-modern and potentially harmonious way of relating. It offers something new.

Adventure at a Time of Social and Environmental Crises

Modern adventurers seeking either transformative or transcendental experiences are both embedded in the historical and cultural contexts of our time. Inevitably, this highlights certain critical issues. Here, we focus on 'privilege' and on the 'relationship with nature'.

Privilege. That the adventure story is also a story told by certain privileged groups is apparent throughout this chapter. In particular, robust ideas of masculinity, expressed by early adventurers and reproduced by some modern adventure experiences draws on the adversarial and exploitative phases of modern human–nature relations. For nature and human relationships with it, this is clearly problematic. William Cronon (1996) problematises American constructions of wilderness in his essay 'The Trouble with Wilderness'. Part of the problem for Cronon lies in the masculinity that undergirds American ideals of wilderness and frontierism.

> The mythic frontier individualist was almost always masculine in gender: here, in the wilderness, a man could be a real man, the rugged individual he was meant to be before civilization sapped his energy and threatened his masculinity. ... [T]he comforts and seductions of civilized life were especially insidious for men, who all too easily became emasculated by the feminizing tendencies of civilization.
>
> *(p. 78)*

Adding to these masculine ideals were also those of privilege:

> The dream of an unworked natural landscape is very much the fantasy of people who have never themselves had to work the land to make a living—urban folk for whom food comes from a supermarket or a restaurant instead of a field, and for whom the wooden houses in which they live and work apparently have no meaningful connection to the forests in which trees grow and die. Only people whose relation to the land was already alienated could hold up wilderness as a model for human life in nature, for the romantic ideology of wilderness leaves precisely nowhere for human beings to actually make their living from the land.
>
> *(p. 80)*

Nash also acknowledges the role of privilege woven through the ideal of romantic wilderness: "Appreciation of wilderness began in the cities. The literary gentleman wielding a pen, not the pioneer with his axe, made the first gestures of resistance against the strong currents of antipathy" (2001, p. 44). This 'nature elsewhere' concern we address more fully below.

Further criticised by Nash is the effect of American colonialism as European pioneers sought to tame the 'hideous and desolate wilderness' they encountered in the New World.

> For the first Americans, as for medieval Europeans, the forest's darkness hid savage men, wild beasts, and still stranger creatures of the imagination. In addition, civilized man faced the danger of succumbing to the wildness of his surroundings and reverting to savagery himself.
>
> *(p. 24).*

These early frontiersmen were tasked with the responsibility of civilising this new world, a manifest destiny which meant subjugating both wild human and wild nature.

Beyond the obvious concerns for equity, diversity and inclusion that adventure institutions might want to address, Cronon concludes with the claim that American constructions of wilderness (rooted in masculinity, colonialism, and privilege) have created a dangerous reductionism and false dichotomy of humans outside-of nature, which does more harm than good when it comes to responsibility to the natural world.

Nature elsewhere. As we mentioned early on, protective approaches to human–nature relations can also be anthropocentric and therefore also problematic in supporting any equitable reconstruction of human–nature relations. The two terms most commonly used to describe the outdoor environment, particularly in the context of adventure, are wilderness and nature. In contrast to simply saying outdoors or out-of-doors, these terms are meant to describe a type of outdoors – one that is wild and in its natural state. Many voices have endeavoured to deconstruct our modern notions of wilderness and nature (Cronon, 1996; Nash, 2001; Oelschlaeger, 1991; Shepard, 2002). Nash (2001) and Oelschlaeger (1991) both outline a history of how humans have understood nature, with Oelschlaeger going as far back as history will allow, and Nash focusing on the settling of the New World and the American frontier. Both recognise the role that social construction and human experience play on our understanding and interaction with the more-than-human world. The anthropocentric perspective portrayed in these works is telling. With some exceptions, wilderness and nature are described through a lens of causal determinism with little acknowledgement of the agency and affect of the more-than-human world. Moreover, the more-than-human world is described by the urban dweller as elsewhere, behind the boundaries of national parks and protected areas set aside as destinations for temporary encounters.

An alternative way of relating to the natural world has been suggested metaphorically as 'nature as friend' (Martin, 1999, p. 465). As Martin contends, 'One distinctive and worthy path is for (adventure) to concern itself primarily with establishing or perhaps re-establishing, a sense of personal relatedness to nature'

(p. 465). Martin suggests that the metaphor of nature as friend can provide language for understanding the natural world in terms of subject–subject, rather than subject–object. As subjects, the relationship is based on care and respect for the 'other.' Rather than relating to nature from an objective, rational paradigm, this type of relating is based in experiential, tacit, and intuitive ways of knowing. Martin is quick to acknowledge, however, that rational/cognitive knowledge is also important in balancing out the relationship, so it is neither a distanced, objective relationship nor that of blind romanticism. This seems to us to align closely with Brymer's (2009) understanding of the experience and meaning making of transcendental adventurers.

Using the nature as friend metaphor can be helpful as we seek to understand what a subject–subject relationship might actually look like. It is also important to acknowledge that the word friend is also a rather amorphous word. Just as we can have a vast array of different relationships, friendship can also vary drastically from a neighbourly acquaintance to a deeply intimate friendship, from everyday encounters to occasional far off visits. One thing that the word friend does for us, however, is paint the relationship in positive terms. Here it's acknowledged that having a positive relationship with nature, rather than adversarial, is a possibility and, we suggest, exemplified by transcendental adventures.

Subsequent to Martin's discussion about nature as friend, he conducted a qualitative study to trace the changes in human/nature relationships based on a "nature as friend" approach (Martin, 2004). Martin found that adventure experiences that were focused on nature connections and less focused on skill development led students to develop an emotional and spiritual attachment to the natural world that resulted in eco-friendly behaviours. Martin contends, "'It is my argument that adventure activities are a powerful medium to elicit emotional connections to the natural world.' (p. 27). Mullins' (2014) research with fly fishing and canoeing supports this claim. He suggests that, as an outdoor sports person travels from novice to expert, a key defining shift in attention is from the activity to the environment, including a sense of the need to care for that environment.

There remans the problem of the twitcher compulsion, completing lists of routes completed or destinations attained. This can become obscene when it is linked to the environmental crises as the 'last chance to see/do, etc package'. However, there is a counter argument that could mitigate some of this harm. Asfeldt and Hvenegaard (2014) studied groups going to uninhabited parts of northern Canada, and Cheung, Baurer and Deng (2019) researched ecotours to Antarctica, both populations incurring substantial carbon footprints in doing so. They found an offsetting value of a kind in that these places gained advocates that would become activists for the environmental protection of these places, something they lacked without any residents to voice their value.

Conclusions

Modern humans are not typically strongly attached to one place as pre-industrial people were. With modernity has come mobility. Finding new and sublime land and seascapes has stimulated the adventure experience as typically far away. Western cultures have co-opted adventure as character building, transformative experiences with sublime land- and seascapes as the spaces where these occur. Whilst of great value to human development, these forms of adventure may have limited potential for supporting new forms of human–nature relations drawing as they do on adversarial and exploitative anthropocentric constructions. On a more hopeful note, in seeking meaningful encounters with nature, extreme adventurers have sought sublime and transcendental experiences that unite them with a universal, perhaps spiritual, integration with a nature greater than the self. This approach to adventure can lead to respect for nature and a desire to care that operates at a global level non-specific to place. This may facilitate important behaviour changes that help to address the current environmental crises. Neither transformative nor transcendental adventures necessarily support the intimate and sustained knowledge and care for specific places – nature as home.

Note

1 "Man" is used here in order to stay authentic to the terms used at the time. We acknowledge that this can be viewed as inappropriate language. However, the bias this implies was embedded in the performance and accounts of these explorations. It was mainly, though not exclusively, men who undertook adventures and almost exclusively men who subsequently wrote about them.

References

Asfeldt, M., & Hvenegaard, G. (2014). Perceived learning, critical elements and lasting impacts on university-based wilderness educational expeditions. *Journal of Adventure Education and Outdoor Learning*, 2(14), 132–152. https://doi:10.1080/14729679.2013.789350

Brady, E. (2013). *The sublime in modern philosophy: Aesthetics, ethics, and nature*. Cambridge: Cambridge University Press.

Brymer, E., Downey, G., & Gray, T. (2009). Extreme sports as a precursor to environmental sustainability. *Journal of Sport & Tourism*, 14(2–3), 193–204. https://doi:10.1080/14775080902965223

Buber, M. (1958). *Hasidism and modern man*. New York: Holt, Rinehart and Winston.

Buber, M. (1970). *I and Thou*. Translated from the German by W. Kaufmann. New York: Simon & Schuster.

Capaldi, C. A., Dopko, R. L., & Zelenski, J. M. (2014). The relationship between nature connectedness and happiness: A meta-analysis. *Frontiers in Psychology*, 5. https://doi:10.3389/fpsyg.2014.00976

Cheung, W., Bauer, T., & Deng, J. (2019). The growth of Chinese tourism to Antarctica: A profile of their connectedness to nature, motivations, and perceptions. *The Polar Journal*, 1(9), 197–213. https://doi:10.1080/2154896X.2019.1618552

Clewis, R. R. (2019). Editor's introduction. In R. R. Clewis (Ed.), *The sublime reader* (pp. 1–13). London: Bloomsbury Academic.

Cronon, W. (1996). The trouble with wilderness; or, getting back to the wrong nature. In W. Cronon (Ed.), *Uncommon ground* (pp. 69–90). 2nd ed. New York: W. W. Norton & Company.

Ewert, A. & Sibthorp, J. (2014). Outdoor *Adventure Education: Foundations, Theory and Research*. Human Kinetics. https://doi.org/10.5040/9781492595663

Hahn, K. (1960). *Address at the Outward Bound Trust.* KurtHahn.org.

James, S. P. (2019). Natural meanings and Cultural Values. *Environmental Ethics*, 41(1), 3–16. https://doi.org/10.5840/enviroethics20194112

Loynes, C. (2008). Narratives of agency. In P. Becker & J. Schirp (Eds.), *Other ways of learning* (pp. 111–130). Marburg: BSJ.

Loynes, C. (2018). Leave more trace. *Journal of Outdoor Recreation, Education, and Leadership.* Sagamore Publishing, LLC, *10*(3), 179–186. https://doi: 10.18666/jorel-2018-v10-i3-8444

MacDonald, R. H. (1993). *Sons of the empire: The frontier and the Boy Scout Movement, 1890–1918.* Ontario: University of Toronto Press.

Macleod, D. I. (1983). *Building character in the American boy: The Boy Scouts, YMCA, and their forerunners, 1870-1920.* Madison: University of Wisconsin Press.

Martin, B. et al. (2017). *Outdoor leadership: Theory and practice.* 2nd edn. Champaign, IL: Human Kinetics.

Martin, P. (1999). Critical outdoor education and nature as friend. In J. Miles & S. Priest (Eds.) *Adventure Education.* 2nd ed. State College, PA: Venture Publishing.

Martin, P. (2004). Outdoor adventure in promoting relationships with nature. *Australian Journal of Outdoor Education*, 1(8), 20–28.

Mortlock, C. (1987). *The adventure alternative.* Milnthorpe: Cicerone Press.

Mortlock, C. (2001). *Beyond adventure: An inner journey.* Milnthorpe: Cicerone Press.

Mullins, P. M. (2014). A socio-environmentsl case for skill in outdoor adventure. *Journal of Experiential Education*, *2*(37). https://doi.org/10.1177/1053825913498366

Nash, R. F. (2001). *Wilderness & the American mind.* 4th edn. New Haven, CT: Yale University Press.

Oelschlaeger, M. (1991). *The idea of wilderness.* New Haven, CT: Yale University Press.

Phelps, R. (1980). *Being prepared: The application of character building and the beginning of the Boy Scouts of America.* Boston, MA. https://eric.ed.gov/?id=ED201553

Raffan, J. (1993). The experience of place: Exploring land as teacher. *Journal of Experiential Education*, 1(13). https://doi.org/10.1177/105382599301600109

Rawles, K. (2013). Outdoor adventure in a carbon-light era. In E. C. J. Pike and S. Beames (Eds.), *Outdoor adventure and social theory* (pp. 159–170). New York: Routledge.

Roberts, J. W. (2012). *Beyond learning by doing: Theoretical currents in experiential education.* New York: Routledge.

Shepard, P. (2002). *Man in the landscape.* 3rd edn. Athens, GA: University of Georgia Press.

Turner, J. M. (2002). From woodcraft to "leave no trace": Wilderness, consumerism, and environmentalism in twentieth-century America. *Environmental History*, *3*(7), 462–484. https://doi: 10.2307/3985918

13

GIVING BACK

An Autoethnographic Analysis of Adventure Experience as Transformational

Vinathe Sharma-Brymer

From an Adventurer's Point of View: I am Padma

I am Padma. I am a 52-year-old woman, working as a full-time schoolteacher. I am living with my husband and children. As an Indian woman, I am bound by my duties to family, striving my best to fulfil my responsibilities of being a dutiful wife and mother. In my late forties, I aspired to move beyond the traditionally followed 'family and job' routine, choosing pilgrimage-related travel. I and a handful of my colleagues planned and carried out several successful pilgrimages to remote holy shrines in the Himalayas. I found out that this was arduous, involving a high level of inner strength, commitment and skilful management of the unknown, risks and outcomes. Nevertheless, I participated in these travel adventures which required good health, fitness and concerted effort. I experienced the meaning and purpose of adventure through the processes I lived while travelling to remote and challenging holy shrines located on mountains, in thick rainforests and across lakes. Within my group of 5-6 friends and colleagues, our pilgrimages were filled with fear, anxiety and nervousness. Yet, we went by our gut feeling, placing our trust in others, feeling hopeful and believing in our sincere efforts. Every step of our pilgrimage was risky, yet every minute felt fulfilling, bringing satisfaction when we completed it. Outcomes did not matter much to us, the lived experience of our adventure did. Living this kind of adventure is a spiritual experience for an ordinary middle-class, traditional Indian woman like me.

DOI: 10.4324/9781003173601-17

I am Lakshmi

> I am Lakshmi. I am in my late thirties. I am a mother of two children. I have been into outdoor and extreme adventure from my teen years. Currently, I identify myself as an extreme overlander, leading expeditions worldwide. I have embodied adventure through nature treks, water sports, and driving 4-wheel cars in extreme terrains such as the upper Himalayas, rainforests and extremely cold regions of Russia. Just following my passion of outdoor and extreme adventure itself was a big deal in my youth. Traditional family and society demanded that I followed their normative model of higher education, job, marriage and family. So, it was a constant feeling of living my dream with anxiety, tension, dilemma and compromises. Moving through the steps of finding money, traveling to the mountains, trekking and staying with strangers involved untold risks and fear. Overcoming the obstacles to pursue adventure itself has been a huge adventure for Indian girls and women like myself. I have felt deeply emotional and confronted at every stage yet I have moved forward with hope and confidence. That is so meaningful for me.

Giving Back: An Autoethnographic Analysis of Adventure Experience as Transformational

Background

This chapter explores how adventure experiences facilitate a desire to give back to nature. To illustrate this, I focus on adventure experiences as lived by adventurers from traditional, non-western societies in India. From this perspective, adventure is encountered through (1) religious or spiritual experiences such as pilgrimages to the remote Himalayan shrines, (2) structured outdoor adventure programmes and, (3) adventures such as four-wheel drive overlander expeditions in extreme terrains. The adventure experience is revealed as profoundly transformational for women, affecting the adventurer's ways of knowing, being and doing. The knowing is through connection, feeling, relating, and sensing the processes of adventure, the being is through building on our relationship with outdoor adventure through values and beliefs such as care and respect and, the doing through actions, attitudes and practices (Sharma-Brymer, 2018). The ways of deep contemplation and reflexive practice bring about a conscious change in the mundane routine way of life (Brymer et al., 2020; Nicol, 2013). These transformative experiences nurture a sense of well-being that reinforces the importance of a positive relationship with nature.

In many parts of the world, adventure is synonymous with outdoor activities where the adventurer undertakes an adventurous activity such as mountaineering or kayaking either for its own sake or to achieve a goal such as summiting a mountain or paddling a river. The adventurer is often modelled as young, fit and healthy; men and women who are trained to navigate through hazardous outdoor environments with skill sets acquired for outdoor adventure activities. For the most part this image reflects a western ideal depicting structure and systemic operationalisation of adventure (Buckley, 2015).

This chapter explores the adventure experience from very different perspectives grounded in diverse sociocultural factors. In a traditional society such as in India there is another type of adventurer. This adventurer may have never been interested in outdoor activities per se or developed the skills to effectively climb a mountain in the Western Ghats or kayak River Ganga. These adventurers are women, middle income group, married with children and leading a culturally normalised life negotiating their identity in a patriarchal system. They could be working age adults, middle aged, close to retirement from employment or retired and find their adventure through participating in short-term structured adventure programmes or pilgrimages associated with religious ideals. These adventurers are not necessarily physically fit or skilled in any outdoor activity. Another type is women undertaking extreme adventure. For example, conducting overland 4WD expeditions. In this example, the female adventurer is trained, physically and mentally fit for outdoor adventure, and confident, while still heralding from a traditional Indian patriarchal sociocultural system where women are oppressed.

For these different types of adventurers, the process of involving oneself in adventure influences and/or enhances self-awareness, triggers personal growth and transforms ideas of what is meaningful in life. For the pilgrims setting out to visit holy shrines in remote regions, this is experienced as a realisation of a deeper connection to nature and valuing nature. Pilgrimages to remote holy shrines take place outdoors and can motivate ordinary people to care for the natural environment (mountains, rivers, ecosystems). The adventurous pilgrim takes inspiration from the environment, has their values challenged and transformed, and chooses to give back to nature. This can further enhance their subjective well-being. For the pilgrim, one adventure experience may be enough to influence their values and attitudes and trigger simplicity, humility, respect and acceptance. For the ordinary person taking part in a short-term adventure programme, this is experienced as liberation from everyday mundane life, may orient the adventurer to connect with nature and impact on their values of respecting and giving back to nature. For the 4WD overland adventurer travelling through extreme environments, the experience facilitates the same sense of respect and care for nature, motivating the desire to give back to nature.

To explicate this experience, the lived experience of these different types of adventurers is examined through autoethnography, specifically focusing on how the participants' understanding of their experiences influence their attitudes and behaviours. For this chapter, I present three very different adventure experiences, including women's pilgrimages in remote regions and a woman's extreme overland 4WD driving expeditions. I explore the participants' meaning-making process of deep awareness of nature facilitating transformative engagement with life satisfaction through adventure.

Conceptual Reflections on Linking Adventure with Giving Back to Nature

Traditional notions of adventure seem to centre around activities involving risk, specific outcomes, methodical processes, and intentional involvement that take place in a variety of outdoor environments. While adventure has the potential for disastrous outcomes, they are considered positive for personal development (Loynes, 2003). Beames and Spike (2013) referred to adventure as lifestyle sports taking place outdoors eliciting excitement in participants (also see Beames et al., 2017). In the last two decades, research into adventure related fields (e.g., adventure sports, adventure education, outdoor recreation, extreme sports) has grown (Beames et al., 2017). While research to date has not directly examined the link between adventure and giving back to nature there are two particular research foci in related fields that provide possible direct and indirect conceptual pathways for how adventure might trigger the desire to give back to nature.

The indirect pathway links to the benefits of nature connection for human health and examines the disconnection between nature and humans due to increased urbanisation (Frumkin et al., 2017). This pathway shows how nature-based activities, including nature-based adventure, might facilitate giving back to nature indirectly through providing avenues for personal growth and improved well-being, especially in children (Sharma-Brymer & Bland, 2016; Sharma-Brymer et al., 2018). For example, the concept of Forest Schools implemented in many schools across the UK integrates adventure, nature and emotional well-being (O'Brien, 2009). Other studies emphasise how exposure to risky and challenging activities in nature impact positive personal growth, meaning and purpose (Bragg & Atkins, 2016). Improvements in positive psychological experiences such as well-being promote non-materialistic attitudes and pro-environmental attitudes and behaviours (see Sharma-Brymer & Brymer, 2019).

The direct route to giving back to nature stems from research in related fields such as extreme sports, outdoor recreation and nature-related engagement with direct experiences. Research in these areas has shown that intense experiences in nature enhance the adventurer's innate relationship (unrelated to feelings of well-being) with nature. This change in relationship includes how people behave in relation to nature. For the most part this change enhances pro-environmental behaviour including giving back to nature (Brymer et al., 2009; Brymer et al., 2019; DeVille et al., 2021; Sharma-Brymer et al., 2018). In line with these conceptual frames, through the presentation of autoethnographic accounts later in this chapter, I show how adventure facilitates the 'oneness with nature' (Humberstone, 2011) where such realisation is profound and spiritual. The 'oneness with nature' experience likely stems from the dissolution of nature as other.

Revisiting Adventure and the Dissolution of Nature as Other

In traditional patriarchal non-western societies such as in Asian countries, the ways of feeling adventurous represent a broad range of personal factors that are tightly coupled within local sociocultural spaces. For example, going out as a group to a nature resort may feel adventurous for urban Indian middle-aged women given the patriarchal norms of their sociocultural and religious environments. Hence more commonly acceptable experiences such as pilgrimages to the remote Himalayan region may be experienced as a once in a lifetime adventure.

For people living in rural and remote regions, adventure is woven into their everyday lives through activities such as farming, collecting natural resources for their livelihood and living at nature's 'mercy'. Most of these activities involve a range of risks and challenges. These everyday micro and macro adventures are essential, not leisure or recreation choices, and successful implementation is dependent on a profound experiential knowledge of nature. Contrastingly, modern day urbanites tend to benefit from access to outdoor adventure programmes such as trekking, nature walks, water sports, leisure and recreation. These examples of the diverse ways that people engage in adventure often reflect values, personal development, affiliation with nature and therefore, valuing nature in spiritual terms (Passarelli et al., 2010). This reflects 'adventure-with-nature' experience as personal, prompting individual agency of self-awareness as well as relating to the natural world (Kramm, 2020). This resonates with 'one with nature' experience and is linked to life satisfaction and well-being.

In recent times, researchers have reiterated the interconnectedness of human health with the conservation and protection of nature (Murage et al., 2021). The efficacy of nature-based interventions for human health and well-being is echoed by global organisations such as the United Nations (UN, 2021). There have also been efforts to value nature for its multi-dimensional economic and non-economic values (van Heezik & Brymer, 2018). These perspectives assume a separation between humanity and nature and value nature only for how 'it' benefits humans.

However, there is another perspective that accepts humans are part of nature and innately drawn to nature. Participants who undertake expedition to extreme and remote locations have reported that the experience is spiritual and 'with-nature' (as differentiated, for example, from conquering nature (Brymer & Gray, 2010)). From this perspective, adventure could be an avenue to relive our oneness with nature, as a central force reminding us of an eco-centric way of life. In this context, what we experience as adventure-with-nature can be autonomous, purposeful and relatable (Ryff, 2021).

Broadening the Adventure Experience

As noted above, for people living in non-western societies the notion of adventure may be different and influenced by traditional religious and sociocultural factors. For example, prior to the globalisation process which started in the late 1990s, urban Indian society had very few private organisations and government-sponsored bodies specialising in outdoor adventure. Adventuring was the dream and reality of a very few individuals who followed in the steps of the colonial British. For ordinary urban Indians, engagement in specific adventures was novel and / or was less relevant to their everyday life (Sharma-Brymer, 2018). Instead, community development works such as planting trees, constructing lakes for water storage, community woodlands and developing urban parklands were deemed adventurous as they were out of the ordinary experiences. Individual well-being was embedded within community well-being, reflecting collective agency. Globalisation ushered in individualised-outdoor adventure experiences offered via well-marketed programmes.

In recent decades, formalised adventure programmes – originally developed in western countries – have rapidly spread to several non-western countries (Chang et al., 2016). These programmes teach and train participants in outdoor adventure and education (OAE). However, Chang et al. (2016) underlined in their analysis of such programmes the lack of, and therefore the need for, cross-cultural sensitivity and relevance. Interestingly, they stated that adventure in traditional Asian countries is perceived more as exploration and discovery rather than an approach towards risks and challenges. Typically, such programmes follow the philosophy of building relationships through adventurous activities in the outdoors. They would incorporate personal development as a component of the programme. Participants are taught personal agency and how to apply self-determination towards the activity, process and experience. Contextualising these aspects of personal development should incorporate cultural responsiveness.

Personal agency, in the case of Indian women, may be linked to life transformation because it facilitates enhanced awareness of life choices, autonomy, and control over outcomes (Kabeer, 1999; Nussbaum, 2000). Women realise their active agency for gaining control over resources, and becoming strategic about result-oriented outcomes (Sharma-Brymer, 2018). These aspects – choice and control over resources and outcomes – influence participants' experience of adventure.

Adventure here could include group activities such as hill walks to holy shrines where collective agency is more apparent than individual agency. On the other hand, in contemporary globalised times, individuals may undertake extreme adventures as opportunities for personal growth and development. Adventurers in these examples might describe the experience as meaningful, facilitating a person-environment relationship that is dependent on their own capabilities and capacities to utilise resources. Importantly, women living in traditional patriarchal societies also need to overcome obstacles, barriers and hindrances impacting on their participation in adventure. For example, urban, middle-aged women may have to convince their male family members to allow the women to take part in nature walks or water sports.

Women undertaking adventure activities can experience a collective sense of spirituality. This spirituality seems to be directly connected with individual well-being grounded within the experience of collective relationships and relationship with nature (Ryff, 2021). However, this spirituality could be expressed very differently at individual and collective level. The premise is that in ancient wisdom societies such as India, nature seems to have a permanently inherent presence in everyday life playing a powerful role in nurturing human understanding and experience of spirituality. For example, nature is worshipped with different perspectives in Hindu and Buddhist religions. The western world also has recognised similar spiritual feelings whilst undertaking adventure and education programmes (Loynes, 2003). This is also linked to enhanced personal development (Humberstone, 2011).

In the next section, I present and discuss autoethnographical accounts of women's experiences of nature-related adventure. Autoethnographical research is increasing towards adventure, leisure and nature-based experiences, and outdoor education (see for example, Anderson & Austin, 2012; Asfeldt & Beames, 2017; Mackenzie & Kerr, 2014; Nicol, 2013; Orams & Brown, 2021). Autoethnography was employed here for the analysis of experience, which led to the delineation of the meaning of adventure; adventure guiding personal development; and adventure impacting well-being.

To analyse the adventure experience, I explore three experiential accounts: (1) the pilgrim's adventure set in remote Himalayan regions with the narrative of 'feeling courageous is adventure'; (2) the adventure of an extreme 4WD overlander where nature is regarded as the mentor of deeply personal experiences, influencing identity, values and self-awareness, and (3) my own experiences of trekking and scrambling. All three adventurers identify adventure as the facilitator of their personal growth and life satisfaction.

Autoethnographical Accounts of Women's Adventure Experience

Qualitative research lends itself to the exploration of subjective experiences. It brings out the participant voice, illuminating the significance of personal connections. In this chapter, I have chosen to narrate the autoethnographical accounts of women's adventures to highlight how adventure influences personal transformation promoting the attitude of giving back to nature. Autoethnography incorporates the researcher's reflexive engagement in the observation of the sociocultural world with a deep self-awareness of the connection between self and context (Ngunjiri et al., 2010). Reed-Danahay (1997, 2017) underlined the importance of the researcher's voice in narrating the stories of others from similar sociocultural contexts. This voice has the authenticity to interpret the phenomena of the social world by using a critical lens (Ellis et al., 2011; Nicol, 2013). In this context, interpreting the experiences of adventure flowed consistently with the meaning-making process and the emergence of themes. It allowed me to reflect on the tensions and contradictions inherent in women's experiences of adventure taking place in patriarchal societies. This reflexive autoethnographic immersion with the data brought to surface emotional intricacies that the three female participants (including myself) had in their lived experience of adventure and the impact it had on their attitudes, values, and well-being.

The three participants are Lakshmi (pseudonym), Padma and myself. Lakshmi is in her late 30s and is an extreme overlander, leading expeditions worldwide. I interviewed Lakshmi whilst following many of her expeditions on social media. Padma is my mother who is now deceased. I was a witness to her experience of outdoor adventure lived through pilgrimages to remote holy shrines in the Himalayas and elsewhere in India. I have also documented her personal narratives besides preserving her journals. I have translated her narratives from Kannada language to English.

The themes for analysis emerged through a reflective process of my engagement with the data - listening, reading, reflecting, relating and re-imagining the participant experience whilst coding the data (interview transcripts, journals, conversations and dialogues). The participant narratives questioned, contemplated, reflected, immersed and delved deep into the meaning of adventure; adventure guiding personal development (especially broadening own perspectives and worldviews); and how adventure impacted on well-being. The following sections elucidate the themes and experiences. The participant text is followed by my interpretative voice.

The Meaning of Adventure

> It feels like a big adventure. We are only 6 people travelling from Bangalore all the way to Ganga Sagar. I feel nervous. Every pilgrimage to remote places feels fearful and anxious. We go by our gut feeling, trust in others, feeling hopeful and believing in our sincere efforts. Still, questions linger in my mind. Every step of our pilgrimage is risky yet every step feels fulfilling and brings satisfaction when we complete it. To collect all the resources, to get permission from husband, ensuring children would be safe in my absence weighs more than the travel… also being in new remote places and managing the unknown. (Padma)
>
> You know, just following my passion of outdoor adventure itself was a big adventure in my youth. Traditional family and society demanded that I followed their model of higher education, job, marriage and family. So, it was a constant feeling of adventure, anxiety, tension, dilemma and compromises. Moving through the steps of finding money, traveling to the mountains, trekking and staying with strangers … everything was risky and fearful. Overcoming the obstacles to pursue adventure itself is a huge adventure for Indian girls and women. You feel your heart pounding, emotional, confronted and yet you move forward with hope and confidence. That is so meaningful. (Lakshmi)

The two women were quite different in their perception of what adventure was, yet their core meaning-making process resonated with sensing adventure within oneself. For example, for Padma, embarking on a long-distance pilgrimage to remote Ganga Sagar which is the confluence of River Ganga and the Bay of Bengal was itself adventurous. As a middle-class traditional woman planning such a tour of several weeks, she had to build a network of people, find appropriate resources and plan every stage with meticulous attention. This was onerous for a schoolteacher when communication was only through postal services and occasional, expensive phone calls. She recorded in her journals (late 1980s) feeling adventurous about the journey and the process which elicited excitement, fear, apprehension of risks, and worries about the outcomes. Trust in people was the key to the success of these adventures as no-one guaranteed a safe, healthy or successful outcome. The sense of adventure was built into every moment of preparation and action, as stepping outside of the mundane everyday life was itself an adventure for women of her generation.

Contrastingly, the meaning of adventure for myself and Lakshmi differed much in terms of choice, access, the structure of adventurous activities, team and resources. Attracted to outdoor adventure from our childhood, we sensed adventure as predominantly nature-related, liberating us amid gender inequalities to spread the message of equality. For example, we would evoke nature and its conservation in our everyday activities to spread the message of valuing nature without discrimination. As for myself, young women promoting pro-nature values, attitudes and behaviours was seen as progressive yet odd in the pre-globalisation period of India. This was adventurous in addition to undertaking outdoor adventure as women. For Lakshmi, choosing outdoor adventure over higher education and thereby a normative pattern of life was very challenging and a difficult experience. Staying strong within herself while pursuing outdoor adventure was itself felt to be adventurous.

In these examples, women participating in non-traditional, unorthodox and unconventional activities was seen as adventurous. Women undertaking adventure felt adventurous not only from the activity-perspective but also from breaking away from sociocultural norms. Overall, for the three women, participation in adventure felt like self-growth (liberating) and gave confidence to motivate others for enriched benefits.

Adventure Experience is Transformational

>Whether I would fulfil the pilgrimage and return home alive was not a question for me. The answer could be in experiencing the entire process and coming to live the experience with conviction and deepest respect for the opportunity, the process of building relationships, the experience and feeling grateful for the outcomes.
>
>When we set out on foot to the holy Amarnath cave on the last leg of our pilgrimage, it brought to my deep awareness that nature was the god. To reach Him, we had to walk on hard snow, sliding and falling yet feeling the raw nature in and around us. However tough it was, it filled me with

deep feelings of who I was in this universe. Look at the vastness of the mountains around me. There is that force in them, in the rivers flowing below in the valleys, in the forests, the snow... it made me feel humble as a human. Respecting everything in our life is the key to happiness. That's gratitude for what we are.

(Padma)

Respect for everything in one's lived world is a core value that was highlighted in participant narratives. Becoming aware of it was transformational for Padma with feelings of humility and gratitude. She reflected on the values of empathy, respect, devotion and belief of caring for both humans and the environment. The details of carrying dry food for the initial days of travel, limited cotton clothing, organic washing products such as soap nut, and giving away clothing, food, kitchen utensils, footwear and so on to local porters were carefully planned. Nothing was to be wasted or discarded out of respect for the natural world and the spiritual journey. That she valued every moment of these phases was journaled with deepest respect for the process and feeling grateful for the experience. Her group members shared similar feelings, emotions and values. Personal agency and collective strength shone bright in dealing with challenges, unexpected twists and turns, resolving problems personally and collectively by mutual support, and strengthening trusting relationships. Everyone respected this experiential learning and living which transformed them, enhancing confidence and motivation.

Adventure is a process and an experience rather than just an activity. Padma's text reflected the essence of valuing the experiential process no matter whether the participant reached the goal or not.

Going to the Himalayan region is an adventure filled with risks and challenges although trips are planned, and a pre-appointed guide assists the traveller. Besides the human-caused risks to personal safety, we were faced with unexpected natural calamities such as floods, landslides, dangerous driving on the mountains, crossing the mighty Himalayan rivers on unsafe bridges, and travelling to places above 3,500 metres of altitude where oxygen would be less. Whilst taking part in two of Padma's pilgrimages, I was excited about those unique experiences. Where possible, I trekked to the shrines on foot accompanied by one or two members of our group. Some treks were arduous and demanding as the altitude increased. Although I had good prior experience in adventure, trekking at higher altitudes was humbling, evoking a feeling of surrendering. I experienced this several times enroute to Gaumukh (origin of River Ganga) and Yamunotri shrine (steep mountain). There were times when I found myself alone on the mountain or in the challenging terrain of Gaumukh. Absolutely new to such experience, I felt I had completely surrendered to nature. Those moments were filled with silence; my mind totally with the natural world around me. There were no emotions, thoughts or memories. I was suspended in 'nothingness' yet 'with-nature' as I could see, sense and feel only nature not even my *self*.

In the following years, I have reflected on these otherworldly experiences and have only come to respect them for what they were without rational reasoning or judgement. This has been transformational for me, influencing my core values of respect and acceptance of things as they are.

Lakshmi also shared that over the years of her extreme overland driving to remote regions of the world, she has realised those profound moments of suspension, surrendering and transformation. She said:

> It's like this. I am sitting there on the mountain. My team, the vehicles, everyone is there. But I feel that moment where nothing exists. Yet I know I am sitting there just watching this vast landscape all around. But I am not focusing or concentrating on anything yet I feel it. I am living it – the moment when nothing exists but everything matters. The surreal silence, the wind across the mountains, the sun ... I just dissolve in those moments. It's just that experience that I am living for ... I am totally in it.

Lakshmi has come to recognise those moments and is able to reflect on them with a conscious attempt of thinking about them. She said she has come to value the experience as defining who she is and the purpose of her life. For example, Lakshmi did a solo journey to the Pole of Cold (in the valley of Oymyakon in Yakutia, Northeast Russia) for a world record. There were moments during the journey (4WD) when she felt the near-death experience:

> You know, there were these feelings. I was driving alone in crazy minus temperature on a frozen river to reach the Pole of Cold and back. Once I just stopped the engine and sat there crying. What if the river broke, what if the engine didn't start, what if the vehicle skidded and fell into a gorge ... I longed to be home, with my kids... then suddenly something clicked. I needed to be alive to go home. Kids should see their mummy returning home from the Pole of Cold. So, I started the engine.
>
> On another occasion again, I stopped the engine. I just wanted to look at the sky filled with bright stars. It was so pure. It felt totally out of the world experience. You know this kind of adventure, it just makes you realise you are so alive. That you are grateful to life. You come to respect that experience. Absolutely in the moment.

Lakshmi shared that the transformative experience had made her a better person with humility as well as open to the possibilities life could offer. She spreads that message to school children in her talks and encourages them to value adventure experience for self-awareness and personal development.

With these narratives, the women affirmed that adventure has a special influence in changing perceptions, attitudes and behaviours. For them, experience of and from adventure becomes the guiding force in their life.

Adventure Influencing Giving Back to Nature

For all three women, adventure provided opportunities for self-growth and development. For Padma, the more pilgrimages she undertook the more visible her values were. For example, after visiting the holy shrine of Swami Ayyappa (God) in Kerala (South India), she gave up materialism. She donated a lot of her belongings to neighbours and the needy in the community. She adopted a simplistic lifestyle such as sleeping on a mat and not buying new sarees. She wrote in her journal:

> When you walk on foot through the thick rainforest to reach the abode of Swami Ayyappa, you let go of everything. Your life is not guaranteed, neither your health nor wealth. To reach His abode successfully you climb those 18 steep steps. That's the time to let go. Of these attachments in life to material. What remains as yours is just the experience of self in this big world. You suddenly realise materials don't matter in life. What you give back is what keeps you going.

This simplicity and giving back resonates with the values of respecting and safeguarding the environment from human acts of materialism, consumerism and economic gain.

My experiences from adventure have illuminated the values of freedom and empowerment. For example, I feel incredibly and deeply liberated when I climb a hill and look at the vast open space around me. I feel empowered with a feeling of unique force filling my soul. Reflecting on these feelings, I have realised that I value freedom including that of all beings. This resonates with my relationship with the natural world. Blending these feelings, I realise every being's freedom is equally important. Unfortunately, human supremacy contradicts my beliefs and values. The escalating issues of climate change, global warming, species extinction and environmental destruction are warning signs of human interference with the natural world. If adventure resonates with feelings of liberation and empowerment, then experience gained from adventure must transform into guiding forces encouraging pro-environmental behaviours in all those who are engaged in adventure in the natural environment. This personal development should lead to happiness and holistic well-being.

Lakshmi's reflections support my above narrative. She said:

> Yes, I see that in my team development. See, people question me about driving in the remote regions, leaving our footprint, carbon print, etc. But, we drive to remote regions that are pretty much inaccessible. We are one with the environment there, cultures of communities we meet … we relate and relive our *self*. On the other hand, we leave no waste, very little human activity outside of our vehicles so that the environment is not touched by us, and we take utmost care in leaving the terrain as it was before except

for our track marks. New members joining our expedition team face a hard learning curve to keep up to our values of 'do no harm'. Giving back to nature is reflected in how we live our life after these expeditions which change us in big ways. Core values in everyday life, in our expeditions, caring for everything … they matter as giving back.

All three women's narratives illuminate the significance of values and practices shown in our everyday life. Caring for everything with respect and having the core experience of humility through adventure were highlighted as the essential aspects of meaning of life. This self-awareness of personal growth is emphasised as important for well-being.

Discussion and Implications

The analysis of participant narratives supports other autoethnographic accounts of adventure, leisure and outdoor education in highlighting emotions, psychological experiences of enhanced confidence levels and the transformative influence on values, attitudes and behaviours (Anderson & Austin, 2012; Asfeldt & Beames, 2017; Mackenzie & Kerr, 2014; Nicol, 2013; Orams & Brown, 2021). The emotions lived were intense; combined with excitement, gratitude, fulfilment, fear and anxiety. For example, Padma's preparatory steps for remote pilgrimages caused her anxiety and apprehension, at the same time eliciting excitement and happiness with courage. Lakshmi faced hard times and difficult moments with fear of the unknown, yet determination and confidence overtook the negative emotions. I opened up to new adventurous experiences with feelings of humility and curiosity. Facing the experience with open-mindedness emphasised our intrinsic motivation, autonomy and choice which are key elements of well-being (Ryff, 2021). These elements also connect to our values of respect, acceptance and freedom.

Similarly, adventure grounded our efforts to build on relationships and give back to nature, heralding a unique spiritual experience of being one with nature (Humberstone, 2011). This in fact enhanced our happiness, life satisfaction and fulfilment.

The autoethnographical analysis of the women's experiences suggests a unique space for understanding cross-cultural adventure experiences. Relationships and sociocultural factors, alongside personal and collective agency, play important roles in impacting participants' personal development (Chang et al., 2016). The voices within the participant narratives provide a valuable analytical framework for future research on examining women's adventure experience in traditional societies.

Conclusion

This chapter explored the adventure experiences of three Indian women from a traditional patriarchal society. Through autoethnography methodology, it provided a cross-cultural lens for the analysis of lived experience in outdoor adventure. The analysis and interpretation demonstrated that adventure becomes more meaningful through its lived process not merely as an activity with the management of risk and challenge. This lived experience is transformational in influencing personal growth and enhancing values, attitudes and behaviours such as giving back to nature and strengthening human-nature relationships. This transformational development is choice-related, revealing personal and collective agency and emphasising autonomy and freedom. Individually, adventure enhances the participant's happiness, fulfilment, purpose of life and well-being.

References

Anderson, L., & Austin, M. (2012). Auto-ethnography in leisure studies. *Leisure Studies, 31*(2), 131–146. https://doi.org/10.1080/02614367.2011.599069

Asfeldt, M., & Beames, S. (2017). Trusting the journey: Embracing the unpredictable and difficult to measure nature of wilderness educational expeditions. *Journal of Experiential Education, 40*(1), 72–86. https://doi.org/10.1177/1053825916676101

Beames, S., Humberstone, B., & Allin, L. (2017). Adventure revisited: Critically examining the concept of adventure and its relations with contemporary outdoor education and learning. *Journal of Adventure Education and Outdoor Learning, 17*(4), 275–279. https://doi.org/10.1080/14729679.2017.1370278

Beames, S., & Spike, E. (2013). Outdoor adventure and social theory. In E. Spike & S. Beames (Eds.), *Outdoor adventure and social theory*. London: Routledge.

Bragg, R., & Atkins, G. (2016). A review of nature-based interventions for mental health care. Natural England Commissioned Reports. UK.

Brymer, E., Downey, G., & Gray, T. (2009) Extreme sports as a precursor to environmental sustainability. *Journal of Sport & Tourism, 14*(2–3), 193–204.

Brymer, E., Feletti, F., Monasterio, E., & Schweitzer, R. (2020). Editorial: Understanding extremes sports: A psychological perspective. *Frontiers in Psychology, 10*(3029), 1–4. https://doi.org/10.3389/fpsyg.2019.03029

Brymer, E., Freeman, E., & Richardson, M. (2019). One health: The wellbeing impacts of human-nature relationships. Frontiers; Environmental Psychology. doi.org/10.3389/fpsyg.2019.01611

Brymer, E., & Gray, T. (2010). Developing an intimate "relationship" with nature through extreme sports participation. *Leisure/Loisir, 34*(4), 361–374.

Buckley, R. C. (2015). Adventure thrills are addictive. *Frontiers in Psychology, 6*(1915), 1–3. https://doi:10.3389/fpsyg.2015.01915

Chang, T.-H., Tucker, A. T., Norton, C. L., Gass, M. A., & Javorski, S. E. (2016). Cultural issues in adventure programming: Applying Hofstede's five dimensions to assessment and practice. *Journal of Adventure Education and Outdoor Learning*. https://doi.org/10.1080/14729679.2016.1259116

DeVille, N. V., Tomasso, L. P., Stoddard, O. P., Wilt, G. E., Teresa, H., Horton, T. H., Wolf, K. L., Eric Brymer, El., Kahn Jr., P. H., & James, P. (2021). Time spent in nature, regardless of the quality of environmental conditions, is associated with increased pro-environmental attitudes and behaviours. *International Journal of Environmental Research and Public Health, 18*(14), 7498, 1–18. https://doi: 10.3390/ijerph18147498

Ellis, C., Adams, T. E., & Bochner, A. (2011). Autoethnography: An overview. *Historical Social Research, 36*(4), 273–290. https://doi.org/10.12759/hsr.36.2011.4.273-290

Frumkin, H., Bratman, G. N., Breslow, S. J., Cochran, B., Kahn, P. H. Jr, Lawler, J. J., Levin, P. S., Tandon, P. S., Varanasi, U., Wolf, K. L., & Wood, S. A. (2017). Nature contact and human health: A research agenda. *Environmental Health Perspectives, 125*(7), 075001. https://doi.org/10.1289/EHP1663

Humberstone, B. (2011). Embodiment and social and environmental action in nature-based sport: Spiritual spaces. *Leisure Studies, 30*(4), 495–512. http://dx.doi.org/10.1080/02614367.2011.602421

Kabeer, N. (1999). Resources, agency, achievements: Reflections on the measurement of women's empowerment. *Development and Change, 30*, 435–464.

Kramm, M. (2020). When a river becomes a person. *Journal of Human Development and Capabilities, 21*(4), 307–319. https://doi.org/10.1080/19452829.2020.1801610

Loynes, C. (2003). Accounts of agency: The hero's journey as a construct for personal development through outdoor adventure. https://doi.org/10.1007/978-3-322-91387-6_9

Mackenzie, S.-H. & Kerr, J. K. (2014). The psychological experience of river guiding: Exploring the protective frame and implications for guide well-being. *Journal of Sport & Tourism, 19*(1), 5–27. https://doi.org/10.1080/14775085.2014.967796

Murage, P., Batalha, H. R, Lino, S., & Sterniczuk, K. (2021). From drug discovery to coronaviruses: Why restoring natural habitats is good for human health. *The BMJ, 375*(n2329), 1–5. https://doi.org/10.1136/bmj.n2329

Ngunjiri, F. W., Hernandez, K. A. C., & Chang, H. (2010). Living autoethnography: Connecting life and research. *Journal of Research Practice, 6*(1), 1–17.

Nicol, R. (2013). Returning to the richness of experience: Is autoethnography a useful approach for outdoor educators in promoting pro-environmental behaviour? *Journal of Adventure Education & Outdoor Learning, 13*(1), 3–17. https://doi.org/10.1080/14729679.2012.679798

Nussbaum, M. (2000). *Women and human development: The capabilities approach*. Cambridge: Cambridge University Press.

O'Brien, L. (2009). Learning outdoors: The Forest School approach. *Education, 3-13, 37*(1), 45–60.

Orams, M. B., & Brown, M. (2021). The dream and the reality of blue spaces: The search for freedom in offshore sailing. *Journal of Sport and Social Issues, 45*(2), 196–216. https://doi.org/10.1177/0193723520928599

Passarelli, A., Hall, E., & Anderson, M. (2010). A strengths-based approach to outdoor and adventure education: Possibilities for personal growth. *Journal of Experiential Education, 33*(2), 120–135. https://doi.org/10.1177/105382591003300203

Reed-Danahay, D. E. (1997). *Auto/ethnography: Rewriting the self and the social*. New York: Berg.

Reed-Danahay, D. E. (2017). Bourdieu and critical autoethnography: Implications for research, writing, and teaching. *International Journal of Multicultural Education, 19*(1), 144–154. https://doi.org/10.18251/ijme.v19i1.1368

Ryff, C. D. (2021). Spirituality and well-being: Theory, science, and the nature connection. *Religions, 12*(914), 9–15.

Sharma-Brymer, V. (2018). Locations of resistance and agency: The actionable space of Indian women's connection to the outdoors. In T. Gray & D. Mitten (Eds.), *The Palgrave Macmillan International Handbook of Women and Outdoor Learning* (pp. 307–319). London: Palgrave Macmillan.

Sharma-Brymer, V., & Bland, D. (2016). Bringing nature to schools to promote children's physical activity. *Sports Medicine, 46*(7), 955–962.

Sharma-Brymer, V., & Brymer, E. (2019). Flourishing and eudaemonic well-being. In W. Filho et al. (Eds.), *Good Health and Well-Being: Encyclopaedia of the UN Sustainable Development Goals.* Switzerland: Springer International Publishing.

Sharma-Brymer, V., Brymer, E., Gray, T., & Davids, K. (2018). Affordances guiding forest school practice: The application of the ecological dynamics approach. *Journal of Outdoor and Environmental Education, 21*(1), 103–115.

Sharma-Brymer, V., Gray, T., & Brymer, E. (2018). Sport participation to create a deeper environmental identity with pro-environmental behaviours. In B. P. McCullough & T. Kellison, (Eds.), *Routledge handbook on sport, sustainability and the environment* (pp. 330–339). New York: Routledge.

United Nations. (2021). https://www.un.org/en/climatechange/cop26

van Heezik, Y., & Brymer, E. (2018). Nature as a commodity: What's good for human health might not be good for ecosystem health. *Frontiers in Psychology, 9*(1673), 1–5. https://doi.org/10.3389/fpsyg.2018.01673

ADVENTURE PSYCHOLOGY

Learnings and Implications

Eric Brymer and Paula Reid

In recent years, the call for health and wellbeing initiatives that suit both planet and people have accelerated. Chapters in this book point to a profound experience that benefits people and planet not captured by any single current psychological discipline. It turns out that adventure is fundamental to the human experience and the learnings in this book extend far beyond the adventure itself. The experience of adventure, and the outcomes for adventure, are far reaching and available to everyone. The limitations inherent in traditional competitive sport constrained by rules, regulations, and manicured environments are not found in adventure. At the very least, adventure could be the key to unlocking the benefits of physical movement for all. Adventure is accessible, non-elitist, non-competitive.

However, what is also very clear from the discussions in this book is that Adventure Psychology is far more than this. Adventure connects people to nature and others, it facilitates transcendence and more harmonious relationships, it frees people from artificial constraints and highlights more productive ways of living. Adventure is open for all ages and abilities and the benefits of adventure are available to everyone. The challenge for society is how best to harness adventure for the benefit of current and future generations and for the benefit of the planet. It may be one of many avenues we use to understand, and have a harmonious relationship with, our precious and threatened natural environment.

This book provides a glimpse into Adventure Psychology however there is clearly more work to be done before Adventure Psychology can truly free itself from the confines of other psychological disciplines. Further research is required to explore the unique role adventure has in facilitating good health and wellbeing. Adventure Psychology requires theoretical frameworks that truly capture the essence of adventure, and in this book, we have encouraged a more relational and systemic perspective on psychology. Research in Adventure Psychology needs to garner more evidence to highlight its uniqueness in ways that make use of traditional and more modern paradigms. For example, there is a need to explicate the nuances of adventure and determine how adventure might be ideal for enhancing positive human–nature relationships.

It is early days in Adventure Psychology; however, there is clear evidence that performance and learning in an adventure context do not align well with other psychology frameworks. The differences are too great. However, the differences in adventure do seem to be well aligned with the human condition more broadly. The impact of this could be important for schools, health practitioners, learning designers, and business psychologists and as such there is a need to find ways to encourage and provide more opportunities for adventure or ways to learn from adventure for the benefit of society and the planet. This book presents clear evidence for the potential of adventure and frame for Adventure Psychology as a relational notion between individual experiences and environmental characteristics.

Adventure is fundamental to the human condition and Adventure Psychology has the capacity to provide the frame for releasing human potential. However, beyond this Adventure Psychology also has the power to enhance the nature-human relationship. Adventure Psychology provides an alternative to the traditional competitive model that seems to be driving so much of modern society. Adventure Psychology also seems to provide the space for relating with the natural world rather than attempting to control or structure it to fit flawed frames. Adventure Psychology points to a more fulfilled way of living that benefits people and planet symbiotically. The impact of this is profound. Human wellbeing is dependent on planetary wellbeing, and the planet's health is dependent on human behaviour. Adventure Psychology should become an ecological, systems psychology unlocking opportunities for maximising the possibility for nature and humans to thrive together. Future research that provides a deeper understanding of the adventure experience may improve global health and international relations.

Recommendations

The research featured in this book can be distilled into a number of recommendations that recognise the importance of collaboration, partnerships, translation of knowledge, accessibility and opportunity, and standardising evaluation frameworks, to better inform policy and practice. Funding to support this research is vital for future development.

1. Translation of knowledge
    The body of knowledge presented in this book should be of great interest to a broad range of governing bodies, organisations, and decision makers, from local to national levels.
    We also suggest that Adventure Psychology, as an explicit and unique discipline, becomes the umbrella term under which this body of knowledge sits, and from where best practices and research can be further shared and

improved upon. It is time to harness the associated practices of adventure tourism, adventure travel, adventure education, adventure therapy, recreational therapy, therapeutic adventure, adventure sports, and adventure recreation together, so that we may collaborate and cooperate, strengthen and evolve, toward a healthy and flourishing ecosphere.

2. Inclusivity and accessibility

    Adventure is a fundamental human experience with the capacity to benefit individuals, communities and the planet. The traditional definitions and mindsets towards adventure are flawed and narrow. As mentioned in Chapter 11 "we must consider who we are including/excluding with our definitions of adventure." Conceptual understanding of adventure, Adventure Psychology and the provision of adventurous opportunities, ought to consider global contexts and needs. Likewise, research should stretch beyond conventional ways of knowing to embrace methodologies and participants that challenge traditional notions of ontology and epistemology.

3. Evaluation frameworks

    An implication of research showing the efficacies of Adventure Psychology is that it can and is having a positive impact on individual and organisational practices. Research needs to identify a wider range of outcomes to evidence the potential human, social, environmental and economic benefits of adventure. There is a need for more consistent metrics and evaluation procedures, using sophisticated tools that are also culturally sensitive. Future research methodologies need to adopt a common system of evaluation so that research in different disciplines and countries can be evaluated as a body of work rather than a collection of disparate findings.

4. Provision of adventure environments

    While there is still a need to better understand the nuances of Adventure Psychology and the implications for the design of opportunities for all, it is not too early to find ways to embed adventure across different social realms. We need to provide appropriate environments for adventure to become part of everyday life. This needs social, political, and policy support.

Call to Action

Finally, we would like to create a call to action from the ground up. The research will continue to evolve, and the discipline is yet to be defined and launched within the worlds of psychology and academia. In the meantime, we can talk about it and share ideas and best practices globally. We can go on adventures, encourage others to go on adventures, and have adventurous mindsets. We can explore together, with open minds and hearts, to improve our physical and psychological fitness and to create a more positive relationship with our planet.

Let's go on a quest – a hero's journey – of extra-ordinary endeavour, with total commitment as we lean in to uncertainty and adversity with courage, curiosity, and humility.

INDEX

adaptability 78–79, 83, 85, 86, 177
adventure education 1, 4, 166, 193–195, 206, 221
adventure recreation 1, 4, 163, 165, 221
adventure sports 1, 4, 54, 105, 109, 111, 123, 136, 181, 206, 221
adventure therapy 1, 4, 104, 179, 221
adventure tourism 1, 4, 16, 193, 221
adventure travel 1, 221
adversity 7, 28, 29, 33, 43, 46, 48, 63, 65, 68, 69, 90–91, 99, 134, 139, 143–144, 146–147, 173–175, 177, 182, 221
altruism 64, 84, 101, 139, 212, 215
Anticipatory Thinking (AT) 81, 82
anxiety 21, 27, 32, 84–86, 146, 163, 215; defined 122–123; and fear, differentiation between 125, 126
autonomy 7, 46, 90, 106, 196, 207–208, 215–216

Baumeister, R. 66
Bergland, C. T. 32
"The Big Five" 20, 21, 38, 84; agreeableness 21; conscientiousness 21, 84; extraversion 21, 84; neuroticism 21; openness to experience 20, 38, 84
bio-ecological model 112
biophilia 79
Bluck, S. 36
Breivik, G. 2
broaden-and-build theory 82
Brunswik, E. 114
Buber, M. 195

Burke, S. 176, 177

Clewis, R. R. 191, 192
cognitive load 81–82
cognitive flexibility 79–82; cognitive reappraisal 64
comfort zone 38, 98
Comte-Sponville, A. 150
conscientiousness 21
consciousness 164–166, 168; defined 161; nature of 161–162; self 163
constraints: defined 108; environmental 108–109; individual 108; task 108
courage 7, 12, 18, 21, 34, 45, 51, 89, 124, 148, 150, 193–194, 215, 221
Cronon, W. 198, 199
Crum, A. J. 31
Csikszentmihalyi, M. 39, 45, 54, 82, 160, 161, 162, 164, 165
curiosity 20, 29, 38, 85

"Death Zone" 54
Deci, E. 101, 161, 162
defining adventure 1, 4, 11, 16, 36, 174, 182
depression 32, 84
Dweck, C. S. 31, 145, 150

ecological dynamics framework 107
endurance 33, 60–75, 99, 146–148
Entropy Model of Uncertainty (EMU) 78
environment: adventure framed through 1, 2–3; crises 198–200; EST 44, 46–47, 51, 55; extreme (*see* extreme environments);

human (*see* human-environment dynamic); individual–environment system 4, 107, 110, 116; natural 6, 20, 137–140, 164, 166–168, 181, 190, 205, 214, 219; performance 106, 108, 109, 111, 113–116, 133; person–environment relationship 4, 106–107, 112, 115, 208
environmental constraint 108–109
extraversion 21
extreme environments 5, 42–59; cognitive and cognitive/emotional process 80; definitions 44–45; ; general considerations 45; motivation of people 84; personality factors 45–46; sensed presence phenomenon 49–50; solo long-distance sailing 53–54; team size and composition 48–49; working in 79
extreme sports 206; cultures 113; frontier version of mountaineering 124; high-risk adventurism 128; nature of fear 124–125

failure 91, 131–141, 146; definition 133, 136–137; expeditions 51; fixed mindsets 31, 33; mismanaged move or mistake 38; repeated 33
fear 46, 54, 120–130, 187, 203, 204, 211; and anxiety, definitions 122–123, 126; and anxiety, differentiation between 125, 215; assumptions about 123–124; of death 68; in extended adventures 121; hardwired fear-based memories 32; of mismanaged move or mistake 38; naturalistic research 124; pilgrimage to remote places 210; stories 93, 94; of uncertainty 135
fixed mindset 31, 33–34
flow 28; 159–171, of action 134; activities 163; and consciousness 161–163; deep 165; defined 39, 54, 160, 161, 165, 166; dimensions 162–163, 164; experiences 161–162, 164, 165, 181; or state of mindfulness 90, 161, 166–168; paratelic 164, 165, 166; and peak experiences 3, 45; psychological 79; telic 164, 165, 166
form of life 107, 110, 111, 113, 115
Fredrickson, B. L. 82

Galonka, S. 147, 148
Gibson, E. J. 148
Gibson, J. J. 109, 114, 148
Glück, J. 36
going knowingly into the unknown 28, 36–38, 67

Green, L. 146
grit 48, 50, 90–91, 99, 146–148, 152
growth 6; personal 47, 90, 91, 133, 137–138, 165, 178, 196, 205, 206, 208–209, 215, 216; post-adventure 3, 47, 179; post-experience 46–47; post-traumatic (*see* post-traumatic growth (PTG)); psychological 3; zone 38
growth mindset 29, 31, 34, 38, 145

Hahn, K. 193, 194
Hämäläinen, R. P. 150–152
Hirsh, J. B. 78
hope 35, 52, 79, 82, 85, 90–91, 94, 99–100, 204, 210
Human-Environment Dynamic 104–119; defined 106; affordances 109; characterisation of skill and skill transfer 113–114; constraints 108–109; ecological context of adventurer 112; ecological perspective 104–105; form of life 107, 110, 111, 113, 115; positive outcomes and motives for participation 105–106; psychological and existential view 106–107; representative design 114–115; research and practice 115–116
human–nature experience 6, 123, 188–192, 194–196, 198–201, 220
humour and laughter 64, 67–68
Humour Coping Scale (HCS) 68

individual–environment system 4, 107, 110, 116
Ingold, T. 29, 38, 111
Isolated, Confined Environments (ICE) environment 43–44

Jackson, S. A. 160–162
James, W. 144, 145, 167, 193, 194, 196

Kant, Immanuel 191, 193
Kashdan, T. B. 38, 39, 85
Klein, G. 82
Kohn, A. 70

Langer, E. J. 30, 34
leadership 3–4, 50–51, 152
"learned helplessness" 33
lived experience 2–4, 18, 31, 91, 133, 144, 203, 205, 210, 216

Mälkki, K. 146
marathons 62–63, 142–143, 147

Maslow, A. H. 20, 21, 162; hierarchy of needs 20
Mayseless, O. 173, 180
meditation 30, 166–168
mental toughness 7, 68–69, 71, 99
Merzenich, M. M. 32
metacognition 64, 71
mindfulness 64, 79; and adaptability 5; and adventures 35; defined 30; knowing 37; and mindlessness 29, 30, 31; or flow 90, 161, 166–168, 181; therapeutic 29
mindset 83, 90–91, 143–144; action 146; adventurous 5, 29, 34–36, 38, 39; automatic 30; challenges 33; cognition 34; defined 31; existence of 32; fixed 31, 33–34; growth 29, 31, 34, 38, 145; mastery 71; position of not knowing 34–36; premature cognitive commitments 32; research on 145; single mindedness 33; stereotypical limits 34; theories 31
Mortlock, C. 194
motivation 5, 17, 19, 29, 66–69, 71, 77, 93, 108, 109, 115, 164, 181; achievement 63; characteristics of adventurers 19; conflict 122; of extreme adventurers 195; flow 161; human 22; intensity theory 64; intrinsic 161, 215; and judgement 133; narrative research 137; potential 64
Muir, John 190, 195

Naor, L. 173, 180
narcissistic personality disorder (NPD) 33
narrative 36, 64, 71, 88–103; chaos 94; cultural 193, 196; discovery 95; dominant 193; examining motivation 137; heroic or relational 90; history 189; and language 90; participant 210, 212, 215; performance 94–95; personal 177–178, 210; quest 94; relational 95; restitution 93–94
narrative theory 89, 92–93
Nash, R. F. 189, 191, 198, 199
natural environment 6, 20, 137–140, 164, 166–168, 181, 190, 205, 214, 219
nature: adventure experience 207–213; adventure influencing 214–215; agentic 4; biological 70; dissolution of 207; of fear 121, 123–125, 128; of flow and consciousness 161–163; as friend 199–200; healing benefits 80; human–nature experience 6, 123, 188–192, 194–196, 198–201, 220; linking adventure with 206; and mindfulness 167; objectification of 189–190; person–nature relationship 6; physical activities 1, 63; relatedness 79–80, 110; revisiting 207; spiritual contact 14; wellbeing of 196
neuroplasticity 31, 32–33
neuroticism 21

Oelschlaeger, M. 199
openness to experience 20
optimal performance 5, 62–63, 148, 161
optimism 31, 83, 85, 89, 90, 101, 179

paratelic flow 164, 165, 166
Paulus, M. P. 148
peak experience 3, 5, 38, 89, 101, 174
peak performance 5, 62–63
perception of effort 64
performance: behavioural 148; competition vs. cooperation 70–71; enduring 61–63; environment 108–109, 111, 114–116, 133; humour and laughter 67–68; mental toughness 68–69; mission performance 50; optimal psychological 79; peak 5, 62–63; perceived effort 64–65; PST (see psychological skills training (PST)); psychological resilience 69–70; regulation 105–106; research into 71; self-control/self-regulation 66–67; self-talk 65–66; skilled or successful 113; task performance 81
performance narrative 94–95
PERMA 90, 98
personal growth 47, 90, 91, 133, 137–138, 165, 178, 196, 205, 206, 208–209, 215, 216
personality: adventurous 10, 18, 134–135; defined 135; differences 22, 23; factors 45–46, 133; of leader 50; sensation-seeking 21; survivor 53; tests 124; thrill-seeking 21; Type T 53; values and motives 19
personality traits 3, 29, 69, 85–86, 105, 108, 123, 135; "The Big Five" 20–21; and context 84–85; defined 84; internal factors 85; measurement tools 123–124; pathological 123
personal narrative 177–178, 210
person–environment relationship 4, 106–107, 112, 115, 208
physical wellbeing 101, 105, 115
physiological survival 20
Pinder, R. A. 114
positive psychology 3, 88–103; and adventures 89–90; and narrative 95–101

post-adventure growth 3, 47, 179
post-experience growth 46–47
post-traumatic growth (PTG) 84, 99–100, 150, 172–177, 179–180, 182
post-traumatic stress disorder (PTSD) 27–29, 46, 84, 178, 180–181
presence 29–30, 49–50, 86, 122, 124–125, 175, 182, 196, 209
problem-oriented *vs.* emotion-oriented coping 22
pro-environmental behaviour 2, 6, 138, 168, 206, 214
psychological skills training (PST) 63–64
psychological wellbeing 80, 89–90, 101, 181

Raffan, J. 197
rating of perceived effort (RPE) 65
recreational therapy 1, 221
representative co-design 114
resilience 3, 12, 33, 48, 51, 68, 85, 89–90, 99, 105; in athletics and music performers 152; defined 177; and growth 150; hope 83; psychological 67, 69–70, 71; to stress and trauma 136
reversal theory 22
risk 1–2, 11, 21, 33, 77, 79–81, 159, 161, 203–204; adventuring 42–43, 45, 48, 52–54; analysing 37; aware 37; and challenging activities 206–208, 212, 216; high-risk 106, 124, 128; individual perceptions 3, 105; managing 37; reduction 163; risk-taking tendency 52, 108, 110, 136, 138, 161, 174; unacceptable 42, 105; underestimating 164
Roberts, J. W. 193, 195

Saarinen, E. 150–152
Sabiston, C. 176, 177
safetyism 16–17
salutogenesis 46–47
"second wind" 144
self-actualisation 20
self-control/self-regulation 66–67
self-determination 162, 208
self-talk 65–66
self-transcendence 6, 113, 135–136, 138–140
sensation-seeking personality 21
sensed presence phenomenon 49–50
Shanker, S. 66
Sheldon, K. M. 167, 168
single mindedness 33

SISU 142–155, adventure with strength and grace 143–144; extraordinary perseverance 144–147; gentle power 148–150; latent strength 147–148; systems intelligence 150–152
spiritual quests 13
state: anxious 125; of being 125; enlightened 125; experiential 4, 39, 163; flow 160, 163, 196; grey 125; meditative 29; of mind 30, 36–37, 39, 90; paratelic 22, 164; positive experience state 161; psychological 160; telic 22; of uncertainty or openness 38
storytelling 90–92
stress 31–32, 46, 50, 67–68, 84–86, 136, 143, 148
stretch zone 38
success 131–140; definition of 136–139; personality and adventure 134–135; TCI (*see* Temperament and Character Inventory (TCI))
survival 61–63, 68, 70, 82–83, 120, 127, 149, 151, 162, 163, 193; physiological 20; psychology 79, 83–84; responses 77; skills 13; training 81
systems intelligence 150–152

telic flow 164, 165, 166
Temperament and Character Inventory (TCI) 135–136
therapeutic adventure 1, 221
thrill-seeking personality 21
thriving/flourishing 6, 82, 89, 182, 196, 221
Tolle, E. 30
transcendence 20, 219; adventure and sublime 188–189, 192–193; adventure as education 193–194; new relations 189–190; protected landscapes 190–192; self 6, 133, 135–136, 138–140; of time 163
transformation 98–99, 174; experiences 106, 139, 211–213, 216; journey 94; properties of adventure 6; and resurrection 100; *see also* post-traumatic growth (PTG)
trauma 6, 29, 94, 136, 150, 173–174–177, 179–182
Type T personality 53

uncertainty 7, 18, 28, 34, 36–38, 46, 50, 68, 76–87, 106, 109–110, 124, 135, 192, 221

Vallerand, R. J. 149
Van Gennep, A. 173

wellbeing: of nature 196; physical 101, 105, 115; psychological 80, 89–90, 101, 181
wilderness 45, 79–80, 82, 173, 176, 178–181, 189–191, 198–199
Wilder, T. 11
Wilson, E. O. 79–80
Wilson, A. D. 147, 148
wisdom 3, 31, 37, 101, 149, 173; foresight (through future assessment) 37; and growth 173, 179, 182; hindsight (from past experience) 37; insight (from present awareness) 37; and knowledge 36, 38

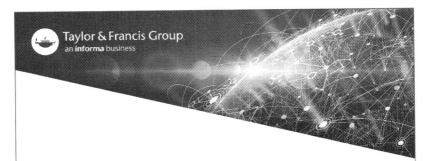

Printed in the United States
by Baker & Taylor Publisher Services